Basic Respiratory Physiology

Basic Respiratory Physiology

Norman C. Staub, MD
Department of Physiology and
Cardiovascular Research Institute
University of California, San Francisco
San Francisco, California

Churchill Livingstone
New York, Edinburgh, London, Melbourne, Tokyo

Library of Congress Cataloging-in-Publication Data

Staub, Norman C., date

    Basic respiratory physiology / Norman C. Staub.

       p.   cm.

    Includes bibliographical references.

    Includes index.

    ISBN 0-443-08755-5

    1.   Respiration.   2. Respiratory organs—Physiology.   I. Title.

    [DNLM: 1. Respiration.   2. Respiratory System—physiology WF

102 S775b]

QP121.S76 1991

612.2—dc20

DNLM/DLC

for Library of Congress   91-11008

                                          CIP

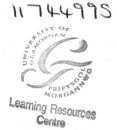
© **Churchill Livingstone Inc. 1991**

Distributed in the United Kingdom by Churchill Livingstone, Robert Stevenson House, 1–3 Baxter's Place, Leith Walk, Edinburgh EH1 3AF, and by associated companies, branches, and representatives throughout the world.

Accurate indications, adverse reactions, and dosage schedules for drugs are provided in this book, but it is possible that they may change. The reader is urged to review the package information data of the manufacturers of the medications mentioned.

The Publishers have made every effort to trace the copyright holders for borrowed material. If they have inadvertently overlooked any, they will be pleased to make the necessary arrangements at the first opportunity.

Acquisitions Editor: *Debra Rapaport*
Developmental Editor: *Margot Otway*
Copy Editor: *Kathleen P. Lyons*
Production Designer: *Jill Little*
Production Supervisor: *Christina Hippeli*

Printed in the United States of America

First published in 1991   7 6 5 4 3 2 1

To Julius H. Comroe, Jr., MD
(1911-1984)

He taught me how to teach.

His books, *The Lung* (1955),
Physiology of Respiration (1965),
and *Exploring the Heart* (1983),
are classic teaching texts
for specific audiences.

Preface

Basic Respiratory Physiology divides naturally into two parts. Chapters 1 through 3 are an introduction and review. They should be read before the first class. A student who has not had much biology background will obtain familiarity with the subject without being bothered by details. The topics in Chapters 4 through 11 develop in a logical sequence but they can be taught in some other order without too much confusion.

I did not plan to write a new textbook on respiratory physiology: I already have seven on my desk. Unfortunately, in teaching basic respiratory physiology to beginning professional students (medical, graduate, dental, nursing, pharmacy, and respiratory therapy) I found that none of these books fulfilled my main teaching objective, which is to provide a concise but thorough explanation of the conceptual and quantitative aspects of medically important respiratory physiology, namely, mechanics, ventilation/perfusion, blood gas transport, and control of breathing. That is about all I expect a first year professional student to learn in a three-week teaching block, such as is allotted in most North American schools.

Nevertheless, respiratory physiology should not be a survey course. A knowledge of quantitative analysis is essential even though modern pulmonary function testing is largely automated and computer-driven. What do we do if the machine stops? A student needs to understand the relation of the numbers on the screen to the underlying physiology.

Upon completion of *Basic Respiratory Physiology* the beginning student will understand normal oxygen and carbon dioxide exchange and transport. Everything else is secondary. Coverage of some traditional areas (pulmonary function tests and high altitude and diving physiology) has been downplayed, which will distress some teachers. But ask yourselves, are those topics not mainly relics from the applied origins of pulmonary physiology in naval and air corps laboratories during World War II?

Nouveau respiratory physiology (lung defense mechanisms, liquid and protein exchange, nonrespiratory functions, molecular biology, and genetics) is very important, but it should be taught later to students in an advanced physiology or clinical course.

Although basic respiratory physiology is a mature field, this book includes considerable new material, for example, information on the function of the chest wall and the importance of the abdomen as part of it; a more modern approach to the regulation of breathing (such as the timing of the breathing cycle); expanded discussion of the pulmonary circulation; and adoption of the new and much clearer teaching of acid-base balance, using Stewart's approach.

I have eliminated nearly all methodologic and historical material but have included a small number of additional readings at the ends of the chapters for those students especially interested.

I have not used any figures showing original experiments, no matter how classic these may be, because they are too difficult to interpret by a beginner, contain irrelevant material, or do not use human subjects. Figures, both new and old, have been redrawn to represent human physiology. They are simplified to stress those features important to the beginning student.

I have adopted the college textbook fashion of including drill questions and problems at the end of each chapter. Working the problems reinforces learning, helps to relieve anxiety, and because some of the questions have clinical relevance, they may even increase student interest in the subject. Do not worry, professors: I have included a chapter containing rather complete approaches, explanations, and answers.

Each chapter begins with a summary called "The Bottom Line." I selected that name because many anxious students have repeatedly asked me for "the bottom line."

Physiology is a quantitative as well as a qualitative science. It is often the first course in which a student is expected to think, synthesize the larger picture from individual facts, and work quantitative problems, in addition to memorizing facts. Students frequently complain about the quantitative aspects of respiratory physiology, yet using equations to solve problems is a considerable part of respiratory physiology. I have introduced quantification but have tried to stick with the essentials.

Finally, there is a great deal of jargon, abbreviations, and symbology in physiology. I think this is a bit too much, but I know how popular it is for the student to be able to give forth a spiel of phrases that identify him or her as part of the "in group." So take your "TEE-EYE OVER TEE-TOTE," add it to the "PEE-AYE-OH-TWO" to "EFF-EYE-OH-TWO" ratio, and you may go far, especially if you know what those phrases mean.

I have used some early drafts of the figures and the text in teaching. I express my gratitude to the many students who forced me to refine, clarify, and simplify the learning of respiratory physiology as much as possible. At one phase of preparation, several anonymous reviewers helped me more than they probably realized; many of their suggestions have been incorporated in this version.

I am particularly grateful to Mary Helen Briscoe, who worked diligently on the figures, both computer-generated and hand-drawn; to Kurt H. Albertine, PhD (Associate Professor of Physiology and Medicine, Thomas Jefferson Medical College of Thomas Jefferson University, Philadelphia, Pennsylvania), for contributing several excellent new figures for Chapter 2; to Dr. Wiltz Wagner, PhD (Associate Professor of Physiology, Indiana University School of Medicine, Indianapolis, Indiana), whose delightful figure on the distribution of pulmonary blood flow (Chapter 7) is the only external figure I have used unchanged; and to Judy White and Bernie Baccay, who typed many of the early drafts.

Norman C. Staub, MD

Contents

1

Respiration and Breathing

THE BOTTOM LINE

The Prime Function of the Lung

The main function of the lung is to bring fresh air into close contact with blood flowing in the pulmonary capillaries so that the exchange of oxygen and carbon dioxide by passive diffusion will take place efficiently.

The basic course on *respiration* in organ system physiology describes the function and regulation of ventilation of the lung and of the flow of blood (perfusion) in the pulmonary circulation, explains how ventilation and perfusion are matched throughout the lung for efficient gas exchange, explains how to assess gas exchange quantitatively, and introduces blood gas transport and acid-base balance from the pulmonary physiologist's and chest physician's point of view. The student is assumed to be familiar with cellular metabolism and respiration from prior biochemistry and general biology courses.

This chapter introduces the general concept of respiration and breathing. Key terms are written in boldface and briefly explained. Other words that may be unfamiliar will be defined and used frequently in the chapters that follow. For now, however, only the general picture is of concern.

Although the title of this book includes the word *respiration*, it is mostly about the phenomenon of *breathing*. **Breathing** is an automatic, rhythmic, centrally regulated mechanical process by which the contraction and relaxation of the skeletal muscles of the diaphragm, abdomen, and rib cage cause gas to move into and out of the terminal respiratory units (the functional alveoli) of the lung. **Respiration** is the overall process of controlled oxidation of metabolites for the production of useful energy by living organisms. It includes breathing.

For successful steady-state respiration to occur in multicellular organisms, **oxygen** (O_2) and other nutrients must be brought to the vicinity of the respiring cells, while **carbon dioxide** (CO_2) and other waste products must be taken away. Large animals, including humans, make use of two systems for this process: a **circulatory system,** which carries whatever is needed to and from the tissue cells in blood, and a **breathing system** (a gas exchanger), which carries oxygen to and carbon dioxide from the alveoli of the lung.

THE PRIME FUNCTION OF THE LUNG

The principal function of the lung is to distribute inspired air and pulmonary blood so that the exchange of O_2 and CO_2 between the alveolar gas and the pulmonary capillary blood occurs efficiently. *Efficiently* means that the exchange is accomplished with a minimal expenditure of energy (the work or power used in breathing and in pumping blood from the right ventricle).

The process of breathing is measured by **ventilation** (rate × depth of breathing). The exchange of O_2 and of CO_2 in the lung is measured by their separate concentration differences between inspired and expired gas. The process of pulmonary blood flow is measured by the **pulmonary vascular resistance** [(pulmonary arterial to left atrial pressure difference)/cardiac output]. The exchange of O_2 and of CO_2 in pulmonary blood is measured by their concentration differences between blood in the pulmonary artery (mixed venous blood) and blood in any systemic artery.

The differences between the O_2 and CO_2 **partial pressures** (the fraction of total gas pressure due to that molecular species) between alveolar gas and systemic arterial blood are useful in determining overall lung function efficiency, which depends on the adequacy of the matching of alveolar ventilation (volume flow rate of fresh air to each part of the lung) to perfusion (volume flow rate of blood to each part of the lung). Ideally, the **ventilation/perfusion** ratios of all parts of the lungs are identical.

The following general rules are worth remembering:

1. The best functional measure of the adequacy of ventilation is the alveolar partial pressure of carbon dioxide.
2. The best functional measure of the adequacy of perfusion (blood flow) is the systemic arterial oxygen transport (cardiac output × arterial oxygen concentration).
3. The best functional measure of the adequacy of ventilation/perfusion matching is the difference of oxygen partial pressure between alveolar gas and arterial blood.

Oxygenated blood leaves the lungs via the pulmonary veins and is pumped by the left ventricle through the systemic arteries to the capillaries associated with all the respiring cells of the body. Likewise, carbon dioxide, the principal waste product of metabolism, is transported away from the respiring cells to the lung for elimination. The process of O_2 and CO_2 transport by the blood is an important part of both pulmonary physiology and respiration.

Diffusion is the passive movement of molecules from regions where they possess more energy to regions where they possess less energy. In respiratory physiology, the energy possessed by oxygen and carbon dioxide is usually stated in terms of partial pressure rather than concentration. This is because diffusional exchange between alveolar gas and blood (liquid), in which the solubilities (hence concentrations) of the respiratory gas molecules are different, is driven by partial pressure differences. Moreover, O_2 and CO_2 molecules in blood are held in chemically altered forms, which further renders comparisons in terms of concentration differences meaningless.

Diffusion occurs at two critical points in the respiration pathway, namely, between gas in the alveoli and the blood flowing through the pulmonary capillaries, and between the blood flowing through the systemic capillaries and the mitochondria of the respiring cells.

The overall process of breathing and of gas exchange—the ventilation/perfusion process—

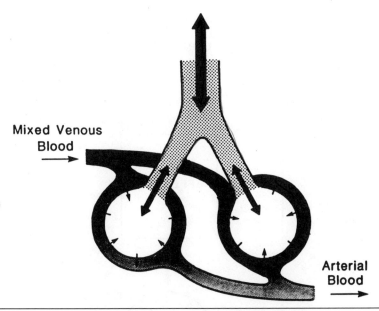

Mixed Venous Blood

Arterial Blood

Fig. 1-1.   Schema of the lungs and pulmonary circulation. The *circles* represent two terminal respiratory units (alveoli); the *shaded tubes* leading to them represent all the conducting airways. The *thick* arrows represent inspired and expired ventilation (tidal volume). *Mixed venous blood* (dark shading) flowing through the pulmonary artery from the right ventricle enters the alveolar wall capillaries, which are in intimate contact with the gas in the alveoli. By the process of diffusion (thin arrows), the capillary blood loses carbon dioxide and picks up oxygen to become *arterial blood* (light shading) in the pulmonary veins and systemic arteries. See Figure 2-8 for a more complete model. (Adapted from Comroe JH: Introduction. p. 1. In Physiology of Respiration. Year Book Medical Publishers, Chicago, 1974)

is shown in Figure 1-1. This diagram is useful for achieving a basic understanding of lung physiology and pathophysiology.

In the description of breathing and of respiration, I have not said anything about the composition of the air that is breathed nor about the composition of the blood within the circulatory system. The lung cannot regulate the composition of the external atmosphere nor is it responsible for the quantity or composition of blood. Although mammals evolved near sea level, they are adaptable and able to exist where there is much less oxygen (high altitude) or the total pressure of gases is markedly different (astronauts, scuba divers). In pulmonary disease, there are distortions of the process of breathing such that alveolar gas or blood may have markedly altered O_2 and CO_2 partial pressures or concentrations.

During the course of evolution, the body has developed ways to adjust, within limits, the gas partial pressures in the alveoli or in blood. This is the part of pulmonary physiology that describes the **regulation** of ventilation, blood flow, and ventilation/perfusion matching by various external agencies (nervous system, humoral substances) and internal agencies (terminal respiratory unit distensibility, resistance to airflow, resistance to blood flow). Figure 1-2 shows the essential components of a regulatory system. In a major way, *regulation of function is the essence of physiology*. It can only be learned from measurements on intact organisms.

The main body mass in humans depends on the lungs (average, 700 g; 1% body mass) for O_2 and CO_2 exchange. But it is not possible for the breathing mechanism alone to regulate the

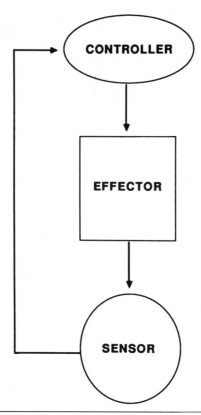

Fig. 1-2. Block diagram of the control of the breathing system. It is a feedback system; that is, the output of each element is the input to the next one. The *controller* is the brain. The *effector* is the muscles of the chest wall (not the lung, which is passive). The *sensor* consists of several elements in the lungs, arterial blood, chest wall, and brain stem that detect various results of the act of breathing and send reports (nerve impulses) to the *controller* to tell it to increase or decrease activity.

concentrations of O_2 or CO_2 in blood, even though it may be able to regulate their partial pressures. For example, if the blood consisted only of plasma, oxygen delivery to the cells would depend on the amount of oxygen dissolved in plasma at the oxygen pressure existing in the lung's alveoli. For (convective) blood O_2 transport, it is concentration not pressure that is important, exactly the opposite of diffusion. Since oxygen is rather insoluble in water, the cardiac output would have to be enormous to supply the oxygen needs (250 ml O_2/min at rest) of the respiring cells using plasma alone, even if every molecule of oxygen could be extracted from the plasma during its transit through the systemic capillaries. Plasma contains about 3 ml O_2/ liter at the normal arterial oxygen partial pressure.

Fortunately, blood contains a special protein, **hemoglobin,** within the erythrocytes. The remarkable property of hemoglobin is its ability to combine *rapidly* and *reversibly* with oxygen (1.34 g O_2/g hemoglobin) to effectively increase its solubility in blood manyfold. The **oxygen-hemoglobin equilibrium curve** (also called the oxygen dissociation curve) (Fig. 1-3) is the empirical (experimental) relationship between the partial pressure of oxygen in blood and the relative amount (percent saturation) bound to normal hemoglobin. Since the normal blood hemoglobin concentration is 150 g/liter (15 g/100 ml blood), hemoglobin is very effective in increasing blood oxygen concentration. Arterial blood contains nearly 200 ml O_2/liter at the normal oxygen partial pressure.

Thus, cardiac output in a resting human adult is about 5 liters/min. Moreover, at rest only about 25% of the oxygen bound to hemoglobin is exchanged between the blood and systemic tissues during each circulation. This has two beneficial effects: (1) it maintains a high oxygen partial pressure difference between systemic capillary blood and tissue cells, which is the driving pressure for oxygen diffusion into the cells, and (2) it provides a reserve of oxygen molecules for use by cells in an emergency (as when capillary blood flow is briefly slowed or stopped by muscle contraction).

Even in the heaviest steady-state exercise sustainable by average normal humans, cardiac output is unlikely to increase to more than three times the resting level (15 liters/min). Since oxygen usage by the body (oxygen consumption) in steady-state exercise may increase sixfold from the resting value (from 250 to 1,500 ml O_2/min), an additional 25% of the O_2 bound to hemoglobin in systemic arterial blood must be unloaded in the capillaries. The threefold increase in blood flow multiplied by the doubling of O_2 removal from blood accounts for the sixfold increase in O_2 consumption. It is possible for some highly trained athletes to increase their exercise cardiac output, ventilation, or oxygen consumption by more than this amount, but such people are not "average normal."

Throughout this text, I stress two components of respiratory physiology: (1) the processes of ventilation, blood flow, ventilation/perfusion, and oxygen transport and how they are regulated for efficient exchange; and (2) the quantitative assessment of these processes under various conditions. It is not enough to understand the concepts of respiration; one must be able to apply that general knowledge to specific instances (problem solving). On the other hand, it is not sufficient to plug numbers into formulas; one must also understand their significance. The process of respiration is completed in living cells when oxygen diffuses out of systemic capillary blood

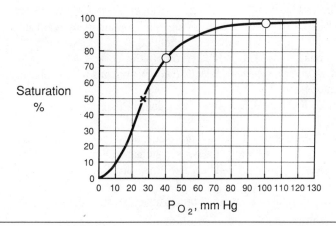

Fig. 1-3.   The standard hemoglobin-oxygen equilibrium curve (dissociation curve) for normal human blood containing hemoglobin A. The curve is an empirical relationship, representing an evolutionary adaptation of the utmost importance to the development of large multicellular animals and an exquisite example of functional utilitarianism (i.e., it works). Although the curve shows the equilibrium condition, it is important to know that the percentage of oxygen bound to the hemoglobin (y-axis) is *rapidly* and *reversibly* changed by altering oxygen partial pressure (x-axis). In this introductory chapter, it is not necessary to understand the detailed use of the curve, but it is important to become familiar with it because of its frequent use in physiology and medicine and later in this book. (See Fig. 8-1 for a more complete description and Questions 6 and 7 of this chapter.)

and through the interstitium to the mitochondria of the individual cells, where it is utilized in the oxidation process. Similarly, the carbon dioxide produced by cellular metabolism diffuses into the systemic capillary blood and flows away to the lung, where it is exhaled.

Although we know a great deal about the chemical processes of respiration within cells, our knowledge of the process of respiration in intact organs and tissue is far less complete. Nevertheless, in discussing the modern view of the physiology of respiration, it is important to keep one's eye firmly focused on the ultimate purpose of respiration, namely, the life and death of individual cells.

READINGS

Books

1. Berne RM, Levy MN (eds): Physiology. CV Mosby, St. Louis, 1983
   Chapters 37 to 41 cover respiratory physiology. Chapter 40 on control of respiration is especially recommended.
2. Forster RE II, DuBois AB, Briscoe WA, Fisher AB: The Lung: Physiologic Basis of Pulmonary Function Tests. 3rd Ed. Year Book Medical Publishers, Chicago, 1986
   Thorough coverage from the clinical physiologic approach. A useful book to read, especially if you are interested in some of the modern methods used to study pulmonary function. See also the 1989 book by Taylor (listed below).
3. Levitzky MG: Pulmonary Physiology. 2nd Ed. McGraw-Hill, New York, 1986
   Chapter 4 on blood flow to the lungs is thorough, and Chapter 10 describes some secondary (nonbreathing) lung functions.
4. Mines AH: Respiratory Physiology. 2nd Ed. Raven Press, New York, 1986
   Has useful questions and answers at chapter ends.
5. Schmidt RF, Thews G: Human Physiology. Springer-Verlag, Berlin, 1978
   Chapters 19 to 21 cover respiratory physiology and contain many good illustrations. Chapter 21 on tissue respiration is especially recommended.
6. Stryer L: Biochemistry. 3rd Ed. WH Freeman, New York, 1988
   Part II, *Generation and Storage of Metabolic Energy*, contains a basic discussion of respiration and energy metabolism.
7. Taylor AE, Rehder K, Hyatt RE, Parker JC: Clinical Respiratory Physiology. WB Saunders, Philadelphia, 1989
   The authors tried to encompass basic and more advanced (clinical) physiology, but emphasized advanced physiology. In some ways this book is similar to Forster et al.'s book (listed above).
8. West JB: Respiratory Physiology—The Essentials. 3rd Ed. Williams & Wilkins, Baltimore, 1985.
   Mainly descriptive. Emphasizes ventilation/perfusion relationships.

Reviews

9. The respiratory section in Annual Review of Physiology presents several mini reviews on different themes. These are oriented to research specialists; there is very little for beginning students, since current pulmonary research is concerned mainly with secondary and tertiary aspects of respiration.
10. State-of-the-art reviews have been appearing since 1974 (with interruptions) in American Review of Respiratory Disease. These are often clinically oriented, but over the years many fine basic physiology reviews have appeared.

QUESTIONS*

1. The process of oxygen transport from the environment to the mitochondria of mammalian cells is the central problem to be solved by the respiratory system. A clear picture of the oxygen transport path will facilitate your overall understanding of respiratory physiology. Describe the main steps in the oxygen transport process (environment to mitochondria). Identify the possible transport-limiting steps.

2. If you could regulate oxygen delivery to all body organs, which organs should have priority in an emergency limitation of oxygen supply? Please explain the order of each choice, including the least important. How does this apply to practical patient care? (*Hint*: Think about what you would do in an emergency, such as helping an accident victim.)

3. If all fresh air were breathed into the right lung and all pulmonary blood flow went to the left lung, what would be the effect on gas exchange? Try to estimate the ventilation/perfusion ratios of the right and left lungs. (*Hint*: Use the model in Fig. 1-1. Knowledge of the exact ventilation or blood flow is not necessary to arrive at the correct answer.)

4. At an oxygen partial pressure (P_{O_2}) of 40 mmHg, what is the percent oxygen saturation of normal hemoglobin in circulating blood? (*Hint*: Use Fig. 1-2.)

5. At an oxygen saturation of 50%, what is the P_{O_2} (oxygen partial pressure) in normal hemoglobin in circulating blood? (*Hint*: Use Fig. 1-2.)

6. What is the limiting feature of Figure 1-2 concerning the relation between blood oxygen concentration and oxygen partial pressure? (*Hint*: Study the labels on the axes.)

7. If you were asked to set up a control system (sensor, controller, effector) to maintain oxygen transport to all the cells of the body, what would you detect? Where would you detect it? What type of a controller would you install? What would the controller do to maintain oxygen transport as close to normal as possible? (*Hint*: Use Fig. 1-3.)

8. Children may threaten their parents by declaring they will hold their breath until they die. Determined children can hold their breath for a minute or even longer, but there is a fail-safe control mechanism that prevents completion of the threat. What is it? (*Hint*: Try to hold your breath indefinitely. What does it feel like just before you breathe?)

* Answers begin on p. 211.

2

Structural Basis for Lung Function

THE BOTTOM LINE

The prime function of the lung—matching of ventilation to perfusion—is reflected by the coordinated branching pattern of the airways and the pulmonary arteries.

Airways

The airways are of two types: cartilaginous bronchi and membranous bronchioles. The alveolar ducts (final branches of the bronchioles) together with the alveoli in their walls form the gas exchange part of the lung.

Pulmonary Circulation

One pulmonary artery branch accompanies each airway and branches with it. To maximize the rate of O_2 and CO_2 diffusional exchange with the pulmonary blood flow, the lung has the most extensive capillary network of any organ; capillaries occupy 70 to 80% of the alveolar surface area. Even during heavy exercise, the erythrocytes remain in the capillaries long enough for gas exchange to reach equilibrium.

Terminal Respiratory Unit

Groups of alveolar ducts and their alveoli together with their supplying arteries are combined into small functional elements called terminal respiratory units. There are about 60,000 of these ventilation/perfusion units in the human lung. The units are arranged in parallel, like the leaves on a tree, thus ensuring the efficient distribution of inspired air and mixed venous blood.

Chest Wall

Functionally, the chest wall includes not only the diaphragm and rib cage but also the abdomen. Coordinated muscle contraction in the chest wall enlarges the thoracic cavity during inspiration, while the lungs expand passively in all directions to fill the cavity.

The lungs of a normal living adult weigh 900 to 1,000 g, of which 40 to 50% is blood. At end expiration, the gas volume (the **functional residual capacity,** or **FRC**) is about 2.4 liters, while at maximal inspiration the gas volume (the **total lung capacity,** or **TLC**) may be 6 liters. Table 2-1 summarizes the mass and volume distribution of the main components of the

9

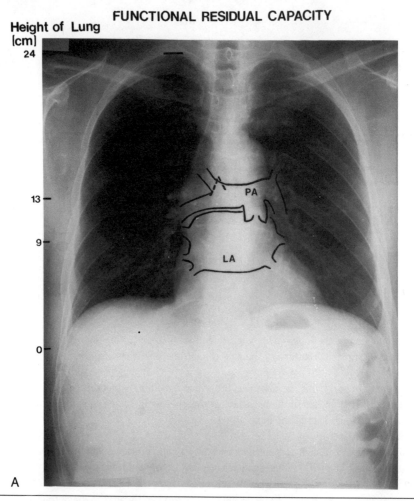

FUNCTIONAL RESIDUAL CAPACITY

Height of Lung [cm]

A

Fig. 2-1.   These chest radiographs taken at (**A**) functional residual capacity (FRC; normal end expiration) and (**B**) total lung capacity (TLC; maximum lung volume), respectively, show the general anatomic relationships among the lungs, heart, and chest wall structures. The outlines of the main pulmonary artery (PA) and the left atrium (LA) are indicated. The left margin of each figure is labeled to show the positions of the various structures relative to the lowest part of the lung. (*Figure continues.*)

human lung. The overall density of the lung (grams per milliliter) at FRC is approximately 0.27 g/ml [900 g/(900 ml + 2,400 ml)], decreasing to 0.14 g/ml at total lung capacity. It is amazing how little tissue, only 250 g, is required for the alveolar wall structures, but it is not difficult to understand the functional importance of this. It is because oxygen must diffuse from the alveolar gas into the erythrocytes flowing along the pulmonary capillaries. In water (the main component of alveolar walls and blood), oxygen diffusion is a rapid transport process over short distances (1 μm, 10^{-6} m) but becomes very slow over longer distances (1 mm, 10^{-3} m).

Figure 2-1 shows two chest radiographs of a normal standing human, whose lung volumes are at functional residual capacity, FRC (Fig. 2-1A), or at total lung capacity, TLC (Fig. 2-1B).

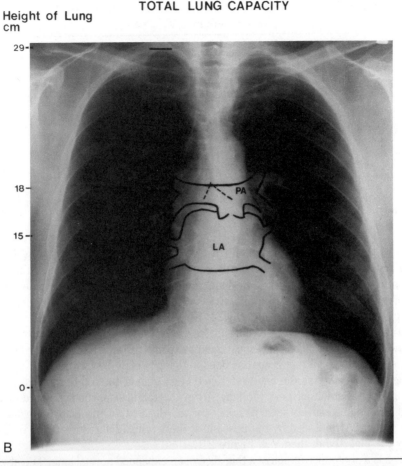

Fig. 2-1 (*Continued*). Notice the downward as well as the outward expansion of the chest cavity with inspiration. Relative to the top of the lung (short horizontal line at the apex of the right chest cavity), the bifurcation of the trachea (dashed line) moves down during inspiration, demonstrating that not only the bottom but also the top portion of the lung expands.

The shadows of the large blood vessels and airways can be seen to radiate out from the hilum (lung root). Although the individual alveolar structures cannot be resolved, the dark areas due to x-ray transmission (overexposure of the film) show that the peripheral parts of the lung are mostly gas. Indeed, the terminal respiratory units are 85% gas by volume, even at FRC.

Inspiration, caused by coordinated neural influences from the respiratory control centers in the brain stem, is the active phase of breathing. It causes the diaphragm and external intercostal muscles to contract. The muscle contraction causes the thoracic cavity to expand, which lowers the pressure in the pleural space surrounding the lungs. As the pressure falls in the pleural space, the distensible lungs expand passively, which causes the pressure in the terminal air spaces (alveolar ducts and alveoli) to decrease. As the pressure decreases, fresh air flows down the branching airways into the terminal air spaces until the pressures are equalized, which marks

Table 2-1. Quantitative Composition of the Normal Human Lung at Two Representative Volumes

Component	Functional Residual Capacity[a]		Total Lung Capacity	
Gas (ml)	2,400		6,000	
Tissue (g)	900		1,000	
Blood	400		500	
Arteries		150		200
Capillaries		70		80
Veins		180		220
Lung	500		500	
Support structures		250		250
Alveolar walls		250		250

[a] Functional residual capacity means at the end of a normal expiration. Total lung capacity means maximal lung volume.

the end of inspiration. During expiration (the mostly passive phase of chest wall motion) the process is reversed, pleural and alveolar pressures rise, and gas flows out of the lung.*

During growth and development, the lung conforms to the shape of the pleural cavities in such a manner as to minimize structural stress (mechanical forces tending to cause distortion of the lung tissue elements). At FRC (Fig. 2-1A), the lungs are about 24 cm high, narrowing at the top (apex; cupola) and at the bottom (costodiaphragmatic recess). With breathing, the lung expands in all directions as the chest cavity expands. Contrary to popular belief, the lung does not "sit" on the diaphragm; neither does it "hang" solely by the trachea. If one uses the apex of the pleural cavity as the fixed reference point (line at the top of right lung in Fig. 2-1), then during inspiration all parts of the lung, even the topmost portion, move downward. The downward movement can be seen not only by the descent of the diaphragm (compare Fig. 2-1B with Fig. 2-1A), but also by the descent of the tracheal bifurcation (carina). The latter is marked by the inverted dashed V in Figure 2-1.

Figure 2-2 is a photomicrograph of a thin slice of an expanded normal lung. The alveolar tissue occupies only a tiny fraction of the total area. Figures 2-3 (low power) and 2-4 (high power) are electron micrographic sections of a group of alveoli and of a single alveolar wall, respectively. The alveolar walls contain a vast network of blood capillaries. The average distance between the alveolar gas and the hemoglobin in the red blood cells is 1.5 μm.

The myriad anatomic alveoli, some of which are shown in Figures 2-2 and 2-3, give the human lung a total internal surface area of approximately 1 m²/kg body weight at FRC. This vast area (70 m² total) is not necessary for the distribution of gas within the lung. Rather, it fulfills the need for distributing the pulmonary blood flow (cardiac output) into a very thin film (one red blood cell thick in Fig. 2-4) in such a manner that even under stressful circumstances (such as exercise) the following are accomplished: (1) the time spent by each erythrocyte flowing along the capillaries is sufficient to permit equilibration of O_2 and CO_2 between blood and gas; (2) the

---

* Less obviously, as pleural pressure decreases during inspiration, so does the pressure in the pericardial sac, which lies in the thoracic cavity surrounded by pleural space. The distensible heart tends to expand, which causes the pressure in the cardiac chambers to fall. As the pressure decreases, venous return increases because of the increased driving pressure from the peripheral venous reservoirs to the right atrium. In that sense breathing "ventilates" the heart as well as the lungs. In cardiopulmonary resuscitation (CPR), the rescuer alternately compresses and decompresses the rib cage, but that does not directly affect the heart. The physiologic effect is to increase (compression) and decrease (decompression) the pressure in the pleural space, which affects venous return and promotes blood flow, even though the heart may not be effectively contracting.

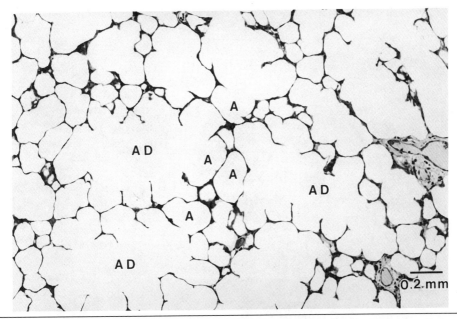

Fig. 2-2.   Low-magnification section of a well-expanded fixed lung. The larger central openings are the final branches of the gas exchange airways, or alveolar ducts (AD). Surrounding the ducts are the anatomic alveoli (A). There is a great deal of gas and very little tissue. The main function of the anatomic alveoli is to greatly increase the gas exchange surface area. (Courtesy of K. H. Albertine, Thomas Jefferson University, Philadelphia.)

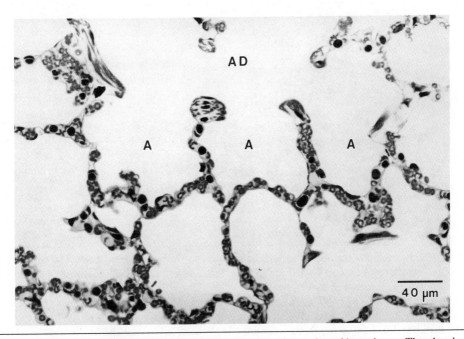

Fig. 2-3.   Low-power electron microscopic view of a very thin section of lung tissue. The alveolar wall capillaries are full of erythrocytes. (Courtesy of K. H. Albertine, Thomas Jefferson University, Philadelphia.)

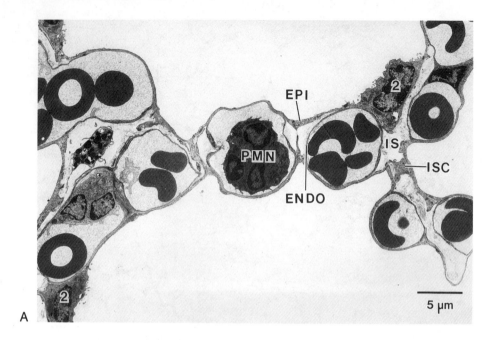

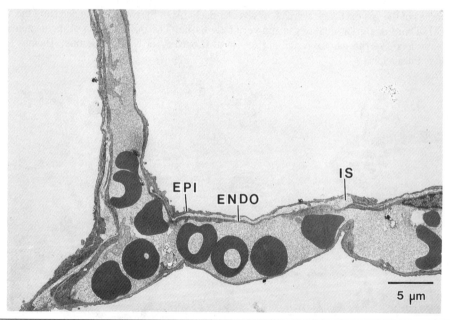

Fig. 2-4. High-resolution transmission electron micrographs of two alveolar walls. The major alveolar wall support structures that are labeled include the thin alveolar epithelium (EPI); a small amount of interstitial space (IS) containing fibroblasts, collagen, and elastin fibers; interstitial cells (ISC); and the capillary endothelium (ENDO). In Fig. A, one can also see a type 2 alveolar epithelial cell (granular pneumonocyte) in the alveolar corner (labeled 2). This is a special cell that appears to be the progenitor of the thin alveolar epithelial cell (type 1) that covers most of the alveolar surface (EPI). The type 2 cell is also the source of the special material known as **surfactant** that lines the alveolar air-liquid interface. Fig. A also shows a polymorphonuclear leucocyte (PMN). (Courtesy of K. H. Albertine, Thomas Jefferson University, Philadelphia.)

tissue phase of gaseous diffusion (air-to-blood distance) is minimized; and (3) the resistance to blood flow is low (large number of parallel pathways).

On the basis of the first effect, the pulmonary physiologist equates the partial pressures of O_2 and CO_2 in the alveoli with the partial pressures of the same gases in the blood leaving the pulmonary capillaries of those alveoli. Because of the second effect, the process of gaseous diffusion is not rate-limiting in the normal lung, even under stressful conditions, such as exercise. Because of the third effect, the power requirement of the right heart for pumping blood is much less than that of the left heart.

AIRWAYS

Figures 2-5 and 2-6 show the two main types of conducting airways: cartilaginous **bronchi** and membranous **bronchioles.** Since these conducting airways do not generally participate in gas exchange, their portion of each breath is wasted (**anatomic dead space**). Their combined length and cross-sectional area is such that the dead space represents about 30% of each normal breath, while resistance to airflow is low.

In addition to their supporting cartilage plates, the bronchi (Fig. 2-5) are characterized by a pseudostratified columnar epithelium, which rests on spiral bands of smooth muscle. The bronchi are able to dilate or constrict independently of lung volume. In fact, the pressure outside these airways is closer to pleural pressure than to alveolar pressure. Among the numerous cell types in the epithelium are a large number of cells with cilia, whose rhythmic beating in a thin liquid layer effectively transports the surface film of mucus and particles out of the lung, by way of the trachea.

The bronchi decrease in diameter and length with each successive branching, but the sum of the cross-sectional area of the two "child" bronchi is greater than that of the "parent." The cartilage support also gradually disappears. In airways about 1 mm in diameter, the cartilage disappears completely; by convention, all subsequent airways are called bronchioles. Figure 2-6A shows several bronchioles in a frozen lung section and Figure 2-6B shows a terminal bronchiole in cross section. The bronchioles have a simple cuboidal epithelium. There is an important functional difference between bronchioles and bronchi, namely, the bronchioles are embedded directly into the connective tissue framework of the lung so that their diameter depends on lung volume.

The airways, from the trachea to the terminal bronchioles, receive their blood supply via the bronchial arteries, a systemic source. Bronchial blood flow is normally about 1% of cardiac output. The bronchial circulation provides nutrition to the airways and larger pulmonary blood vessels, warms and adds water vapor to condition inspired air, and provides substrate for airway cellular metabolism and secretions.

Not seen in standard histologic sections are the motor and sensory nerves of the airways, which participate in the reflex regulation of breathing, airway caliber, and glandular secretion and in bronchial vasomotor control. The subepithelial smooth muscle bands (Figs. 2-5B and 2-6B) receive their motor innervation via the parasympathetic branch of the autonomic nervous system (vagus nerve). When the airway smooth muscle contracts, the lumen is narrowed, thereby reducing the anatomic dead space and increasing airflow resistance.

Sensory fibers are located beneath and within the intercellular junctions of the epithelial cells. The best understood sensory receptors, located in the bronchi (chiefly the trachea and main stem bronchi), are sensitive to physical distortion (stretch) and to chemical substances (irritants). All along the airways, particularly in the bronchioles and in the alveolar walls, are small, non-myelinated, slowly conducting C fibers. Although these fibers are nonspecific, they occur in great numbers and can be stimulated by a variety of chemical mediators, by which various

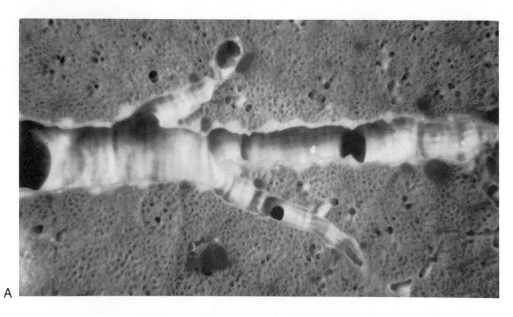

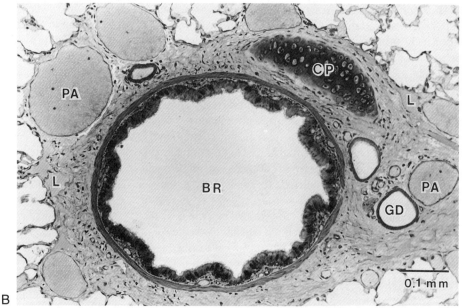

Fig. 2-5. Cartilaginous bronchi shown **(A)** in longitudinal section and **(B)** in cross section. In both pictures, the prominent cartilage supporting structures can be seen. There are frequent branchings whose diameters and angles are not uniform (irregular dichotomous branching). The volume of gas within the bronchus (BR) is part of the **anatomic dead space** (wasted ventilation). The cross section in Fig. B shows, in addition to the piece of a cartilage plate (CP), some pulmonary arterial branches (PA). Lining the bronchus is the pseudostratified columnar epithelium, whose ciliated surface can be barely resolved at this magnification. Surrounding the epithelium is a layer of smooth muscle, which actively regulates airway diameter. The smooth muscle cells are arranged in a spiral conformation, which allows the airways to shorten as well as to narrow. In the surrounding loose connective tissue are some glands and their ducts (GD) and lymphatic vessels (L).

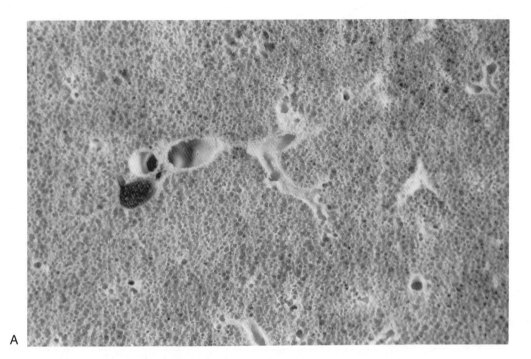

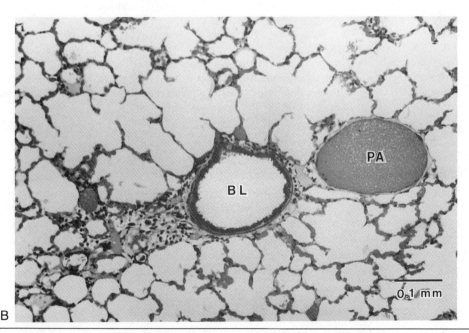

Fig. 2-6. Frozen lung sections **(A & C)** showing longitudinal sections of bronchioles and **(B)** a chemically fixed cross section. The main difference between bronchi and bronchioles, other than size, is that bronchioles have no cartilage and no secretory glands and are directly attached to the connective tissue structure of lungs. In cross section, bronchioles (BL) show a simple cuboidal epithelium, which is surrounded by a thin band of spirally arranged smooth muscle. (*Figure continues.*)

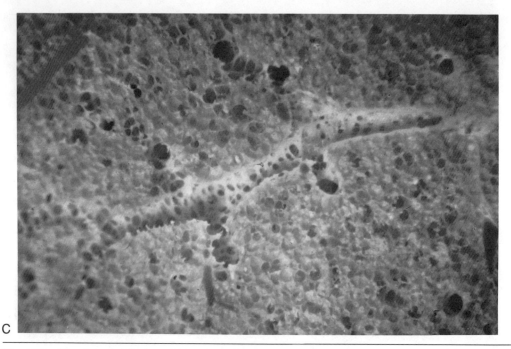

C

Fig. 2-6   (*Continued*). The bronchioles generally are not named except for the last generations (terminal bronchioles, respiratory bronchioles, and alveolar ducts). A respiratory bronchiole is a terminal bronchiole with primitive alveoli, as shown in Fig. C. Alveolar ducts (AD) are bronchioles whose walls have become almost completely replaced by alveolar openings. Although the bronchioles are part of the airway system through which gas flows, they are also part of the gas exchange volume. In Fig. C, each branch of the airway is accompanied by a pulmonary artery branch. The relationship between the airway (ventilation) and pulmonary artery (perfusion) is maintained. A **terminal respiratory unit** consists of all alveolar ducts and alveoli distal to the first generation respiratory bronchiole. (Fig. B courtesy of K. H. Albertine, Thomas Jefferson University, Philadelphia.)

pulmonary-cardiac reflex responses are elicited. The role of these fibers in normal regulation of the lungs and heart, however, is not well understood.

Eventually, the bronchioles develop outpouchings, which are the primitive alveoli (Fig. 2-6C). The first bronchioles with alveoli are called **respiratory bronchioles** to convey the concept that they participate in gas exchange. With successive branching (generations) of the respiratory bronchioles, the number and size of the anatomic alveoli increase until the walls of the bronchioles are almost completely replaced by the mouths of the alveoli. These final airway branches are called **alveolar ducts** (see Figs. 2-2 and 2-6C).

PULMONARY CIRCULATION

Not only the chest radiograph (Fig. 2-1) but also the histologic sections (Figs. 2-5 and 2-6) reveal the close relationship between the airways (ventilation) and the pulmonary arteries (perfusion) at all levels down to the respiratory bronchioles. Thus, the physiologic theme of *ventilation/perfusion matching for efficient lung function* is reflected in the anatomic pattern of the bronchovascular system. The distribution of the pulmonary veins is different. The veins lie within the interlobular and interlobar connective tissue septae, where they receive blood from many terminal respiratory units.

Pulmonary arteries and veins larger than about 50 μm in diameter in the normal adult human contain smooth muscle and actively regulate their diameter, thus altering resistance to blood flow. The pulmonary vasculature is richly innervated. The motor nerve to the smooth muscle comes from the sympathetic branch of the autonomic nervous system. However, in contrast to the systemic circulation, the normal pulmonary circulation shows little evidence of active external regulation. The extensive sensory innervation, located in the adventitia surrounding the blood vessels, can be stimulated by vascular pressure changes (stretch) and by various chemical substances, but its role in regulation of pulmonary and cardiac events is unclear. Most active regulation is caused by local metabolic influences.

The walls of the larger conducting arteries and veins are supplied by vasa vasorum from the bronchial arteries. As with the airways, this systemic supply disappears in the small muscular arteries at the level of the respiratory bronchiole. There are no functional connections between the bronchial circulation and the pulmonary arteries in normal humans, but the intrapulmonary bronchial venules anastomose with small pulmonary veins. Thus, intrapulmonary bronchial blood returns mainly to the left heart, forming part of the venous admixture (venous blood that effectively bypasses the pulmonary gas-exchange capillaries).

A simple way to remember the distribution of the bronchial circulation is to remember that it is the **nutritive** supply to all lung support structures (airways, vessels, connective tissue septae, and pleura). The pulmonary circulation is the nutritive supply to the alveolar walls.

The pulmonary capillaries form an extensive interdigitating network within the alveolar walls. Indeed, some anatomists describe the capillary network as a sheet of blood. Figure 2-7 shows two alveolar walls as they might be seen by an oxygen molecule in the alveolar gas space. When the capillaries are full, most of the alveolar wall (70 to 80%) overlies red cells. The total capillary surface area thus is nearly as great as the alveolar surface area.

In the living lung under resting conditions, the capillaries are not completely filled with blood. Anatomically, the maximal capillary volume of the human adult lung is about 200 ml, whereas at rest the effective volume is about 70 ml (1 ml/kg; 40 ml/m^2 body surface area) at FRC. Capillary volume may be increased by opening of closed vessels (recruitment, as with increased blood flow in exercise) or by enlargement of open vessels as their internal pressure rises (distension, as when the lungs are congested in left heart failure). Figure 2-7A shows a relatively normal capillary network in a single alveolar wall. Figure 2-7B shows a congested capillary network. As Table 2-1 shows, increasing lung volume by natural breathing increases capillary volume modestly.

Another feature of the alveolar capillary network is that the capillaries are continuous over several alveoli. Red blood cells travel an average of 600 to 800 μm through pulmonary capillaries before they enter the venous drainage system. Interestingly, in the normal upright human, the blood within the pulmonary capillaries at any instant (the capillary blood volume) is about equal to the stroke volume of the heart. That means that at an average heart rate of 75 beats/min, red blood cells will remain within the capillaries for one cardiac cycle of 0.8 second (60 s/75 beats). This is more than enough time for the diffusion of O_2 and CO_2, which occurs rapidly (<0.25 second to equilibration), through the very thin (average, 1.5 μm) barrier between the alveolar gas and the red blood cells.

The diffusion of oxygen is only meaningful when the alveolar walls contain red blood cells. Thus, in Figure 2-7, those areas of the alveolar wall that do not contain red blood cells are not contributing to O_2 and CO_2 exchange.

From the top to the bottom of the lung (Fig. 2-1), the hydrostatic pressure in the pulmonary

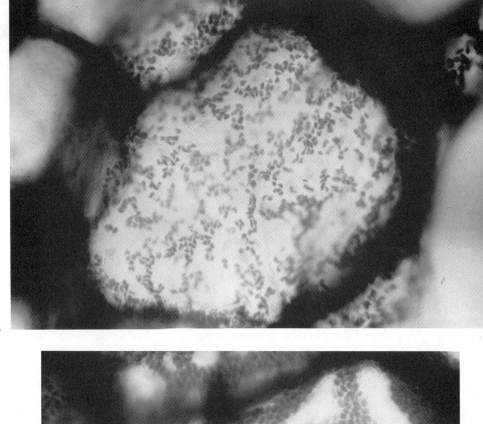

A

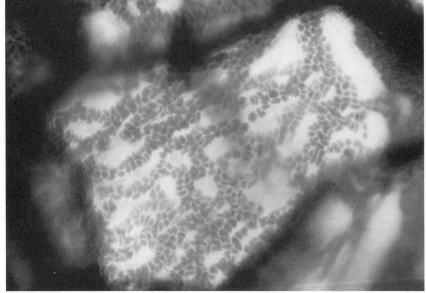

B

Fig. 2-7. Single alveolar walls seen face-on to show the extent of filling of the capillary network. In Fig. A, the capillaries are less well-filled with erythrocytes than in Fig. B. **(A)** Alveolus near top of the lung, where the vascular pressures are low. **(B)** Alveolus near the bottom of the lung, where the vascular pressures are high, so that the capillary network is fully recruited and also distended.

circulation varies by approximately 1 cmH_2O/cm height (in the direction of gravity). Thus, at FRC the pressure in the pulmonary artery is 24 cmH_2O greater near the bottom than near the top (Fig. 2-1A). The pressures in the veins vary in the same manner. Since left atrial pressure (the effective venous outflow pressure) is less than pulmonary arterial pressure (in order for blood flow to occur), the pressure in the veins near the top of the lung may fall below atmospheric pressure (alveolar pressure) at end expiration or end inspiration. The anatomic effect of this compressive (negative*) transmural pressure is that the pulmonary capillaries and venules will collapse and form a Starling resistor (flow-limiting segment), as you may have learned in cardiovascular physiology.

The physiologic importance of the distribution of pulmonary arterial and venous pressures over the height of the lung is that the lung can be divided into functional regions (zones) of blood flow, which depend on the pressures in the pulmonary vessels relative to alveolar pressure (see Chapter 7 for a detailed description). The volume of blood in the pulmonary capillaries represented in Figure 2-7 is the anatomic reflection of the regional vascular pressures and blood flow. Figure 2-7A is from the upper part of a normal lung, where venous pressure is less than alveolar pressure. Both blood flow and capillary filling (blood volume) are reduced in comparison with Figure 2-7B, which is of a congested alveolar wall near the bottom of the lung, where vascular pressures are high and the capillaries are distended with blood.

The distribution of blood flow throughout the lung is complicated. The important thing to learn at this point is that there are functional anatomic variations in the pulmonary microcirculation that can be explained on a mechanical (passive) basis. This effect is important for understanding the normal distribution of ventilation/perfusion ratios in the lung.

Finally, the pulmonary vessels can be divided into those that are directly affected by alveolar pressure and those that are not. These are referred to as **alveolar** and **extra-alveolar** vessels, respectively. The alveolar vessels include most of the capillaries. If the lung is forcibly expanded by gas at high pressure, it is possible to squeeze most of the alveolar capillaries so that they contain no blood (and therefore no flow), but it is not possible to squeeze the blood out of the arteries and veins because the surrounding lung tissue elements effectively pull them open as lung volume increases. In Table 2-1, notice the large increase in arterial and venous volumes as the lung expands. The effect of alveolar pressure on cardiac output and pulmonary vascular resistance becomes important when mechanical devices (ventilators) are used to assist breathing.

THE TERMINAL RESPIRATORY UNIT

When physiologists or chest physicians use the term alveolus, they are not usually referring to the anatomic alveoli, of which there are 300 million in the normal human lung. They are referring to a *functional* unit which behaves in terms of oxygen and carbon dioxide exchange as if it were one large alveolus. Anatomically, this unit is called the **terminal respiratory unit.** For simplicity and because it is difficult to change common usage, I will sometimes refer to it as the alveolus, but the student must clearly understand that I do not mean the anatomic structure of that name.

In the human adult lungs, there are some 60,000 terminal respiratory units. Each unit contains about 5,000 anatomic alveoli and 250 alveolar ducts. All components of the terminal respiratory

---

* Pressure (P) across the walls of distensible hollow organs is always measured as $P_{inside} - P_{outside}$.

unit participate in volume changes. Nearly one-third of the total "alveolar" gas volume is located in the alveolar ducts, not in the anatomic alveoli. As the terminal respiratory unit expands (inspiration), the gas in the alveolar ducts (left over from the previous exhalation) enters the anatomic alveoli, and fresh air fills the alveolar ducts. The anatomic alveoli are not ventilated with fresh air during tidal breathing. This process, known as sequential ventilation, means that the oxygen molecules in fresh air must diffuse into the anatomic alveoli and that the carbon dioxide molecules in the alveolar gas from the previous breath must diffuse into the alveolar ducts. However, this happens so rapidly (several thousandths of a second in the gas phase) that for practical purposes the partial pressures throughout the gas phase of a terminal respiratory unit are in equilibrium.

ANATOMIC MODEL

Figure 2-8 is a model of the relationships among the various structural elements of the lung. It has the same general design as the schema shown in Figure 1-1 but illustrates some functions of the lung that cannot be understood using the simpler model. For example, in Figure 1-1 the pulmonary arteries do not have any relationship to the airways, whereas in Figure 2-8 they are shown accompanying the bronchi and bronchioles down to the terminal respiratory units. The

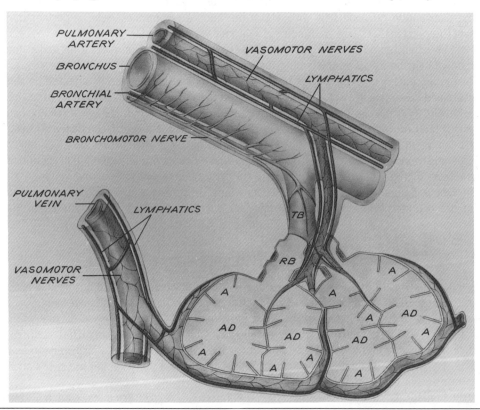

Fig. 2-8.   Compare this model with the simplified schema in Figure 1-1. The main difference between the two pictures in terms of structure-function relations is the close relationship between the pulmonary arteries (perfusion) and airways (ventilation), which is necessary in order to understand the local regulation of ventilation/perfusion. (From Gray TC, Nunn J (eds): General Anaesthesia. 4th Ed. Butterworth, London, 1980)

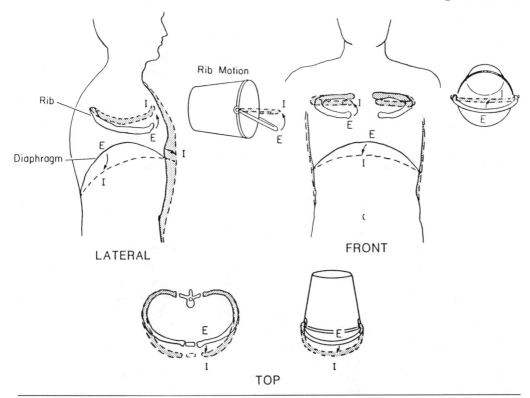

Fig. 2-9. Model demonstrating the motion of the chest wall between end expiration (E) and end inspiration (I). The movements are exaggerated compared with normal breathing. The ribs may be likened to a **pail handle,** as shown in the lateral, front, and top views. The diaphragm descends as it shortens. The anterior chest wall moves outward due to the rib motion over the thorax and the increasing pressure within the abdomen.

local regulation of ventilation/perfusion by alveolar gas composition depends on knowing the correct anatomy.

CHEST WALL

The functional chest wall includes not only the rib cage and diaphragm but also the abdominal cavity and anterior abdominal muscles. Since the lungs are passive during breathing, it is up to the muscles of the chest wall—principally the diaphragm—to expand the thoracic cavity and thus cause inspiration.

The shape of the lungs is necessarily the same as that of the thoracic cavity. The **visceral** and **parietal** pleurae cover the surfaces of the lungs and thoracic cavity, respectively. These surface structures help to keep the pleural space open, probably by inhibiting fibroblast migration. The lung and the chest wall pleurae are coupled together by a thin film of liquid (about 20 μm thick). This liquid coupling is better than a direct anatomic attachment because it allows the lung to move relative to the chest wall during breathing and thereby to accommodate with minimum stress to changes in thoracic configuration.

The thoracic cavity enlarges in all dimensions as the rib cage rotates upward and outward (pail-handle motion) and the diaphragm simultaneously descends into the abdomen (Fig. 2-9).

The diaphragm is the main muscle of the chest wall. In chest radiographs it appears as a dome-shaped structure separating the thoracic and abdominal cavities (Fig. 2-1). The diaphragm is a *musculotendinous sheet.* It consists of muscle bundles that originate along the lower ribs and insert on a flat central tendon. The caudal rim of the rib cage marks the attachment of the diaphragm. Thus, the diaphragm is higher in front (sternum) than behind (spinal column).

The blood supply to the diaphragm is from branches of the intercostal arteries. The veins drain centrally into the inferior vena cava. The diaphragm is innervated by two phrenic nerves, which originate from the third to fifth cervical (spinal cord) segments and descend laterally in the mediastinum to the right and left leaves of the diaphragm.

The human rib cage consists of 12 ribs on each side articulating with the thoracic vertebrae. Each rib can be thought of as part of a pail handle or hoop, as shown schematically in Figure 2-9. Normally, each rib is tilted some 30° below the horizontal plane. The only motion permitted the ribs is rotation upward toward the horizontal plane. This motion increases the cross-sectional area of the thorax viewed along its cephalocaudal axis.

The principal inspiratory muscles of the rib cage are the **external intercostals,** which are so oriented that as they contract, the rib hoops rotate upward toward the horizontal. The **internal intercostals** are expiratory muscles that are so oriented that when they contract, the rib hoops rotate downward away from the horizontal. The **accessory muscles** include the sternocleidomastoid and the scalene muscles, which are attached to the first two ribs and to the sternum. When these muscles contact, they pull up on the rib cage, thereby assisting inspiration. The rib cage muscles are supplied by intercostal arteries and veins and are innervated by intercostal nerves (motor and sensory).

An important characteristic of the rib cage is its stiffness. In normal quiet breathing, the rib cage may contribute up to one-half of the active inspiratory volume change; the diaphragm produces the rest. The rib cage also contributes passively to inspiration because it prevents any inward (paradoxical) movement of the thoracic wall. This inward movement can be seen in the newborn, whose cartilaginous rib cage is soft. In conditions in which the diaphragm is paralyzed, the rib cage must do all the work of breathing. As pleural pressure decreases in such individuals, the diaphragm is sucked up into the thorax (paradoxical motion of the diaphragm).

The diaphragm and chest wall muscles are of the fast, nonfatiguing variety. At low lung volume (i.e., at **residual volume,** RV), it is possible to generate very negative intrathoracic pressure (− 80 mmHg) by attempting to inspire against a closed glottis (Müller's maneuver). The Müller's maneuver produces an unpleasant sensation and sucks blood from the peripheral veins into the thoracic cavity. Near the total lung capacity (TLC), the ability of the chest wall muscles to generate further negative pleural pressure decreases rapidly to zero as the lungs become less compliant. This effect limits maximal inspiratory volume.

Many diseases involve an increase in end-expiratory lung volume (FRC) (for example, asthma with marked expiratory airway resistance or emphysema, characterized by destruction of lung elastic tissue). Under these conditions, the muscles of inspiration operate at a disadvantage, and their ability to reduce pleural pressure to cause lung expansion is reduced.

The work of taking a breath is done by the inspiratory muscles. This work is low under normal conditions (high lung distensibility and low resistance to airflow), so that the respiratory muscles have a large reserve capacity. In certain diseases, fatigue of the chest wall muscles, especially the diaphragm, may occur and be the immediate cause of serious disability (respiratory failure).

READINGS

Books

1. Miller WS: The Lung. 2nd Ed. Charles C Thomas, Springfield, 1947
   Several important special aspects of lung anatomy are described.
2. Von Hayek H: The Human Lung. Hafner, New York, 1960
   The classic modern reference of human lung anatomy.
3. Weibel ER: Morphometry of the Human Lung. Academic Press, San Diego, 1963
   The classic description of quantitative lung histology.

Reviews

4. Staub NC: The interdependence of pulmonary structure and function. Anesthesiology 24:831–854, 1963
   A physiologist uses lung anatomy to describe function.
5. Staub NC, Albertine KH: The structure of the lung relative to its principal function. In Murray JF, Nadel JA (eds): Textbook of Respiratory Medicine. Chapter 2. WB Saunders, Philadelphia, 1988
   Up-to-date view of lung structure for physicians.

QUESTIONS*

1. What is the main anatomic difference between the pathways of ventilation and perfusion in the lung?
2. Alveolar surface area is 1 m^2/kg body weight, and the alveolar wall thickness is 8 μm at FRC. What is the volume (in cubic centimeters) of the alveolar tissue (blood and alveolar walls) in a 50-kg woman?
3. Describe the major structural differences between bronchi and bronchioles in humans.
4. When a pulmonary artery branch is completely obstructed by a blood clot (pulmonary embolus), the lung tissue served by that artery is metabolically depressed for days or weeks, but the involved lung tissue does not usually die. What pathways for nutritional blood supply sustain life in the obstructed lung segment?
5. In heavy steady-state exercise, the cardiac output may be 15 liters/min. If the capillary blood volume expands to 150 ml, how long does the average erythrocyte remain in the gas exchange vessels (capillaries) of the alveolar wall?
6. Use Figure 2-1 to calculate pulmonary arterial pressure at the top and bottom of the lung at total lung capacity, when the mean arterial pressure at the level of the left atrium is 20 cmH_2O.
7. What is the volume of the average terminal respiratory unit at an FRC of 2,400 ml? What is its volume at a TLC of 6 liters?

---

* Answers begin on p. 211.

3

Some Fundamental Concepts

THE BOTTOM LINE

Respiratory Nomenclature

Although the symbols, abbreviations, and conventions of pulmonary physiology are confusing at first, they simplify writing equations. It is also important to learn some of the normal pulmonary function variables at rest and during steady-state exercise.

Universal Gas Law

The following equation is used to convert gas volumes, V, between different conditions of pressure, P, and temperature, T: $V_2 = V_1 \times (P_1/P_2) \times (T_2/T_1)$.

Partial Pressure

Ideally, the fraction of the total gas pressure exerted by each kind of gas in a mixture is proportional to the fractional concentration of the gas. Thus, in dry air at sea level, $P_{O_2} = 0.21 \times 760 = 160$ mmHg. *Water vapor pressure* in the lungs at 37°C is fixed at 47 mmHg and must be subtracted from the total pressure to obtain the dry gas pressure. Thus, normal $P_{A_{CO_2}} = (760 - 47) \times 0.056 = 40$ mmHg and $P_{A_{O_2}} = (760 - 47) \times 0.143 = 102$ mmHg.

Blood Gas Concentrations

The solubility coefficient α of O_2 in blood is low ($\alpha = 0.03$ ml O_2/[liter $\times$ mmHg]). The red protein hemoglobin (Hb) in erythrocytes binds O_2 rapidly and reversibly. Fully oxygenated hemoglobin carries 1.34 ml O_2/g Hb. Normal blood contains 150 g Hb/liter; thus, the oxygen capacity of normal blood is 201 ml O_2/liter.

Conservation of Mass

The fundamental concept of conservation of mass is widely used in the form of volumes of dilution. For example, to measure cardiac output by the Fick principle, $\dot{Q} = \dot{V}_{O_2}/(Ca_{O_2} - C\bar{v}_{O_2})$.

Graphs

Physiologists often show relationships by graphs. The hemoglobin-oxygen (HbO_2) equilibrium curve, the pressure-flow curve of the pulmonary circulation, and the pressure-

(Continues).

27

(*Continued*).
volume curve of the lung or chest wall are important graphs, the use and physiologic significance of which must be understood.
Concept of Independent Streams
A conceptual device often used to simplify complex problems (such as ventilation/perfusion problems) is to consider the problem "as if" it were composed of separate simpler parts.

RESPIRATORY NOMENCLATURE

In the average healthy adult, VC = 4 liters, BTPS, at a resting $\dot{V}_{O_2}$ of 250 ml/min, STPD. What do these terms mean? VC is shorthand for **vital capacity**, the maximum volume of air that can be breathed out after taking in as large a breath as possible. Vital capacity is measured at *body temperature* and *pressure*, using air *saturated* with water vapor (BTPS). Such a designation is reasonable because the physiologist or physician is interested in the volume of gas moved into and out of the lungs under the conditions that exist at the time.

In contrast, the **oxygen consumption** $\dot{V}_{O_2}$—the volume of oxygen consumed by the body per minute—is measured under uniform conditions called *standard temperature* (273 K) and *pressure* (760 mmHg), *dry* (STPD). Why is $\dot{V}_{O_2}$ measured this way? Because the physiologist or physician wants to know the moles of oxygen (number of O_2 molecules) used per minute, not the volume occupied by the oxygen.

A dot (·) over a symbol should be read as *quantity per unit time* or *rate*; for example, $\dot{V}$ means gas volume per unit time, that is, gas flow. A bar ($-$) over a symbol should be read as *mean* value; for example, $C\bar{v}_{O_2}$ is the mean venous blood oxygen concentration. Appendix 1 explains and lists all the standard respiratory symbols and abbreviations used in this book and gives examples. Although it is not necessary to memorize these symbols and abbreviations, the student will find it helpful to know and use them. Appendix 2 lists many of the commonly used respiratory variables together with their values for a normal adult under resting and steady-state exercise conditions.

Expressing values in correct units is important for communication. The quantity with the most units is pressure. The following conversion equations are used:

$$1 \text{ cmH}_2\text{O} = 0.74 \text{ mmHg (torr)} = 0.1 \text{ kPa}$$

$$1 \text{ mmHg (torr)} = 1.36 \text{ cmH}_2\text{O} = 0.136 \text{ kPa}$$

$$1 \text{ kPa} = 10 \text{ cmH}_2\text{O} = 7.4 \text{ mmHg (torr)}$$

The units mmHg (millimeters of mercury) and torr are equivalent. The torr was introduced to get around the fact that millimeters of mercury and centimeters of water are lengths not pressures (pressure is force per unit area).* Because of the density difference between mercury and water, millimeters of mercury has to be multiplied by 1.36 to obtain centimeters of water. The unit kilopascal (kPa) is part of a system of units called SI (Système Internationale), which

---

* A torr is the force generated by a column of mercury 1 mm high and 1 cm^2 in area; that is, 1 torr is equivalent to 1 mmHg.

is used widely in Europe but less in the United States. Since there is confusion enough in getting through a basic course in respiratory physiology, I will use only cmH_2O and mmHg as pressure units in this book.

Pulmonary vascular pressures (arterial, venous, left atrial) are usually expressed in cmH_2O by chest physicians but in mmHg by cardiologists. For example, normal left atrial pressure (Pla) = 11 cmH_2O × 0.74 mmHg/cmH_2O = 8.1 mmHg.

Gas phase pressures and blood gas tensions (the partial pressures exerted by gases dissolved in blood) are expressed in mmHg, never cmH_2O. For example, the partial pressure of carbon dioxide in alveolar gas (P_{ACO_2}) is 40 mmHg and the partial pressure of oxygen in systemic arterial blood (Pa_{O_2}) is 100 mmHg.

UNIVERSAL GAS LAW

The equation of state for ideal gases relates three variables—pressure (P), temperature (T), and volume (V)—to the number, n, of moles of gas. These quantities are related by a proportionality factor, R, called the **gas constant**:

$$n\text{R} = PV/T \tag{3-1}$$

where R = 62.4 (liters × mmHg)/(mole × K).*

This law is mainly used to convert volume between different conditions. If the number of moles of gas is constant, the volume under various conditions of pressure and temperature can be calculated. For example, if the gas exhaled from a person's lungs (condition 1) is collected in a large container (condition 2), it is clear that the number of moles of gas stays the same. Therefore, one can relate the three variables (pressure, volume, temperature) under the two conditions as follows:

$$\frac{V_1 \times P_2}{T_1} = n\text{R} = \frac{V_2 \times P_2}{T_2}$$

For volume conversion, the useful form of this equation is

$$V_2 = V_1 \times \frac{P_1}{P_2} \times \frac{T_2}{T_1} \tag{3-2}$$

As an example, consider a person with a vital capacity (VC) of 4.0 liters, BTPS. How is VC measured? One way is for the subject to breathe through a valve into a device called a **spirometer** (Fig. 3-1), which measures the volume of gas breathed. The gas in the spirometer is at sea level atmospheric pressure (760 mmHg) and room temperature (21°C) and is saturated with water vapor because it was humidified by the lungs and because the spirometer has water in it. In the spirometer, VC is measured as liters, ATPS. ATPS is a new set of conditions: *a*mbient (surrounding) *t*emperature and *p*ressure, *s*aturated with water vapor. Ordinarily, ATPS means atmospheric pressure at sea level and room temperature, but it does not have to. It is important

---

* At 273 K (0°C), 1 mole of an ideal gas at 760 mmHg (one standard atmosphere pressure) occupies 22.4 liters. Substituting these numbers into Eq. 3-1 yields R. Other values for R are obtained when other units are used. The most common substitution is using 1 atm (atmosphere) instead of 760 mmHg. In that case, R = 0.82 (liters × atm)/(mole × K).

to be alert to ambient conditions. To calculate VC as recorded on the spirometer, we use the gas law (Eq. 3-2) as follows:

$$VC, \text{ATPS} = 4.0 \text{ liters} \times \frac{(760 - 47) \text{ mmHg}}{(760 - 19) \text{ mmHg}} \times \frac{(273 + 21) \text{ K}}{(273 + 37) \text{ K}}$$

$$= 4.0 \times 713/741 \times 294/310$$

$$= 4.0 \times 0.962 \times 0.948$$

$$VC, \text{ATPS} = 3.6 \text{ liters}$$

The source of some of these numbers requires explanation. The total gas pressure in the alveoli of the lung (P_A) is equal to the total pressure in the spirometer (P_B; 760 mmHg), because the vital capacity maneuver begins with the alveoli in continuity with the outside air through the open airways (Fig. 3-1). In the lungs at 37°C, the water vapor pressure is always $P_{H_2O} = 47$ mmHg. In the spirometer, however, the lower temperature causes some of the water to condense out of the gas. Thus, at 21°C, $P_{H_2O} = 19$ mmHg.*

The loss of some water vapor, of course, violates the fundamental tenet of the universal gas law as expressed in Eq. 3-1, in which it is required that the number of moles of gas be constant. The pulmonary physiologist is only interested in *dry* gas volume. Thus, for the respiratory gases other than water vapor, the universal gas law does hold. In the above example, I corrected pressure to that of dry gas by subtracting the appropriate P_{H_2O} from each total pressure (alveolar and spirometer). For temperature, one always uses absolute temperature: (K) = 273 + (°C).

In the example, both the pressure and temperature ratios are slightly less than 1. That makes sense because there is less water vapor pressure in the spirometer, so the dry gas pressure is greater than in the lungs. If the pressure is greater, the volume must be less. Likewise, spirometer temperature is less than in the lungs. If the temperature is less, the volume must be less.

As a second example, let us convert oxygen consumption ($\dot{V}_{O_2}$) as measured in a spirometer to standard conditions (STPD). Assume the normal resting subject rebreathes (breathes the same gas in and out) for several minutes from a spirometer filled with oxygen and equipped with a carbon dioxide absorber (Fig. 3-2). The utilization of oxygen by the subject's body shows up as a steady decrease in the volume of the spirometer with time. Suppose the volume in the spirometer decreases by 2,760 ml, ATPS, in 10 min and that the subject's lung volume does not change (an important assumption). To convert from the conditions in the spirometer—ATPS—to standard conditions—STPD—we use Eq. 3-2 as follows:

$$\dot{V}_{O_2}, \text{STPD} = 2,760 \frac{\text{ml } O_2}{10 \text{ min}} \times \frac{(760 - 19) \text{ mmHg}}{760 \text{ mmHg}} \times \frac{273 \text{ K}}{(273 + 21) \text{ K}}$$

$$= 276 \times 741/760 \times 273/294$$

$$= 276 \times 0.975 \times 0.928$$

$$\dot{V}_{O_2}, \text{STPD} = 250 \text{ ml } O_2/\text{min}$$

The pressure and temperature ratios are again less than 1 because the gas is compressed by increasing the dry gas pressure and contracted by lowering the temperature.

---

* Between 21°C and 37°C, P_{H_2O} changes by about 2 mmHg/°C.

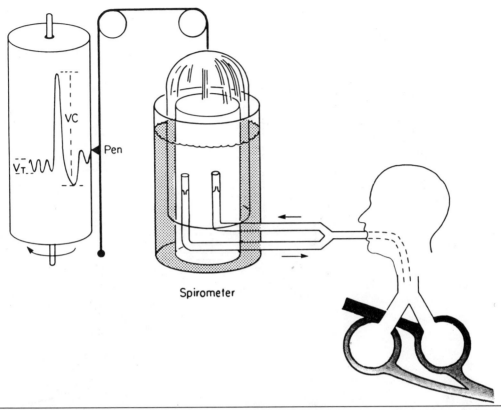

Fig. 3-1. Working diagram of a spirometer, a device for measuring volumes of gas. The spirometer contains a central compartment from which the subject inspires and into which the subject expires. The direction of breathing is controlled by one-way valves in the tubes. Surrounding the gas compartment is a water barrier, which seals the movable part of the spirometer, a lightweight, well-balanced dome. The dome moves up and down in proportion to the volume of gas entering or leaving the spirometer. The dome is connected by pulleys to a pen which writes on a vertical drum rotating at a fixed speed. In the figure, after several normal breaths (tidal volumes, V_T) the subject took a breath to total lung capacity and then breathed out as much as possible (vital capacity, VC). The subject then resumed normal tidal breathing.

Remember: If one converts from a high dry gas pressure to a low dry gas pressure or from a low temperature to a high temperature, volume *increases*. If one converts from a low dry gas pressure to a high dry gas pressure or from a high temperature to a low temperature, volume *decreases*.

PARTIAL PRESSURE

The concept of the **partial pressure** or **tension** of a gas is important. In any volume, the total gas pressure of all molecular species is the sum of the individual pressures *that would exist if each species were alone in the same volume.* This law of partial pressures is based on the assumption that the gas molecules do not interact; an assumption that is nearly true for the

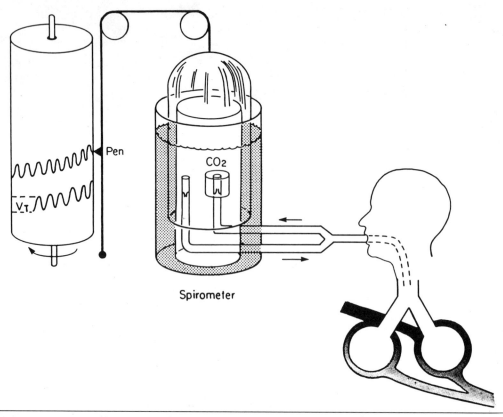

Fig. 3-2.   Configuration of a spirometer used to measure oxygen consumption. A CO_2 absorber has been added to the end of the tube which carries expired gas back to the spirometer. This markedly changes the tracing of spirometer volume (breathing). The tidal volumes (V_T) are no longer on an even line; rather, there is a continuous loss of spirometer volume. The slope of the end-expiration points (functional residual capacity, FRC) is the rate of oxygen utilization, ATPS. Conversion of the slope to STPD gives $\dot{V}_{O_2}$.

respiratory gases (O_2, CO_2, N_2, and H_2O). The law of partial pressures is a direct consequence of the universal gas law (Eq. 3-1), as can be seen by keeping volume and temperature constant and relating n (moles of gas) to pressure P.

In 100 liters of dry room air there are 21 liters of O_2 and 79 liters of N_2. For practical purposes, $[CO_2] = 0$ in ambient air. Thus, room air is 21% O_2 and 79% N_2. If all the nitrogen is removed and the remaining oxygen allowed to fill the 100 liter volume at constant temperature, the universal gas law requires that the pressure of oxygen (P_{O_2}) be

$$P_{O_2} = 0.21 \times P_B$$

$$= 0.21 \times 760 \text{ mmHg}$$

$$= 160 \text{ mmHg}$$

By the same reasoning, $P_{N_2} = 600$ mmHg. Table 3-1 lists the normal partial pressures of the respiratory gases at various physiologically important locations in the body.

Table 3-1. Total and Partial Pressures of Respiratory Gases in Ideal Alveolar Gas and
Blood at Sea Level Barometric Pressure (760 mmHg)

	Ambient Air (Dry)	Moist Tracheal Air	Alveolar Gas (R = 0.80)	Systemic Arterial Blood	Mixed Venous Blood
P_{O_2}	160	150	102	102	40
P_{CO_2}	0	0	40	40	46
P_{H_2O}, 37°C	0	47	47	47	47
P_{N_2}	600	563	571[a]	571	571
P_{total}	760	760	760	760	704[b]

[a] P_{N_2} is increased in alveolar gas by 1% because R < 1 normally.
[b] P_T in venous blood is reduced because P_{O_2} has decreased more than P_{CO_2} has increased.

Water Vapor Pressure

When air is inspired, it is warmed to 37°C in the nasal passages, throat, and trachea. As the air is warmed, water evaporates from the respiratory surfaces, and the air becomes saturated with water vapor at 37°C. The warming and saturation of inspired air is obligatory and rapid; no one can breathe fast or deeply enough, even on a very cold day, to prevent complete temperature and water vapor equilibration by the time the inspired air reaches the alveoli. The heat and water vapor are supplied by the airway submucosal (bronchial) blood flow. The water vapor exerts a mandatory partial pressure P_{H_2O} of 47 mmHg. That does not change the percentage of O_2 or N_2 in the dry gas mixture. Thus, about 6% of the inspired air (47/760 mmHg) is water vapor.

The total quantity of water in expired gas is not trivial. It is about 40 mg/liter, which over 24 hours accounts for a large fraction of the insensible (obligatory) water loss from the body. Room air (inspired gas) varies in its water vapor content (relative humidity) from near 0% (a summer day in Phoenix, Arizona) to 100% (a summer day in Washington, DC). In beautiful San Francisco where I live, it is about 50% year round. Pulmonary physiologists ignore the water vapor partial pressure in inspired gas by considering gas only after it has been saturated with water vapor at 37°C (referred to as **tracheal gas**). The fractions (F) of respiratory gases in inspired air (and in all gas volumes) are always dry. For example, for ambient air, $F_{I_{O_2}}$ = 0.21 regardless of location or weather.

Because the water vapor added during inspiration *dilutes* the inspired air, the concentrations of O_2 and N_2 must decrease. But, as already mentioned, respiratory physiologists prefer to say that the total dry gas pressure decreases. That must be so because in normal breathing there is no total pressure difference between room air and the moist, warm inspired air in the trachea. The dry gas pressure in the trachea is 760 − 47 = 713 mmHg, and the partial pressures of O_2 and N_2 in tracheal air are reduced to

$$P_{O_2} = 0.21 \times (760 - 47) \text{ mmHg} = 150 \text{ mmHg}$$

and

$$P_{N_2} = 0.79 \times (760 - 470) \text{ mmHg} = 563 \text{ mmHg}$$

> **Remember:** Always subtract P_{H_2O} from P_B before converting gas fractions to partial pressures.

In the alveoli, some oxygen diffuses into the pulmonary capillary blood, further reducing the partial pressure of the oxygen in alveolar gas. At a normal respiratory exchange ratio (R) of 0.80, the O_2 concentration of alveolar gas is 14.3%. For use in calculations, the oxygen concentration is usually expressed as the fraction F of O_2 in alveolar gas: $F_{A_{O_2}} = 0.143$. Thus, normally, alveolar P_{O_2} $P_{A_{O_2}} = 0.143 \times (760 - 47) = 102$ mmHg. The deficit in O_2 between inspired air and alveolar gas $(0.21 - 0.143 = 0.067)$ is made up by the CO_2 entering from the blood $(F_{A_{CO_2}} = 0.056)$ and by the slight increase in N_2 concentration caused by the fact that more O_2 is removed than CO_2 is added, while total pressure remains constant. Normally, $P_{A_{CO_2}}$ (alveolar P_{CO_2}) is closely regulated. It is the main controlled variable in breathing, as I will describe in Chapter 11.

$$P_{A_{CO_2}} = 0.056 \times (760 - 47) \text{ mmHg} = 40 \text{ mmHg}$$

The partial pressures of gases dissolved in water (such as blood plasma and interstitial or intracellular liquid) are equal to the partial pressures in the gas phase that is in equilibrium with the liquid. In the normal resting human, blood leaving the pulmonary capillaries has come to equilibrium with the alveolar gases: $P_{A_{O_2}} = P_{pv_{O_2}}$, $P_{A_{CO_2}} = P_{pv_{CO_2}}$, $P_{A_{N_2}} = P_{pv_{N_2}}$, $P_{A_{H_2O}} = P_{pv_{H_2O}}$. However, small quantities of venous blood from the bronchial venules and the thebesian veins of the heart contaminate pulmonary venous outflow so that the partial pressure of O_2 $(P_{a_{O_2}})$ in systemic arterial blood (a) is normally slightly less than that in "ideal" alveolar gas:

$$P_{a_{O_2}} = 100 \text{ mmHg}$$

$$P_{a_{CO_2}} = 40 \text{ mmHg}$$

BLOOD GAS CONCENTRATION

From the hemoglobin-oxygen (HbO_2) equilibrium curve (Fig. 1-3) one reads that at $P_{O_2} = 100$ mmHg the saturation of blood (S_{O_2}) = 97.4%. However, there is more oxygen in blood than is chemically bound to hemoglobin. Some oxygen is dissolved (is in physical solution) even though oxygen is not very soluble in water (blood). The quantity in solution is tiny compared with the quantity chemically bound to hemoglobin. The concentration of dissolved oxygen is determined by the solubility coefficient α. For oxygen in blood, $\alpha = 22.8$ ml/(liter $\times$ 760 mmHg). Thus, 1 liter of blood dissolves 0.03 ml O_2 for each 1 mmHg increase in P_{O_2}. The concentration, C, of dissolved oxygen in blood at any partial pressure is calculated as follows:

$$C_{O_2, \text{dissolved}} = \alpha \times V \times P \qquad (3\text{-}3)$$

where V is in liters and P is partial pressure.

Thus, at $P_{a_{O_2}} = 100$ mmHg, blood contains in solution

$$C_{O_2, \text{dissolved}} = 0.03 \text{ ml } O_2/(\text{liter} \times \text{mmHg}) \times 1 \times 100 \text{ mmHg}$$

$$= 3.0 \text{ ml } O_2/\text{liter}$$

Hemoglobin is able to chemically bind 1.34 ml O_2/g and the normal "ideal" [Hb] in blood is 150 g/liter. We now define a new term, the *O_2 capacity of hemoglobin*, which is the maximum quantity of oxygen that can be chemically bound to hemoglobin in blood when the oxygen saturation (S_{O_2}) is 100%. This quantity is computed as follows:

$$O_{2,\text{capacity}} = 1.34 \text{ ml } O_2/\text{g} \times [\text{Hb}] \text{ g/liter}$$

$$= 1.34 \times 150$$

$$= 201 \text{ ml } O_2/\text{liter}$$

In normal aortic blood, $S_{O_2} = 97.4\%$ because $Pa_{O_2} = 100$ mmHg (Fig. 1-2). This means that the bound oxygen content is 97.4% of capacity. To obtain the *total* O_2 concentration in blood, one adds the chemically bound O_2 to that in physical solution at the appropriate P_{O_2}. For systemic arterial blood, this is

$$Ca_{O_2} = (0.974 \times 201 + 0.03 \times 100) \text{ ml } O_2/\text{liter}$$

$$= 196 + 3$$

$$= 199 \text{ ml } O_2/\text{liter}$$

CONSERVATION OF MASS

A physical principle widely used in physiology (but often disguised by special names) is the *law of conservation of mass*. This law states that in a closed system (such as the whole body) the total number of atoms remains constant.

Let us examine this law in the context of a person with a normal $\dot{V}_{O_2}$ of 250 ml/min, STPD. That means that during 1 minute, the O_2 content of expired gas will be less than that of inspired gas by an amount equal to the oxygen consumption (Fig. 3-2). We can write the conservation of mass for lung oxygen exchange as

$$\dot{V}_{O_2} = F_{I_{O_2}} \times \dot{V}_I - F_{E_{O_2}} \times \dot{V}_E$$

If this equation is mysterious, the student should review part I of Appendix 1 and try to figure out the meaning of each symbol before resorting to the footnote below.*

Since oxygen is entering the body at the rate of 250 ml/min, conservation of mass requires that the same quantity of oxygen leave the body. As a steady-state, closed system, the body is not allowed to accumulate oxygen.

In physiology, a **steady state** means that over a sufficiently long period (the duration of which is deliberately left vague), the fluctuations of the variables under consideration average out. Over short periods, of course, there can be an imbalance; we will avoid such transient phenomena by dealing only with the steady state. A steady state is not necessarily an *equilibrium*. In fact, the most interesting steady state—our own state of life—is not an equilibrium. The moment of our death is time enough to consider the equilibrium condition.

The $\dot{V}_{O_2}$ is not generally constant on a minute-to-minute basis, what with eating, talking,

---

* The volume flow rate of oxygen $\dot{V}_{O_2}$ into the body from the lung (oxygen consumption) equals the fraction of inspired oxygen, $F_{I_{O_2}}$, multiplied by the inspired volume flow rate $\dot{V}_I$ (inspired minute ventilation) minus the fraction of expired oxygen $F_{E_{O_2}}$ times the expired volume flow rate $\dot{V}_E$ (expired minute ventilation). The $\dot{V}_{O_2}$ must, of course, be corrected to STPD.

exercising, sleeping, etc. Averaged over 24 hours, however, $\dot{V}_{O_2}$ is constant, so that one may make very accurate predictions about long-term oxygen utilization. If a person sits, stands, or lies quietly, awake but relaxed, the $\dot{V}_{O_2}$ measured minute by minute is reasonably constant (reproducible). Such a resting steady-state oxygen consumption is usually measured during a steady-state period about 10 min long.

Oxygen leaves the body as carbon dioxide or water vapor (conservation of mass permits chemical reactions). The ratio of carbon dioxide production ($\dot{V}_{CO_2}$) to oxygen consumption ($\dot{V}_{O_2}$) has metabolic significance. It is called the respiratory exchange ratio R*:

$$R = \dot{V}_{CO_2}/\dot{V}_{O_2} \qquad (3\text{-}4)$$

R in the steady state ranges between 0.7 and 1.0. The variability in the respiratory exchange ratio is due to variations in the metabolic fuel being burned by the body, which determines the number of CO_2 molecules produced for a given number of O_2 molecules consumed, as explained in any textbook of biochemistry. Appendix 2 lists the average respiratory quotient as 0.80, which is a reasonable value for a person living on a mixed diet of carbohydrates, protein, and fat.

Thus, if resting $\dot{V}_{O_2} = 250$ ml/min,

$$\dot{V}_{CO_2} = 0.80 \times \dot{V}_{O_2} = 0.80 \times 250 \text{ ml/min}$$

$$= 200 \text{ ml/min}$$

Normally, the volume of gas inspired is slightly greater (by about 1%) than the volume expired. The missing oxygen atoms are consumed in the production of water in the body. This slight inequality is usually ignored; physiologists generally assume that $V_I = V_E$. The only condition in which inspiratory and expiratory volumes are exactly equal is when R = 1.

Since $\dot{V}_{O_2}$ represents the oxygen disappearing into the body, this oxygen must be taken up by the blood flowing through the pulmonary capillaries. The flow of blood perfusing the pulmonary capillaries, $\dot{Q}_T$, is equal to the cardiac output.[†] Applying the law of conservation of mass again, we equate the oxygen consumption with the blood flow multiplied by the oxygen concentration difference between blood entering and leaving the pulmonary capillaries:

$$-\dot{V}_{O_2} = \dot{Q} \times (Cpa_{O_2} - Cpv_{O_2})$$

where Cpa_{O_2} and Cpv_{O_2} are the oxygen concentrations in pulmonary arterial (pa) and pulmonary venous (pv) blood, respectively (see Appendix 1). By convention, the *uptake* of a substance into blood is a *negative* consumption and therefore takes a minus sign. It is understood that STPD conditions hold, because O_2 consumption and CO_2 production are never referred to in any other way. It is also important to recall that blood in the pulmonary artery is *mixed venous blood* (denoted by $\bar{v}$), whereas blood in the pulmonary vein normally is nearly the same as in the aorta (or any systemic artery; denoted by a). When all these considerations are included, we end up with the famous Fick equation for measuring cardiac output:

FICK EQUATION

$$\dot{Q} = \frac{\dot{V}_{O_2}}{(Ca_{O_2} - C\bar{v}_{O_2})} \qquad (3\text{-}5)$$

---

* Not to be confused with the gas constant R (p. 29), which will not be used again.

[†] Although $\dot{Q}_T$ is the correct symbol for cardiac output, nearly all physiologists omit the T. Thus, $\dot{Q}$ is understood to be cardiac output in the context of the latter.

The minus sign in front of $\dot{V}_{O_2}$ was eliminated by multiplying the right-hand side by $-1/-1$, which also changed the order of terms in the denominator.

If the fundamental concept is clear, it ought to be obvious that one can also measure the pulmonary blood flow using $\dot{V}_{CO_2}$. An even broader interpretation is that the Fick equation can be applied to *any* organ and to *any* substance in the blood, as long as a concentration difference can be measured between blood flowing into and out of the organ, and regardless of whether the blood concentration difference is positive (consumption) or negative (excretion).

To return to the example, the normal resting $C\bar{v}_{O_2} = 150$ ml/liter and the normal $Ca_{O_2} = 200$ ml/liter whole blood.* Therefore, the normal resting pulmonary blood flow (cardiac output) $\dot{Q}$ is

$$\dot{Q} = \frac{250 \text{ ml } O_2/\text{min}}{(200 - 150) \text{ ml } O_2/\text{liter}} = \frac{250}{50} = 5 \text{ liters/min}$$

GRAPHS

Let us briefly review what graphs represent to physiologists. In general, graphic relationships are not to be interpreted as *cause* and *effect* (that is, as independent and dependent variables). The graphic form is used because it clearly displays rather complex relationships (whether or not their significance can be understood).

The Hemoglobin-Oxygen Equilibrium Curve

A classic graph in respiratory physiology is the hemoglobin-oxygen (HbO_2) equilibrium curve (Fig. 1-3). That graph is a plot of the HbO_2 saturation (S_{O_2}; the amount of oxygen bound to hemoglobin as a percentage of the maximum possible amount) as a function of the partial pressure of O_2 (P_{O_2}). This graph is used mainly to determine one of the variables when the other is known. It is obvious that the relationship between S_{O_2} and P_{O_2} is complex.

What cannot be seen in the graph is that, even at equilibrium, very rapid dissociation and association chemical reactions are continuously occurring. In other words, any point on the equilibrium curve corresponds to the situation where $O_2 + Hb \rightarrow HbO_2$ exactly equals $HbO_2 \rightarrow Hb + O_2$. The speed (kinetics) of these two simultaneous reactions must be known to fully understand the physiologic value of the hemoglobin-oxygen equilibrium curve in life.

Pressure-Flow Curve

Another commonly used graphic relationship is the pressure-flow curve (P–$\dot{Q}$) for the pulmonary circulation, shown in Figure 3-3. In this equation, the variables are related by the well-known equation for steady flow resistance, $R = \Delta P/\dot{Q}$, where ΔP is the difference between the inflow and outflow pressures. Much useful information will be gleaned from this graph in Chapter 7. Here I limit its interpretation to practice in reading total pulmonary vascular resistance.

There are some important differences between Figure 3-3 and Figure 1-3. First, Figure 3-3 has two lines. These lines represent different conditions, which must be specified before the graph can be fully interpreted. Second, there are no numbers or dimensions on the axes, so the graph represents a general relationship. Third, the origin, O, and the arrows on the axes imply that cardiac output $\dot{Q}$ and driving pressure (Ppa − Pla) increase as a point moves away

---

* Earlier in this chapter I gave normal systemic arterial total oxygen concentration as 199 ml O_2/liter. Here I round it off to 200 to avoid decimal fractions.

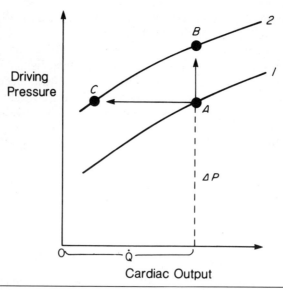

Fig. 3-3. Generalized graph of pulmonary vascular pressure-flow relationships. There are no scales, but both axes begin at the origin, with increasing cardiac output along the x-axis and increasing pressure along the y-axis. Lines 1 and 2 represent two pressure-flow curves that were obtained experimentally. At point A the driving pressure (ΔP) divided by the cardiac output ($\dot{Q}$) gives the calculated pulmonary vascular resistance, PVR = (Ppa − Pla)/$\dot{Q}$. Line 2 is displaced above but is nearly parallel to line 1. Points B and C on line 2 represent changes at constant cardiac output and constant driving pressure, respectively.

from the origin within the axis boundaries. Fourth, the curves are incomplete. That means that interpretations should be restricted to the solid portions of the lines.

On curve 1, point A represents a certain flow, $\dot{Q}$, and driving pressure, ΔP. The total **pulmonary vascular resistance** (PVR) can be read as the slope of a straight line drawn from the origin to point A: PVR = ΔP/$\dot{Q}$. Pressure-flow graphs are sometimes drawn with the driving pressure on the x-axis (abscissa) even though that makes reading the resistance awkward.

The defined part of curve 1 is reasonably straight. When extrapolated to zero flow, it intercepts the x-axis at a positive P. It would be a mistake, however, to assume that this would invariably happen if the flow were measured at lower driving pressures.* Since the slope, ΔP/$\dot{Q}$, of any straight line from the origin to curve 1 decreases gradually as ΔP increases, the pulmonary vascular resistance also decreases steadily. In other words, flow, $\dot{Q}$, rises more rapidly than does ΔP. This is characteristic of distensible systems such as the pulmonary vascular bed.

Curve 2 is above and appears to be parallel to curve 1. The arrows to points B and C represent two changes in the status of the pulmonary circulation. A → B shows increased driving pressure at constant flow; A → C shows decreased flow at constant driving pressure. Since PVR = ΔP/$\dot{Q}$, the pulmonary vascular resistance must be greater at B than at A because the pressure difference has increased, and greater at C than at A because flow has decreased.

What about the resistance at B relative to that at C? The total pulmonary vascular resistance

---

* In fact, this curve comes from a real experiment in which the P–$\dot{Q}$ line bent sharply toward the origin at low flows.

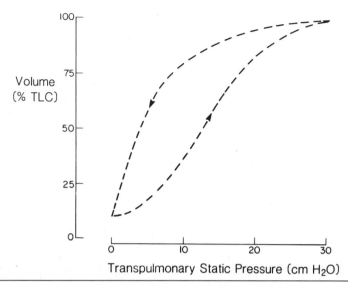

Fig. 3-4. Normal pressure-volume curve of the air-inflated human lung. The y-axis has been moved to the left to clarify the end points of the curve. The curve is complex and in general does not fit any simple relationship. The curve must be traced in the direction indicated by the arrows.

is less at B than at C because the slope of the straight line from the origin to B is less than that to C.*

Pressure-Volume Curve

The third example of reading a graph is the pressure-volume (P–V) curve of the lung shown in Figure 3-4. This is a complex enclosed curve (loop) with arrows. It can be read only in one direction—that is, by going around in the direction of the arrowheads. The opposite direction is forbidden. The two end points of the graph—(0, 10) and (30, 100)—show discontinuities (sharp changes in direction). Thus, there are two parts of the graph: one for increasing trans-pulmonary pressure and volume (lung inflation) and one for decreasing transpulmonary pressure and volume (lung deflation). The path taken by the lung during inflation is different from the path taken during deflation. For some reason (which is not discernible in the figure) at any given volume—obtained by drawing a horizontal line across the graph at any volume between 0 and 100% TLC (total lung capacity)—the static (zero flow) pressure needed to reach that volume is greater during inflation than deflation. At any pressure between 0 and 30 cmH$_2$O, the lung volume is larger during deflation than inflation. Cyclic functions that graph as loops rather than lines are said to exhibit *hysteresis* (from Greek *hysterein*, 'to lag behind or fall short'). The curve in Figure 3-4 will be explained in much more detail in Chapter 5.

CONCEPT OF INDEPENDENT STREAMS

In some situations, in which actions are occurring in opposite directions or in several parallel compartments, it may be useful to break the process down into two **independent streams**.

---

* In general, resistance is not the slope of the pressure-flow line itself. In some textbooks, the slope is used that way for what is called *incremental resistance,* but that is a special case.

In Chapters 7 and 8, for example, we will learn that blood flowing past some terminal respiratory units equilibrates with less oxygen than the blood flowing past other units because the units are not all ventilated equally in relation to their perfusion. Although there are very complex ways to determine the distribution of ventilation/perfusion ratios, for practical purposes physiologists usually think of two independent streams of blood—one flowing through the lung and equilibrating with ideal alveolar gas and one bypassing the lung completely (venous admixture or shunt flow).

The concept of independent streams belongs to the category of "as if" applications. The function in question behaves *as if* part of the system is doing all the activity and the other part is doing nothing. In Chapters 9 and 10 on oxygen and carbon dioxide transport, I will show some other examples of independent streams that simplify understanding of the process.

READINGS

Books

1. Barcroft J: The respiratory function of the blood. Cambridge University Press, Cambridge, 1925
   An old but excellent general discussion of the HbO_2 equilibrium curve and its importance to blood oxygen transport.
2. Macklem PT: Symbols and Abbreviations, p. ix and endpapers. In Fishman A (ed): Handbook of Physiology. Section 3: Respiration. American Physiological Society, Bethesda, MD, 1985
   The complete list of internationally recognized respiratory shorthand symbols and abbreviations.
3. Ruppel G: Manual of Pulmonary Function Testing. 3rd Ed. CV Mosby, St. Louis, 1982
   Chapter 9 on pulmonary function testing equipment describes and illustrates several modern spirometers.
4. Stryer L: Biochemistry. 3rd Ed. WH Freeman, New York, 1988
   One of several modern biochemistry textbooks.
5. West JB: Respiratory Physiology—the essentials. 3rd Ed. Williams & Wilkins, Baltimore, 1985
   The excellent chapter on ventilation/perfusion relations makes use of conservation of mass in terms of volumes of dilution and mixing volumes as well as the concept of independent streams. It also gives an inkling of how complex the ventilation/perfusion relationships really are.

Reviews

6. Green JF: Mechanical Concepts in Cardiovascular and Pulmonary Physiology. p. 116. Lea & Febiger, Philadelphia, 1977
   Chapters 2 and 7 give a clear exposition of the strictly passive mechanical view of pressure-flow relations.
7. Roughton FJW: Transport of oxygen and carbon dioxide. In Fenn WO, Rahn H (eds): Handbook of Physiology. Section 3: Respiration. Vol. 1. American Physiological Society, Bethesda, MD, 1964
   An elegant but difficult discussion of all aspects of oxygen and carbon dioxide transport in blood. Especially helpful are the sections on the normal oxyhemoglobin equilibrium (dissociation) curve and on the kinetics of the reactions between O_2 and Hb.

QUESTIONS*

Drill

1. Using Appendix 1, write the respiratory symbols for the following: (a) alveolar volume; (b) alveolar ventilation; (c) alveolar fractional concentration of oxygen; (d) pulmonary arterial pressure; (e) transpulmonary pressure; (f) mixed venous oxygen partial pressure; (g) systemic arterial carbon dioxide concentration; (h) barometric pressure; (i) pressure difference between the airway opening and alveoli; and (j) pleural pressure.

2. Using Appendix 1, write out the English meaning of the following respiratory symbols: (a) P_{AO}; (b) Ca_{O_2}; (c) $F_{E_{CO_2}}$; (d) V_D; (e) V_T; (f) Prs; (g) S_{O_2}; (h) $R = \dot{V}_{CO_2}/\dot{V}_{O_2}$, (i) T_E; (j) $P_A - P_B$; and (k) C_W.

3. Convert from the volume at condition 1 to the volume that would be present at condition 2. For each example, specify condition 1 (STPD, ATPS, BTPS).

| | Condition 1 | | | Condition 2 | | |
Volume	P_B (mmHg)	T (°C)	P_{H_2O} (mmHg)	P_B (mmHg)	T (°C)	P_{H_2O} (mmHg)
a. 2 liters	760	0	0	760	37	47
b. 4.5 liters	760	20	0	760	37	47
c. 800 ml	760	25	24	760	0	0
d. 3 liters	600	37	47	760	0	0
e. 2,700 ml	760	0	0	1,500	21	19
f. 6 liters	450	37	47	450	15	13
g. 10 liters	760	0	0	760	−100	0

Problems

4. Calculate the respiratory exchange ratio given that oxygen utilization and carbon dioxide production, measured separately ATPS (T = 21°C, P_B = 747 mmHg), are 350 and 298 ml, respectively.

5. What is the pulmonary blood flow of a normal person exercising at a steady state at sea level and 21°C, if $\dot{V}_{O_2}$ = 1,200 ml/min, ATPS; the systemic arterial O_2 concentration is 200 ml/liter; and the mixed venous O_2 concentration is 125 ml/liter?

6. What is the oxygen consumption of a newborn baby if its cardiac output is 600 ml/min and the O_2 concentrations in systemic arterial and mixed venous blood are 200 ml/liter and 160 ml/liter, respectively?

7. Use the data in Chapters 1 through 3 to calculate normal pulmonary vascular resistance at rest and during exercise. What can you conclude about the effect of exercise on the pulmonary circulation?

8. Lung compliance C_L is defined as the slope of the volume-pressure curve ($\Delta V/\Delta P$) for any stated changes in volume. In Figure 3-4, which volume ranges during inflation show the highest and the lowest values of C_L? Calculate the average C_L between minimum volume and total lung capacity, if TLC = 4.5 liters.

---

* Answers begin on p. 211.

4

Lung Volumes and Ventilation

THE BOTTOM LINE

Total Ventilation Versus Alveolar Ventilation

Breathing is measured as total minute ventilation ($\dot{V}_E$), defined as the volume of gas moved in each breath (V_T) times the number of breaths per minute (f): $\dot{V}_E = V_T \times f$. The main purpose of ventilation is to maintain an optimal composition of alveolar gas. Alveolar ventilation ($\dot{V}_A$) is the useful (fresh air) portion of minute ventilation that reaches the gas exchange units.

Anatomic Dead Space and Tidal Volume

The portion of each breath that fills the airway is called the dead space (V_D). Normally, $V_T - V_D = 500 - 150$ ml $= 350$ ml, the normal alveolar ventilation per breath. For alveolar ventilation per minute, $\dot{V}_A = f \times (V_T - V_D)$ or $f \times V_T(1 - V_D/V_T)$. The V_D/V_T ratio is normally 0.25 to 0.35.

Lung Volumes and Capacities

The total lung capacity (TLC) is 6.0 liters in a 70-kg normal adult. TLC is composed of several separate volumes and overlapping capacities; the most important are residual volume (RV) (1.2 liters) and tidal volume (0.5 liter); functional residual capacity (FRC) (2.4 liters) and vital capacity (VC) (4.8 liters). Except for RV, all volumes and capacities can be readily measured.

Alveolar Ventilation

$P_{A_{CO_2}}$ or its equivalent, $P_{a_{CO_2}}$, describes the adequacy of $\dot{V}_A$. The normal $P_{a_{CO_2}}$ is 40 mmHg. Hyperventilation is defined as $P_{A_{CO_2}} < 40$ mmHg, and hypoventilation as $P_{A_{CO_2}} > 40$ mmHg. The *alveolar ventilation equation* describes the relation among $\dot{V}_A$, $P_{a_{CO_2}}$, and metabolism ($\dot{V}_{CO_2}$):

$$\dot{V}_A, \frac{\text{liters}}{\text{min}} = \frac{\dot{V}_{CO_2}, \text{ml/min}}{P_{A_{CO_2}}, \text{mmHg}} \times 0.863, \frac{\text{mmHg} \times \text{liters}}{\text{ml}}$$

(Continues).

(*Continued*).

The *alveolar gas equation* permits the calculation of mean $P_{A_{O_2}}$ (mmHg):

$$P_{A_{O_2}} = F_{I_{O_2}} \times (P_B - P_{H_2O}) - P_{A_{CO_2}} \left[F_{I_{O_2}} + \frac{(1 - F_{I_{O_2}})}{R} \right]$$

Normal $P_{A_{O_2}}$ is 102 mmHg. The $O_2 - CO_2$ *diagram* is a graphical method for relating all possible alveolar oxygen and carbon dioxide partial pressures under given physiologic conditions.

Wasted Ventilation

In the real world some ventilation goes to alveoli that do not receive sufficient blood flow. Thus, not only the anatomic dead space but some portion of alveolar ventilation is wasted. Use of $P_{a_{CO_2}}$ instead of $P_{A_{CO_2}}$ in the alveolar ventilation equation yields the effective alveolar ventilation.

This chapter describes the process of breathing by describing the components of lung volume, using these to measure ventilation qualitatively and quantitatively, and evaluating the adequacy of alveolar ventilation in terms of alveolar (A) and arterial (a) partial pressures of CO_2 ($P_{A_{CO_2}}$; $P_{a_{CO_2}}$) and O_2 ($P_{A_{O_2}}$; $P_{a_{O_2}}$). Because tissues engaged in aerobic metabolism use O_2 and produce CO_2, they remove O_2 from systemic capillary blood and add CO_2 to it. This lowers the P_{O_2} of mixed venous blood ($P\overline{v}_{O_2}$) to below that of alveolar gas and raises the P_{O_2} of mixed venous blood ($P\overline{v}_{CO_2}$) to above that of alveolar gas. The partial pressures of the common respiratory gases in ideal systemic arterial and mixed venous (pulmonary arterial) blood are listed in Table 3-1.

Half of the process of ventilation/perfusion matching involves ventilating the alveoli in such a way as to increase the $P_{A_{O_2}}$ well above that of mixed venous blood ($P\overline{v}_{O_2}$). This causes oxygen to diffuse along its partial pressure gradient and loads oxygen into the pulmonary capillary blood. Ventilation lowers the $P_{A_{CO_2}}$ below that in mixed venous blood ($P\overline{v}_{CO_2}$). This causes CO_2 to diffuse along its partial pressure gradient and reduces the CO_2 content of the pulmonary capillary blood.

When body metabolism rises, as in exercise, $P\overline{v}_{O_2}$ will decrease and $P\overline{v}_{CO_2}$ will increase as the body consumes more oxygen and produces more carbon dioxide. To keep the arterial blood gases ($P_{a_{O_2}}$; $P_{a_{CO_2}}$) at steady levels, the lungs—by the process of **alveolar ventilation**—must supply to the alveoli an amount of O_2 equal to the amount removed from the blood by the metabolizing tissues and must remove from the alveoli the amount of CO_2 that was added to venous blood by the systemic tissues.

The main purpose of ventilation, then, is to *maintain an optimal composition of alveolar gas*. Think of alveolar gas as a buffer (stabilizing) compartment of gas lying between room (ambient) air and pulmonary capillary blood. Oxygen is continuously removed from alveolar gas and carbon dioxide is continuously added to it by blood flowing through the alveolar wall capillary network. Oxygen is supplied to the alveolar gas and carbon dioxide is removed from it by the process of ventilation—the inspiration of fresh air followed by the expiration of alveolar gas. The cyclic nature of ventilation suggests the importance of the buffering effect of a large alveolar gas volume.*

---

* In the course of evolution, the flowthrough ventilation system of the gilled fishes, in which gill water P_{O_2} is maintained as high as possible and consequently gill water P_{CO_2} is very low, has been replaced by a system in which the alveolar partial pressures of these gases are not the same as in ambient air but are stable. The concentration of O_2 in air is more than 40 times that in water at the same P_{O_2}, so that flowthrough ventilation is not necessary for an adequate supply of O_2 to alveolar gas.

TOTAL VENTILATION VERSUS ALVEOLAR VENTILATION

Total ventilation is the volume of air entering or leaving the nose or mouth during each breath or each minute. It can be measured from breath to breath by volume recorders, such as the spirometer shown in Figure 3-1.

The volume of each breath is called the **tidal volume** (VT) because like the tide it moves back and forth over the same path. Tidal volume varies with age, sex, body position, and metabolic activity. The average normal value for a resting adult is 0.5 liter (500 ml). The largest possible tidal volume is the **vital capacity** (VC).

Alveolar ventilation is the volume of *fresh* air entering the alveoli in each breath or in each minute. The symbol $\dot{V}A$ can be used for both the minute alveolar ventilation and the alveolar ventilation per breath. Ordinarily, $\dot{V}A$ is understood to mean *minute* alveolar ventilation.

Alveolar ventilation is always less than total ventilation; how much less depends on the anatomic dead space and tidal volume.

ANATOMIC DEAD SPACE AND TIDAL VOLUME

Fresh air does not go directly to the terminal respiratory units. It first goes through the conducting airways (nose, mouth, pharynx, larynx, trachea, bronchi, and bronchioles). As there is no significant exchange of O_2 and CO_2 between gas and blood in the conducting airways, that portion of the fresh inspired air is called the **anatomic dead space** (VD).

The volume of the anatomic dead space in healthy humans varies with age, sex, body position, and lung volume. Although this volume can be measured, most physiologists and physicians estimate it from standard tables. An easily remembered estimate is that VD is approximately 2 ml/kg of ideal body weight.

At the end of a normal expiration (just before the next inspiration begins), the conducting airways are filled with *alveolar* gas, which has an ideal P_{O_2} of 102 mmHg and a P_{CO_2} of 40 mmHg (Table 3-1). Let us say that VD = 150 ml (70-kg adult) and that the next tidal volume will be 500 ml, a normal value. Although the alveoli will receive 500 ml, the gas composition will differ somewhat from that entering the nose or mouth because the alveoli must first receive the 150 ml of gas that was in the anatomic dead space from the last exhalation. This gas does not raise alveolar P_{O_2} or lower alveolar P_{CO_2}, since it has the same composition as the alveolar gas. Finally, the alveoli receive 350 ml of fresh air. The remaining 150 ml of fresh air remains in the conducting airways at end inspiration. This process is diagramed in Figure 4-1.

The volume of the dead space VD and the tidal volume VT are important factors in determining the amount of alveolar ventilation per breath. The VD/VT ratio is a simple and useful index of adequate ventilation. Normal values range between 0.25 and 0.35. In the example illustrated in Figure 4-1, VD/VT = 0.30 (150 ml dead space/500 ml tidal volume).

The VD/VT ratio is sensitive to the tidal volume: increased lung volume tends to increase dead space. For example, in Figure 4-1, if tidal volume had been 1,000 ml and if the anatomic dead space had increased to 175 ml due to the increased VT, then VD/VT = 0.175 (175 ml/ 1,000 ml). On the other hand, if tidal volume had been only 200 ml and the VD had been 125 ml, then VD/VT = 0.625.

LUNG VOLUMES AND CAPACITIES

The lungs do not collapse to the airless state with each expiration partly because the chest wall (ribs, intercostal muscles, diaphragm) becomes more rigid (stiff, noncompliant) at the end of expiration. Indeed, the lungs cannot be emptied of gas, even by the most forceful expiration; some gas, the **residual volume** (RV), still remains. Figure 4-2 shows all of the named lung volumes.

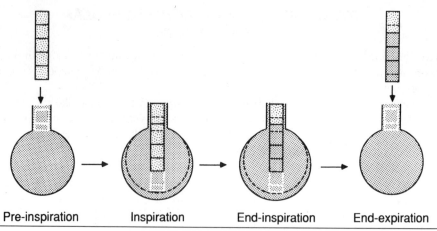

Pre-inspiration   Inspiration   End-inspiration   End-expiration

Fig. 4-1.   Alveolar ventilation and anatomic dead space. Each square block represents 100 ml of gas. Dotted blocks represent inspired air; shaded blocks represent alveolar gas. During inspiration, 150 ml of dead space gas (white outlining) plus 350 ml of inspired air enter the terminal respiratory units (alveoli); by end inspiration this has mixed with and become alveolar gas. One and one-half blocks of inspired gas fill the anatomic dead space at end inspiration and are washed out by alveolar gas during expiration. Dashed lines show end-expiratory lung volume. (Modified from Comroe JH Jr: The Lung. 2nd Ed. Year Book Medical Publishers, Chicago, 1962, with permission.)

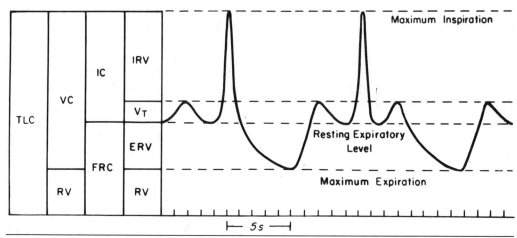

Fig. 4-2.   Lung volumes, capacities, and the normal spirogram. To the left are four bars showing the various ways in which lung volume may be apportioned. The volumes as they appear in a normal spirogram are shown to the right, corresponding to tidal volume (V_T), *i*nspiratory *r*eserve *v*olume (IRV), and *ex*-piratory *r*eserve *v*olume (ERV). The sum of these three volumes, that is, the volume between maximum inspiration and maximum expiration, is the *v*ital *c*apacity (VC). The spirogram is drawn in real time. The normal (first) tidal volume shown takes 5 seconds (frequency = 12/min). The vital capacity maneuver is an inspiration to TLC (about 1 second), followed by an expiration to residual volume (about 5 seconds), although most of the expiration occurs in the first second. (Modified from Comroe JH Jr: The Lung. 2nd Ed. Year Book Medical Publishers, Chicago, 1962, with permission.)

The **functional residual capacity** (FRC) is the volume of air remaining at the end of a normal expiration. FRC is not actively regulated; it is determined by the passive mechanical relationship between the chest wall and the lungs, although airflow dynamics may contribute in some conditions.

The FRC acts as a buffer against large changes in alveolar P_{O_2} with each breath (the bagpipe bellows principle*). If FRC was very small, Pa_{O_2} would fluctuate markedly with each breath, decreasing toward that of mixed venous blood in the pulmonary capillaries at end expiration ($P\bar{v}_{O_2}$ = 40 mmHg) and rising toward that of moist tracheal air (P_{O_2} = 150 mmHg) with inspiration. The advantage of cyclic ventilation of a relatively large space (FRC = 2.4 liters; 40% of total lung capacity [TLC] normally) by a small volume of alveolar ventilation per breath (V_T − V_D) is that fluctuations of Pa_{O_2} and Pa_{CO_2} and, consequently, of Pa_{O_2} and Pa_{CO_2} are minimal, about 4 mmHg for the former and 3 mmHg for the latter. For practical purposes, physiologists and physicians tend to ignore breath-to-breath fluctuations in alveolar and blood gas tensions in normal people, but in some circumstances the fluctuation may be important for the control of breathing.

The various static lung volumes and capacities are shown in Figure 4-2, which also includes the tracing of a normal spirogram. Four nonoverlapping volumes are shown together with several capacities, each of which includes two or more volumes. It is important to know how the volumes and capacities relate to each other (some normal values are listed in Appendix 2). Of the four named volumes, all except residual volume can be measured directly by volume recorders, such as the spirometer shown in Figure 3-1.

Diseases of the lungs or chest wall affect lung volumes and capacities in various ways. The most frequent change is in the vital capacity (VC) which may be greatly reduced. The reduction may be due to limited expansion (restrictive disease) or to an abnormally large RV (obstructive disease). Because knowing the RV is important to the assessment of lung function and because it illustrates the law of conservation of mass, I will briefly describe a common procedure for measuring it.

This method is called the single-breath volume of dilution. The *concept* is to take into the lungs a known volume of gas of markedly different composition from normal alveolar gas and to use the law of conservation of mass to obtain the result of mixing two volumes of different composition. One gas used is 100% O_2, but more commonly an insoluble inert tracer gas such as helium (He) is used. From a suitable sample of the expired gas one can measure the tracer gas concentration and compute the unknown volume. The idea is simple, but the measurement and computation are complicated by temperature and water vapor corrections and, conceptually, by the tendency of students to confuse sample volume with the volume of interest, namely, RV.

Before measuring RV, we will review how the concept of volume of dilution works. Suppose we mix 1 liter of air with 1 liter of 100% oxygen and measure the oxygen concentration of a 100-ml sample of the mixture. What will it be? We proceed by equating the sum of the quantity of O_2 (concentration × volume) in each liter of gas before mixing to the total volume of the system and the average concentration (C) after mixing as follows:

$$(V_1 \times C_1) + (V_2 \times C_2) = V_{total} \times C$$
$$(1 \text{ liter} \times 0.21) + (1 \text{ liter} \times 1.00) = 2 \text{ liters} \times C_{O_2} \qquad (4\text{-}1)$$
$$C_{O_2} = (0.21 + 1.00)/2 = 0.605$$

Substituting the known values, we obtain the average O_2 of approximately 60% (F_{O_2} = 0.60).

---

* The piper blows into a large bag kept under pressure by his arm. The air flowing out the pipes to make the sound is not the air being blown into the bag at that moment. The bag acts as the buffer (FRC).

Note that the *sample* volume has nothing whatsoever to do with the computation. The sample volume could have been 1 ml or 2,000 ml; it would have made no difference, as long as the sample was *representative*, so that we obtained the correct average concentration in the space whose volume we are calculating.

Now let us apply the volume of dilution method to the measurement of residual volume (RV) as illustrated in Figure 4-3. It is important not to lose sight of the general principle amid all the correction factors. From RV, a normal subject inspires 4.4 liters, ATPS, of a mixture of 10% helium ($F_{I_{He}} = 0.100$) in oxygen from a spirometer at 21°C (Fig. 4-3). On expiration, a 1-liter sample of alveolar gas (not contaminated by dead space gas) is collected in which the helium concentration is 8.0% ($F_{A_{He}} = 0.080$). To compute RV, we set up the mixing equation as above (Eq. 4-1):

$$[RV \times F_{A_{He,i}}] + [V_I \times F_{I_{He}}] = V_{total} \times F_{A_{He,f}}$$

where the subscripts i and f designate the *i*nitial and *f*inal alveolar helium concentrations, respectively.

The advantage of using a foreign gas is that its normal alveolar concentration is zero: $F_{A_{He,i}} = 0$. Thus,

$$V_I \times F_{I_{He}} = V_{total} \times F_{A_{He,f}} \qquad (4\text{-}1A)$$

We can omit the f because there's only one $F_{A_{He}}$.

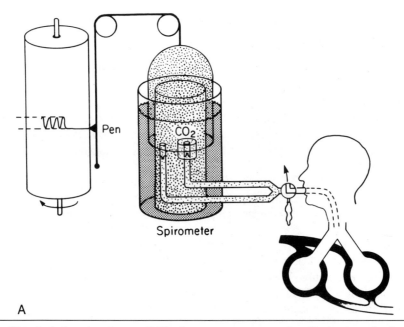

A

Fig. 4-3.   The single-breath **volume of dilution measurement** of residual volume is shown in three figures. Watch the spirometer tracing at the left and the multidirectional valve near the mouth. **(A)** The spirometer is filled with oxygen containing 10% helium (dots), an insoluble gas not normally present in the lungs. As in Figure 3-2, there is a CO_2 absorber (labeled CO_2). There is an empty sampling bag attached to the valve. In the first maneuver, the valve is turned so that the subject can breathe out to residual volume into the room air (arrow). The spirometer does not show this event having been switched out of the circuit at end expiration. (*Figure continues.*)

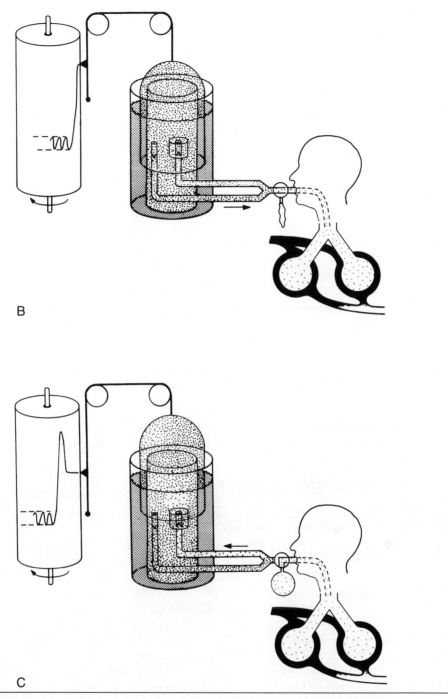

B

C

Fig. 4-3 *(Continued)*. **(B)** The valve is turned and the subject inspires from the spirometer. The inspired volume is shown on the tracing. We must know the inspired volume to compute the volume of dilution. Helium molecules enter the lung and are diluted by the residual volume. **(C)** The subject expires into the spirometer as shown in the tracing at the left until sufficient volume has cleared the dead space. Then a representative sample of alveolar gas is taken in the bag for analysis.

Remembering that $V_{total} = RV + V_I$, the equation becomes,

$$V_I \times F_{I_{He}} = (RV + V_I) \times F_{A_{He}} \qquad\qquad (4\text{-}1B)$$

Before going further we must remember that residual volume is measured at BTPS, whereas the inspired volume came from a spirometer at ATPS. We have two choices: we can either correct the inspired volume immediately to BTPS, or carry out the calculation, obtain RV at ATPS, and then convert it to BTPS. Either method must give the same result. The second approach is simpler.

$$4.4 \text{ liters} \times 0.10 = (RV + 4.4) \text{ liters} \times 0.080$$

It is not necessary to correct either of the helium fractions (concentrations) for water vapor because gas fractions are always measured *dry*. Continuing the calculation

$$0.44 \text{ liter} = (RV \times 0.080 + 0.35) \text{ liter}$$

$$RV = (0.44 - 0.35)/0.08$$

$$RV, \text{ATPS} = 1.10 \text{ liters}$$

Finally, we correct RV to BTPS:

$$RV, \text{BTPS} = 1.10 \text{ liters} \times \frac{(760 - 19) \text{ mmHg}}{(760 - 47) \text{ mmHg}} \times \frac{(273 + 37) \text{ K}}{(273 + 21) \text{ K}}$$

$$RV = 1.10 \times 1.039 \times 1.054$$

$$RV, \text{BTPS} = 1.20 \text{ liters}$$

Functional residual capacity (or any lung volume) can be computed in the same manner, or we can add the expiratory reserve volume (ERV) to the residual volume to get FRC (Fig. 4-2). For example

$$FRC = ERV + RV = 1,200 \text{ ml} + 1,200 \text{ ml} = 2,400 \text{ ml, BTPS}$$

In practice, FRC is usually measured and the expiratory reserve volume, measured by spirometry, is subtracted to obtain residual volume.

$P_{A_{O_2}}$ is the main determinant of the rate of diffusion of O_2 from alveolar gas to pulmonary capillary blood. The *amount* of alveolar ventilation is more important in determining $P_{A_{O_2}}$ than is the size of the FRC. Indeed, the FRC mainly acts as a buffer. For a resting $\dot{V}_{O_2}$ (oxygen consumption) of 250 ml/min, only 250 ml O_2 needs to be added to alveolar gas each minute by the process of ventilation to maintain $P_{A_{O_2}}$; this is independent of the size of the FRC. In the normal lung, because of rapid and uniform distribution of gas within each terminal respiratory unit, the volume of the lung is unimportant in determining the steady-state $P_{A_{O_2}}$.

On the other hand, the size of the FRC is important when there is a rapid *change* in inspired alveolar gas composition. For example, if a person breathes 100% O_2 instead of air at any given tidal volume, a new steady-state alveolar O_2 concentration will be achieved more rapidly if the initial lung volume is low rather than high.

ALVEOLAR VENTILATION

The alveolar ventilation per breath when multiplied by the frequency of breathing (respiratory rate), f, gives the alveolar ventilation per minute, $\dot{V}_A$, just as tidal volume times frequency gives the total minute ventilation, $\dot{V}_E$. Notice that pulmonary physiologists and physicians use $\dot{V}_E$ (expired minute ventilation) to indicate total minute ventilation. The unstated assumption is that the inspiratory and expiratory volumes are equal. This is not quite true, as we have already seen, because the respiratory quotient is usually < 1.0. Expired volume is slightly less than inspired volume. Practically, this discrepancy may be ignored.

If $V_T = 500$ ml and the normal respiratory frequency is 12/min, then

$$\dot{V}_E = V_T \times f = 500 \text{ ml} \times 12/\text{min} = 6{,}000 \text{ ml/min}$$

We obtain alveolar ventilation ($\dot{V}_A$) by subtracting the volume of the anatomic dead space (V_D) from the tidal volume (V_T) and multiplying by the frequency of breathing.

$$\dot{V}_A = f \times (V_T - V_D) \text{ or } \dot{V}_A = f \times V_T(1 - V_D/V_T) \tag{4-2}$$

The second form of Eq. 4-2 is sometimes more useful because it refers to the dead space/ tidal volume ratio rather than to the actual dead space.

Either form is correct in terms of *ideal* alveolar ventilation. But from the practical point of view, V_D is not often measured. More frequently, physiologists use the volume of dilution principle to compute alveolar ventilation.

The method is the same as for the previous example in which we calculated RV by helium dilution. This time, however, instead of using a foreign gas or O_2, we will use CO_2 with the knowledge that no CO_2 exchange occurs in the anatomic dead space. Therefore, ventilation of the dead space contributes nothing to the expired CO_2, *but* it does contribute to expired volume. In making this computation, we can use either the partial pressures of CO_2 in alveolar, dead space, and expired gas or their fractions (F) (concentrations) of total dry gas pressure, as long as *all* gas concentrations are measured in the same units.

What is the alveolar ventilation of a normal person, if $\dot{V}_E$, BTPS $= 6.0$ liters/min, and $F_{E_{CO_2}} = 0.039$?

In terms of F_{CO_2}, the volume of dilution equation is

$$(\dot{V}_A \times F_{A_{CO_2}}) + (\dot{V}_D \times F_{D_{CO_2}}) = \dot{V}_E \times F_{E_{CO_2}} \tag{4-3}$$

where $\dot{V}_D$ and $F_{D_{CO_2}}$ refer to dead space ventilation and CO_2 fraction, respectively. The dead space by definition does not contribute any CO_2 to expired gas, so the second term in the lefthand side is zero. Notice that on the right side, we use expired ventilation and CO_2 concentration, not alveolar. We must collect all of the expired gas, not an alveolar sample.

Since this is a normal subject, $P_{A_{CO_2}} = 40$ mmHg, but we will convert that to $F_{A_{CO_2}}$ to match the form of the expired gas value.

$$F_{A_{CO_2}} = 40 \text{ mmHg}/(760 - 47) \text{ mmHg} = 0.056$$

Normal alveolar gas contains 5.6% CO_2. Substitute the known values into the equation above to obtain

$$\dot{V}_A \times 0.056 = 6.0 \text{ liters} \times 0.039$$

$$\dot{V}_A = (6.0 \times 0.039)/0.056$$

$$\dot{V}_A = 4.2 \text{ liters, BTPS}$$

I simplified the calculation by giving $\dot{V}_E$ at BTPS. If the expired ventilation had been collected in a spirometer, ATPS, then corrections similar to those used with the residual volume calculation would have been required.

Because the main purpose of ventilation is to maintain an optimal concentration of alveolar gases, alveolar ventilation is in balance (steady state) for O_2 when it matches O_2 use with O_2 supply.

For example, using the normal values of 500 ml for tidal volume and 150 ml for dead space volume, the alveolar ventilation per breath is 350 ml. If a normal person breathes 12 times/min, the alveoli are supplied with an alveolar ventilation, $\dot{V}_A$, of 4,200 ml/min. Since $F_{IO_2} = 0.21$, the amount of O_2 supplied is 882 ml/min, BTPS. Of this, a $\dot{V}_{O_2}$ of 250 ml/min, STPD (303 ml/min, BTPS) diffuses into the pulmonary capillary blood for distribution to the systemic tissues. The individual, however, is not overventilating with respect to oxygen, because during expiration the 579 ml/min, BTPS of excess O_2 is breathed out. The useful O_2 supply to the alveoli per minute is the *difference* between the quantity inspired and the quantity expired.

As will be discussed in Chapter 11, it is not the oxygen supply to the alveoli but the partial pressure of CO_2 in arterial blood, Pa_{CO_2}, that is closely regulated. If the Pa_{CO_2} is held at 40 mmHg, which can be equated with the average PA_{CO_2} of 40 mmHg, then the Pa_{O_2} is maintained at 102 mmHg while breathing air at sea level.

Therefore, normal alveolar ventilation means that $PA_{CO_2} = 40$ mmHg. *Hyperventilation* (overventilation) for a particular metabolic state means that the alveolar gas is being replaced at a rate greater than necessary. That must mean that PA_{CO_2} is < 40 mmHg. *Hypoventilation* (underventilation), which is the more common condition encountered in patients with lung disease, means that the supply of fresh air to the alveoli is less than is needed to maintain the PA_{CO_2} at 40 mmHg.

When a person has abnormal lungs, a normal PA_{O_2} of 102 mmHg may not be sufficient to oxygenate the blood (because of poor matching of ventilation to perfusion, anatomic shunts around the lungs, or, rarely, interference with the process of gaseous diffusion between the alveoli and blood in the pulmonary capillaries). Under such conditions neither the alveolar nor the arterial P_{O_2} is a satisfactory guide to the adequacy of ventilation. Besides, it is easy to alter the inspired oxygen concentration, either lowering it (as we normally experience when we go to higher altitudes) or raising it (breathing enriched oxygen mixtures).

Remember: Physiologists describe the adequacy of ventilation in terms of PA_{CO_2}. Increased PA_{CO_2} means hypoventilation, and decreased PA_{CO_2} means hyperventilation.

Alveolar Ventilation Equation

The alveolar ventilation equation makes use of PA_{CO_2} rather than PA_{O_2}. Let us pick up the last numbered equation for alveolar ventilation (Eq. 4-3). If there is no CO_2 in inspired air, as is normally the case, we can delete the dead space ventilation term on the lefthand side

$$\dot{V}_A \times F_{A_{CO_2}} = \dot{V}_E \times F_{E_{CO_2}} \tag{4-3A}$$

This equation is correct if both $\dot{V}_A$ and $\dot{V}_E$ are measured under the same conditions (BTPS, ATPS, or STPD). We will use BTPS because $\dot{V}_A$ is always measured that way. Either side of Eq. 4-3A, when converted to STPD, equals CO_2 production ($\dot{V}_{CO_2}$). We will convert the righthand term to CO_2 production by using the appropriate temperature and pressure corrections and at the same time convert $F_{A_{CO_2}}$ to its equivalent form in terms of partial pressure.

$$\dot{V}_A \times \frac{PA_{CO_2}}{P_B - P_{H_2O}} = \dot{V}_{CO_2} \times \frac{760}{P_B - P_{H_2O}} \times \frac{(273 + 37)}{273}$$

If the correction factors on the righthand side of the equation seem to be upside down, go back and set up the conversion of $\dot{V}_E$, BTPS to $\dot{V}_E$, STPD.

Conveniently, $P_B - P_{H_2O}$ appears in the denominator on both sides and can be canceled. If the barometric pressure is 760 mmHg and alveolar (body) temperature is 37°C, then the correction factor term can be evaluated as 0.863 mmHg × liters/ml, when $\dot{V}_A$ is given in liters/min and $\dot{V}_{CO_2}$ is given in ml/min.

Thus, the alveolar ventilation equation, under normal conditions, is:

ALVEOLAR VENTILATION EQUATION

$$\dot{V}_A,\ \text{liters/min} = \frac{\dot{V}_{CO_2},\ \text{ml/min}}{P_{ACO_2},\ \text{mmHg}} \times \frac{0.863,\ \text{mmHg} \times \text{liters}}{\text{ml}} \tag{4-4}$$

Many beginning textbooks do not show the derivation of the alveolar ventilation equation. Why have I? *The reason is that the derivation is basic to understanding what the equation means.* Equation 4-4 is nothing but a manipulation of Eq. 4-3, under the conditions specified; namely, $F_{ICO_2} = 0$, $P_B = 760$, and $T = 37°C$.

The student will use Eq. 4-4 frequently in pulmonary physiology problems. It is simple and convenient. But occasionally, a problem will be encountered which deviates sufficiently from the two conditions listed above, so that the correct relationship between alveolar ventilation and alveolar CO_2 partial pressure can only be obtained from Eq. 4-3. The most likely condition is when the inspired CO_2 is not zero.

Examine Eq. 4-4 and note the following points. It is correct for any CO_2 production, even heavy exercise, where $\dot{V}_{CO_2}$ may be six times the resting value. The equation carries with it the implication that P_{CO_2} is the controlled variable for the regulation of alveolar ventilation, which is true (see Ch. 11).

Alveolar Gas Equation

Once P_{ACO_2} has been calculated, one can calculate P_{AO_2} by the alveolar gas equation. If the respiratory exchange ratio, $R = 1$, each molecule of oxygen removed from the alveoli is replaced by one molecule of CO_2. Therefore, the alveolar P_{O_2} equals the P_{O_2} in moist tracheal air minus the alveolar P_{CO_2}:

$$P_{AO_2} = P_{IO_2} - P_{ACO_2}$$

when $R = 1.0$. Unfortunately, R is seldom 1.0. The average normal value is 0.80. Thus, the normal P_{AO_2} is slightly less than one might expect. The exact equation for computing P_{AO_2} (mmHg) is:

ALVEOLAR GAS EQUATION

$$P_{AO_2} = F_{IO_2} \times (P_B - P_{H_2O}) - P_{ACO_2} \times \left[F_{IO_2} + \frac{1 - F_{IO_2}}{R} \right] \tag{4-5}$$

P_{AO_2} should *always* be calculated by using this equation. To solve it one must know F_{IO_2}, P_B, P_{H_2O}, P_{ACO_2}, and R. When $R = 1$, the complex term in the square brackets equals 1, and Eq. 4-5 becomes the same as the simplified equation listed above it. If one breathes 100% oxygen ($F_{IO_2} = 1.0$), the correction factor in the square brackets also reduces to unity because there is no nitrogen to be concentrated in the alveoli.

Equation 4-5 is too complex to be easily remembered, especially if it is used only occasionally. Therefore, although most respiratory physiologists memorize Eqs. 4-3 and 4-4, they rarely memorize Eq. 4-5.

O_2-CO_2 Diagram

There is a tight relationship between Pa_{CO_2}, R, and PA_{O_2} when breathing air. The relationship is not linear because of the correction factor in Eq. 4-5, but it has been carefully worked out and presented in graphic form as the O_2-CO_2 diagram. The O_2-CO_2 diagram in its basic form (Fig. 4-4) is useful and easy to read. It fell into disuse, however, because it was made too complicated. An entire book has been written on how to use the O_2-CO_2 diagram. But in basic pulmonary physiology, the line shown in Figure 4-4 is about all one needs. The line begins on the x-axis at a point labeled I, the inspired P_{O_2} in moist tracheal air at sea level. The point labeled A represents normal alveolar gas at R = 0.80. PA_{CO_2} is = 40 mmHg and Pa_{O_2} = 102 mmHg. The line continues to the left with a fairly flat trajectory ending at a point labeled $\bar{v}$, which represents the normal mixed venous blood gas tensions: $P\bar{v}_{O_2}$ = 40 mmHg and $P\bar{v}_{CO_2}$ = 46 mmHg. If some alveoli receive no ventilation, the blood passing through their capillaries exits into the venules with the same gas tensions as mixed venous blood. Every possible combination of Pa_{O_2} and Pa_{CO_2}, under the conditions described, lies on the line in the figure. The points on the line to the left of A represent hypoventilation, while all points to the right represent hyperventilation.

WASTED VENTILATION (PHYSIOLOGIC DEAD SPACE)

Until now, we have considered "ideal" ventilation, namely, when all alveoli receive ventilation and blood flow in the same proportion (ideal $\dot{V}A/\dot{Q}$). This ideal condition does not actually exist even in the healthiest individuals, and ventilation may be markedly abnormal in diseased lungs. The concept of **wasted ventilation** or **physiologic dead space** is used as a measure of the deviation from ideal of ventilation relative to blood flow.

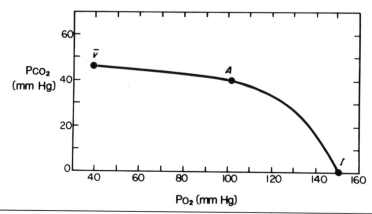

Fig. 4-4. The O_2-CO_2 diagram in its simplest form. Every possible pair of alveolar O_2 and CO_2 partial pressures for a given condition is shown on this line. I, the inspired P_{O_2} point, is on the x-axis, since normally there is no CO_2 in inspired air. This represents the P_{O_2} in moist tracheal gas during inspiration. The point labeled A represents normal alveolar gas, which in this example is exactly correct for a respiratory exchange ratio of 0.80. One can read that the PA_{O_2} = 102 mmHg and the PA_{CO_2} = 40 mmHg.

Let us return to Eq. 4-3, which describes alveolar and anatomic dead space ventilation. Ventilation of the dead space is necessary but is wasted because no useful gas exchange occurs. *Suppose* that one lung has an obstructed pulmonary artery (embolus) so that that lung does not receive any pulmonary blood flow (see Question 1-5). The alveolar ventilation to that lung would be wasted, since it does not participate in any useful exchange. The physiologic dead space would be the sum of V_D and the portion of $\dot{V}_A$ per breath going to the lung with no blood flow.

Equation 4-3 can be used to calculate the total wasted ventilation, which includes the anatomic dead space and that portion of alveolar ventilation that behaves *as if* (concept of independent streams) it does not contribute to CO_2 exchange. To use Eq. 4-3 for such a purpose, however, one must know what F_{ACO_2} is in the normally exchanging alveoli. This is obtained by assuming that measured Pa_{CO_2} equals PA_{CO_2} in the effectively ventilated part of the lung.

$$\dot{V}_A \times \frac{Pa_{CO_2}}{P_B - P_{H_2O}} = \dot{V}_E \times F_{ECO_2} \qquad (4\text{-}6)$$

Equation 4-6 may appear to be identical to Eq. 4-3A but that is not the case. Equation 4-3A was set up using the law of conservation of mass to account for all of the CO_2 molecules in expired gas. The F_{ACO_2} or its equivalent $[P_{ACO_2}/(P_B - 47)]$ was the ideal alveolar CO_2 concentration. In real life, however, there is no easy way to measure P_{ACO_2}. It must be assumed or estimated by using the P_{CO_2} in the last portion of expired gas (end-tidal P_{CO_2}); otherwise, Eq. 4-3A will have two unknowns, namely, $\dot{V}_A$ and F_{ACO_2}.

Equation 4-6, on the other hand, uses the important identity

$$Pa_{CO_2} \equiv \text{effective } PA_{CO_2}$$

Equation 4-6 gives the effective $\dot{V}_A$, which will always be *less than* ideal $\dot{V}_A$.

Clinical pulmonary physiologists use Eq. 4-6 to compute the wasted ventilation as an index of the efficiency of ventilation. If we rearrange the terms slightly, we can see that alveolar ventilation is equal to the minute ventilation times the ratio of expired to arterial P_{CO_2}. The wasted ventilation, of course, is the minute ventilation minus the effective alveolar ventilation ($\dot{V}_E - \dot{V}_A$). Normally, it is less than 35% of $\dot{V}_E$. That is similar to the anatomic dead space/tidal volume ratio, which means that normally there is not much physiologic dead space in excess of V_D.

At this point, we must also revise our interpretation of Eq. 4-4, the alveolar ventilation equation. If we use Pa_{CO_2} instead of PA_{CO_2}, then $\dot{V}_A$ will be the *effective* alveolar ventilation, which is actually what the pulmonary physiologist wants. Likewise, if we substitute the Pa_{CO_2} for PA_{CO_2} in the alveolar gas equation (Eq. 4-5), we obtain the PA_{O_2} for the *effectively* ventilated lung.

It is not necessary to learn two sets of equations, one for the total alveolar ventilation and one for the effective alveolar ventilation, as long as you know the source of the numbers used.

READINGS

Few recent references deal with the basic topics of this chapter because it was all worked out long ago. However, if you are interested in some of the background and basis for the ventilation equations, the following four references are comprehensive.

Books

1. Fenn WO, Rahn H (eds): Handbook of Physiology, Section 3. Respiration. Vols. 1 and 2. American Physiological Society, Washington, 1964–1965

Especially significant chapters are: Bouheys A: Respiratory dead space (Chapter 28); Briscoe WA: Lung volumes (Chapter 53); Hyatt RE: Dynamic lung volumes (Chapter 54); and Otis AB: Quantitative relationships in steady-state gas exchange (Chapter 27).

2. Forster RE II, Dubois A, Briscoe WA, Fisher AB: The Lung: Physiologic Basis of Pulmonary Function Tests. 3rd Ed. Year Book Medical Publishers, Chicago, 1986
Chapters 2 and 3 describe some of the commonly used tests to measure lung volumes and ventilation. The Appendix is a review of the various equations.

3. Rahn H, Fenn WO: A graphical analysis of the respiratory gas exchange: the O_2-CO_2 diagram. p. 38. American Physiological Society, Washington, 1955
More than anybody ever wanted to know about the subject. A brilliant analysis that sank under its own weight. Still, it is the bible on gas exchange. All the ventilation equations are derived in detail.

Reviews

4. Rossier PH, Buehlmanns A: The respiratory dead space. Physiol Rev 35:860–870, 1955
A thorough review of what at the time was still controversial.

QUESTIONS*

Drill

1. Calculate $\dot{V}_A$, P_{ACO_2}, or $\dot{V}_{CO_2}$ as appropriate, assuming $P_B = 760$ mmHg and $T = 37°C$. Then state the adequacy of alveolar ventilation for each.
   a. $\dot{V}_A = 2$ liters/min, $\dot{V}_{CO_2} = 240$ ml/min, STPD
   b. $P_{ACO_2} = 28$ mmHg, $\dot{V}_{CO_2} = 650$ ml/min, STPD
   c. $\dot{V}_A = 8$ liters/min, $P_{ACO_2} = 40$ mmHg
   d. $P_{ACO_2} = 84$ mmHg, $\dot{V}_{CO_2} = 175$ ml/min, STPD
2. Calculate P_{AO_2} in each of the conditions shown in question 1, using the following additional information:
   a. $F_{IO_2} = 0.50$, $R = 0.75$
   b. $F_{IO_2} = 0.21$, $R = 0.80$
   c. $F_{IO_2} = 0.21$, $R = 1.0$
   d. $F_{IO_2} = 1.00$, $R = 0.85$

Problems

3. In steady-state exercise $P\bar{v}_{CO_2}$ is increased. Does P_{ACO_2} (Pa_{CO_2}) rise? Explain your answer in words based on an important equation.
4. A person with chronic obstructive pulmonary disease may have $V_D/V_T = 0.60$. What must V_T be at normal breathing frequency to maintain $P_{ACO_2} = 40$ mmHg, assuming $\dot{V}_{CO_2}$ is normal?
5. In order to measure TLC by the volume of dilution principle, must the test breath begin at RV or FRC? Please explain.
6. In the measurement of FRC by the volume of dilution principle, would FRC be overestimated or underestimated if the gas sample included some of the dead space gas? Please explain. (*Hint*: Make the calculation including all of the dead space, as a worse case analysis.)
7. A subject inspires 3 liters of 100% O_2 at 21°C (ATPS) and then expires through a drying agent before 0.5 liter of alveolar gas is collected, whose $F_{O_2} = 0.60$. Compute FRC, BTPS, given that $P_{H_2O} = 19$ mmHg at 21°C.
8. If a normal subject at rest stops breathing at FRC, how much time will elapse before the P_{AO_2} falls to 30 mmHg? What else will be occurring in alveolar gas and arterial blood during the breath hold? Are there any advantages to breath holding at TLC rather than FRC?
9. (This question is difficult.) Normal alveolar P_{O_2} is 102 mmHg and FRC $= 2,400$ ml, BTPS. How many 1-liter breaths of 100% O_2, ATPS at normal frequency will be required to raise Pa_{O_2} to 600 mmHg or above? In this example, the inspired gas has constant composition and the expired gas is breathed out into the room (open circuit; non-rebreathing system). Assume uniform instantaneous mixing in alveolar gas and a normal dead space. What is the P_{AO_2} after all the nitrogen is washed out? (Careful, a trick is involved.)

---

* Answers begin on p. 211.

5

Mechanical Properties in Breathing: Statics

THE BOTTOM LINE

Lung Distensibility
The normal lungs are easy to distend at low volume (FRC), i.e., they are compliant, but become stiffer (reduced compliance) at high volume (TLC).

Measure of Lung Distensibility
Lung compliance is calculated as $C_L = \Delta V/\Delta P_L$, where ΔV is the change in volume and ΔP_L is the change in translung pressure, $\Delta(P_A - P_{pl})$. The resistance to distension is the elastance, $E_L = 1/C_L$. The pressure-volume curve of the lung inscribes a wide loop (hysteresis), which means that its distensibility during inflation is different from its distensibility during deflation.

Surface Forces and Lung Recoil
The main cause of pressure-volume hysteresis is the variable air-liquid surface tension in the alveoli. Since the alveoli have a small radius (r), averaging 110 μm at FRC in humans, surface tension (T) is a potent force. Surface tension has the units of force per unit length. The surface tension in the lung alveoli is related to the transmural pressure by the LaPlace equation for spheres, $P = 2 \times (T/r)$. P is that portion of translung pressure (P_L) attributable to surface tension. Alveolar surface tension varies as the surface area changes, ranging between 50 dynes/cm at TLC to <5 dynes/cm at FRC. During normal tidal breathing, surface tension slowly approaches its equilibrium value of 28 dynes/cm. The reason for the variable surface tension is a special surface-active material whose main component is dipalmitoyl phosphatidylcholine. The lung surfactant is secreted by type 2 alveolar epithelial cells.

Chest Wall Distensibility
The chest wall has a different passive pressure-volume curve from the lung. At FRC, after deflation from TLC, pleural pressure averages -3.5 cmH$_2$O. The lungs are re-coiling to a smaller volume, but the chest wall is recoiling in the opposite direction

(Continues).

(Continued).

toward a larger volume. This is what accounts for the FRC volume and the subatmospheric pleural pressure. The pressure across the chest wall, Pw, = Ppl − Pbs, i.e., pleural pressure minus body surface pressure. Even though the chest wall is normally under compression in the range of tidal breathing, chest wall compliance (Cw) is a positive number. The diaphragm and abdominal wall are important functional components of the chest wall. The pressure difference across the diaphragm-abdominal wall must equal Pw at any lung volume.

Elastic Recoil of the Total Respiratory System

The lungs and chest wall move together. The total compliance of the respiratory system (Crs; lung + chest wall) is less that of either part alone. The simplest way to determine Crs is to add the elastance of the lung (EL) to the elastance of the chest wall (Ew), i.e., to add the reciprocals of their individual compliances: Ers = EL + Ew, where Ers = 1/Crs.

Statics refers to the treatment of stationary properties; the properties of the breathing apparatus that are independent of movement during breathing. The static mechanical properties of the lung (L) and chest wall (w) encompass an enormous part of modern respiratory physiology and have important clinical manifestations in such diverse diseases as emphysema, fibrosis, and respiratory distress syndromes. In Chapter 6, I discuss the mechanical properties of the lung in motion (dynamics).

The main point to remember about static respiratory mechanics is that we must treat the lungs and chest wall as passive; that is, they must be displaced by an external force. That is easy to comprehend for the lungs because they are always passive, but normally the chest wall, by contracting the diaphragm and intercostal muscles, actively develops all of the pressure difference that distends the lungs. Still, we can study the chest wall when it is passive, as when the lungs and chest wall are ventilated by a pump in a patient who is paralyzed.

LUNG DISTENSIBILITY

Gas, being a fluid, flows from a region of higher pressure to one of lower pressure. When the total pressure in the alveoli is equal to atmospheric pressure, there is no airflow. For inspiration to occur, alveolar pressure must be less than atmospheric pressure, and vice versa for expiration. There are two ways of producing the pressure difference necessary for inspiratory flow: (1) alveolar pressure can be lowered, as in natural ("negative pressure") breathing, or (2) pressure at the airway opening, Pao, can be raised, as is done by most mechanical ventilators ("positive pressure" breathing).

Elasticity

Elasticity is the *property of matter that causes it to return to its original shape or size after being deformed by an external force*. It represents resistance to deformation. The more force necessary to deform a structure, the more elastance it has; the less force necessary to deform a structure, the more compliance it has. Elastance (E) is the reciprocal of compliance (C). Thus, E = 1/C.

Figure 5-1 presents two common analogies concerning the behavior of perfectly elastic bodies. In the top panel and graph is an example taken from physics; namely, a steel spring (one-

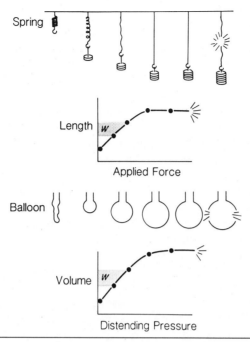

Fig. 5-1.   Hooke's law applied **(A)** to a linear spring and **(B)** to a balloon. For a compliant structure, the increase in length or volume varies directly with the increase in the applied force or pressure until the elastic limit is reached. The work necessary to overcome the elastic recoil of either the spring or the balloon is the necessary applied pressure multiplied by the change in length or volume, as represented by the shaded areas for work (W).

dimensional model) that obeys Hooke's law—the applied force (increasing weight on the spring) causes a deformation (change in spring length). Hooke's law states that the deformation is proportional to the applied force up to the elastic limit. The slope of the line relating deformation to force is equivalent to the compliance and is characteristic for a particular material. Compliance is defined as the strain divided by the stress.

The work, W, necessary to lengthen the spring, l, is expressed as follows:

$$W = F \times \Delta l$$

In the figure, the work done on the spring to lengthen is represented by the area between any two lengths (on the y-axis) and the line.

The lower panel of Figure 5-1 shows the three-dimensional analogue, a distensible balloon. In this case, the applied force is the transmural (distending) pressure ($Ptm = P_{inside} - P_{outside}$) and the deformation is the volume change, ΔV. The pressure-volume (P-V) curve is analogous to Hook's law. We refer to the compliance of the balloon in terms of its distensibility, $\Delta V/\Delta Ptm$.

The work of distending the balloon, by analogy to the linear case, is

$$W = P \times \Delta V \qquad (5\text{-}1)$$

Elastic Recoil of the Lung

The usual analogy applied to the lung is that of a distensible balloon. A new balloon contains essentially no air. To inflate it, you increase the pressure across its wall. By continuing to increase the distending pressure (ΔPtm), the balloon eventually reaches some arbitrary large volume, which we define as its total capacity. Attempting to increase the volume further will cause the balloon to burst (exceed its elastic limit). If one does not exceed total capacity but rather reduces the pressure inside the balloon, it recoils because of the elastic energy stored in its walls. Upon deflation, however, a new balloon will not generally return to its original condition. It remains at a somewhat larger volume than before, even when the transmural pressure becomes zero. This is because the balloon is not a perfectly elastic body. The lung is not a perfectly elastic body either.

After a few inflations and deflations (pressure-volume cycles), the balloon and the lung will achieve steady-state conditions, and either can then be cycled more or less reproducibly. For the balloon this represents a permanent condition. For the lung, however, the steady-state condition is not permanent but depends in part on the turnover of special phospholipid molecules in the alveoli (surface-active material).

The lung, of course, is much more complex than a balloon because of its anatomic structure and because of an important additional force that is not generally of concern in the balloon, namely, alveolar air-liquid surface tension.

The tissues of the lung are not uniform springs; they consist of collagen and elastic fibers, giant glycoprotein molecules in the interstitial matrix, and various cells, such as the alveolar epithelium and capillary endothelium. Some of the lung tissues are compliant (easily stretched): cells, interstitial ground substance molecules, and elastic fibers. These tissues are stretched during inspiration by an applied external force; namely, muscle contraction in the chest wall, which generates the translung distending pressure, P_L. Collagen fibers, however, are not easily stretched. As lung volume increases, they restrict lung deformation more and more. This causes the lung to become stiffer and the pressure-volume curve of the lung to become flatter (lower slope).

THE MEASURE OF LUNG DISTENSIBILITY

The compliance of the lung, C_L, which is the measure of its distensibility, is defined as the slope of the line between any two points on the pressure-volume curve. Compliance is the volume change, ΔV, divided by the translung pressure change, ΔP_L, measured under static conditions:

$$C_L = \Delta V/\Delta P_L \qquad (5\text{-}2)$$

The units of lung compliance are liters/cmH$_2$O.

Since the elastance of the lung, E_L, is the reciprocal of compliance

$$E_L = 1/C_L = \Delta P_L/\Delta V_L \qquad (5\text{-}2A)$$

Pressure Differences

Before going further, let us review the pressure differences across the various distensible portions of the breathing apparatus. These are shown in Figure 5-2, which at first sight looks complex but is straightforward, if you take it bit by bit. Figure 5-2 is a handy reference that can be of use whenever one is confused by pressure relationships, which may be a frequent occurrence until one becomes familiar with lung mechanics.

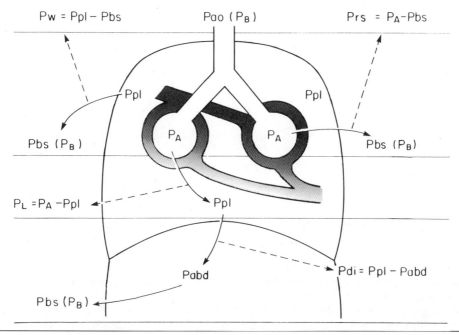

Fig. 5-2. Schema showing stylized lungs and pulmonary circulation in the thorax. All the pressures and pressure differences that are important to the respiratory system are shown. The abbreviations are standard in modern respiratory physiology (see Appendix 1). Around the outside of the diagram are the four main distending pressures: Pw, P_L, Prs, and Pdi (dashed arrows).

In referring to transorgan pressures, the pressure difference across the wall is always measured from the inside to the outside. For the lung, transorgan pressure, P_L, is defined as

$$P_L = P_A - Ppl$$

where P_A is total alveolar gas pressure and Ppl is the average pressure in the pleural space.

In Figure 5-2, translung pressure, P_L, appears only once, along the left-hand side of the figure near the bottom. Become familiar with some of the other distending pressures, such as the chest wall distending pressure, Pw (top line, left-hand side); the distending pressure across the diaphragm, Pdi (right-hand side, bottom); and the pressure across the entire respiratory system, Prs (top line, right-hand side).

The Deflation Pressure-Volume Curve

The static **deflation** pressure-volume curve of an isolated, normal, air-filled human lung is shown in Figure 5-3. Applied transorgan static pressure is zero near the middle of the x-axis (thin vertical line). Pressures to the right are distending pressures; pressures to the left are compressive pressures; that is, the external pressure is greater than the internal pressure.

The left-hand y-axis shows normal absolute volume from 0 to 6 liters (TLC). The y-axis also shows various named lung volumes: residual volume (RV), functional residual capacity (FRC), and tidal volume (V_T). One new volume has been added, minimal volume (MV). It is part of RV. When the chest is opened, as during thoracic surgery, and the lungs are allowed to recoil

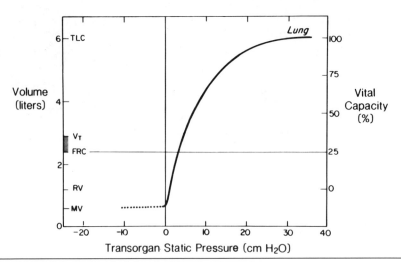

Fig. 5-3. The deflation pressure-volume curve of the lung. The x-axis shows the transorgan static pressure for the normal human breathing apparatus. Translung pressure is zero at the thin vertical line near the middle of the graph. The pressure-volume curve of the lung is normally limited to the positive or distending pressure range. The dashed (theoretical) line to the left is included to show that the lung becomes stiff (resists deflation at compressive pressures). The y-axis on the left shows absolute volume in liters together with the main lung volumes. The tidal volume is shown by the stippled zone, and FRC is shown by a thin horizontal line across the graph. Minimal volume (MV) is the volume of the lung when the translung static pressure is zero. The righthand y-axis shows volume as a percentage of vital capacity between residual volume (0% VC) and total lung capacity (100% VC).

until the translung static pressure equals zero ($P_L = 0$), the lung does not collapse to the airless condition but retains approximately 10% of its total gas capacity. Minimal volume for the lung as a whole does not occur in life normally because the chest wall prevents it. But some regions of the lung may reach minimal volume during normal breathing, especially in older people. In the disease **emphysema** lung elastic tissue degenerates, so that minimal volume ($P_L = 0$) occurs within the normal FRC or V_T range. This may cause residual volume to increase markedly. After all, RV cannot be less than MV, can it?

The right-hand y-axis in Figure 5-3 shows percent vital capacity (% VC). Zero percent equals residual volume; 100% equals TLC. There are two different y-axis labels because there is no standard convention. One must be prepared for both possibilities. The best feature of the left-hand axis is that it is in real numbers, but of course not all lungs have a TLC of 6 liters. The best feature of the right-hand y-axis is that it is correct for all lung sizes, but it does not indicate what those volumes are and gives no information about residual volume.

The static pressure-volume curve shown in Figure 5-3 is for an idealized adult human lung that has been inflated with air to total lung capacity and then allowed to deflate slowly. By convention, static lung compliance is measured during deflation following a maximal inspiration. The purpose of this convention is to ensure reproducible initial conditions.

The deflation pressure-volume curve is alinear. The essential points are that the slope is less (low compliance or high stiffness) over its upper third but steep (high compliance or low stiffness) over its lower portion (between 0 and 10 cmH$_2$O). Thus, it is easy to inflate the lung when the transpulmonary pressure is low, which is a good thing because normally, even in exercise when tidal volumes are larger than usual, we breathe over the lower 70% of the pressure-

volume curve. V_T seldom exceeds half of vital capacity. The work involved in breathing, P ×
ΔV, is less than if one breathed near the top of the curve, as may occur in a person suffering
from asthma, where the narrowed airways lead to increased FRC. Compliance changes as a
function of lung volume because at low transpulmonary pressures the main forces affecting
deflation of the lung are the elastic elements in the walls of the terminal respiratory units but
at high volumes the collagen fibers in the lung's supporting structures are tense and make a
large contribution.

The main operating point of the pressure-volume curve is FRC, represented by the thin
horizontal line in Figure 5-3. The static recoil pressure (P_L) of the lung at FRC averages 3.5
cmH_2O at a standard volume of 2,400 ml (40% TLC; 25% VC). The normal tidal volume (500
ml), shown by the stippled bar on the left-hand y-axis, subtends only a small portion of the
pressure-volume curve.

To calculate the compliance of the lung between any two points on the deflation P-V curve,
one divides the change in volume, ΔV, by the change in the translung pressure, ΔP_L. Thus,
absolute pressure is not important, only relative pressure.

Relative Pressure

Ordinarily, physiologists use P_A to indicate total pressure in the alveoli relative to pressure
at the airway opening (Pao), where Pao = P_B (atmospheric or ambient pressure) (see Fig. 5-2).
Absolute sea level (standard) atmospheric pressure is 760 mmHg but is taken as zero when
used as the reference point for other pressures.

Thus, at FRC in Figure 5-3 the difference between alveolar pressure and pleural pressure
is 3.5 cmH_2O. Since it is only the *pressure difference* that counts, it does not matter whether
pleural pressure is -3.5 cmH_2O and alveolar pressure is zero (natural or "negative pressure"
breathing) or whether pleural pressure is $+6.5$ and alveolar pressure is $+10$ cmH_2O (positive
end-expiratory pressure, as in mechanical ventilation).

Calculation of Compliance and Elastance

Let us compute the compliance of the lung for a volume change between 50% vital capacity
and FRC on deflation. Using Figure 5-3, read from the right-hand y-axis over to the left hand
y-axis at 50% vital capacity (not 50% TLC). At 50% VC, lung volume is 3.6 liters. Read down
to the x-axis from the 3.6-liter point on the P-V curve. The static recoil (transorgan) pressure
(P_L) at that volume is 7 cmH_2O. Now set up the equation for compliance as follows:

$$C_L = \Delta V / \Delta P_L = \frac{50\%\ VC - FRC}{P_{L,\ 50\%\ VC} - P_{L,\ FRC}}$$

$$= \frac{(3.6 - 2.4)\ liters}{(7 - 3.5)\ cmH_2O}$$

$$= \frac{1.2\ liters}{3.5\ cmH_2O} = 0.34\ liters/cmH_2O$$

The convention is to put the higher volume and consequently the higher translung pressure
first, thus avoiding two minus signs.

We should also calculate lung elastance, E_L, so you'll become equally familiar with it.*

$$E_L = 1/C_L = \frac{1\ cmH_2O}{0.34\ liter} = 2.94\ cmH_2O/liter$$

Remember: Lung compliance (or its reciprocal elastance) is always a positive number. To measure compliance or elastance, one must change lung volume by changing translung pressure.

What happens to lung volume when transmural pressure goes negative, that is, when pleural pressure exceeds the alveolar pressure? Figure 5-3 shows a short horizontal dotted line indicating that lung volume should not decrease below minimal volume when the lung is compressed. The line is dotted, meaning it is theoretical, because that portion of the deflation P-V curve cannot usually be measured. The reason is that the compressive pressure causes the airways to collapse (see Ch. 6), so that P_A does not equal P_{ao}.

Specific Compliance and Elastance

Lung compliance (elastance) is in part dependent on the size of the lung. In a child, whose vital capacity is 3 liters, compliance will be half that calculated using absolute volumes on the left-hand y-axis of Figure 5-3. If one always calculated compliance using the volume change as a fraction of the starting volume, the size of the lung would not matter. This is called *specific compliance*, the compliance per unit lung volume.

A newborn baby has a vital capacity (when crying lustily) of 120 ml. If we computed the compliance of the baby's lungs, it would be a very small number, not because there is anything wrong with the infant's lungs but because of their small size. It is meaningless to compare the absolute compliances or elastances of lungs of different sizes. Compare specific compliances or specific elastances.

For example, in our previous calculation we obtained a compliance of 0.34 liter/cmH$_2$O for a normal adult. Since the average lung volume over which that measurement was made was 3.0 liters [(2.4 + 3.6)/2], the specific compliance, $SpC_L = 0.11$ liter/(cmH$_2$O × liters) = 0.11/ cmH$_2$O, and $SpE_L = 1/SpC_L = 9.1$ cmH$_2$O.

Compute both the total compliance and the specific compliance of the newborn, given that FRC = 60 ml and lung volume at 50% VC = 80 ml but the change in the transpulmonary pressure is the same as in the adult:

$$C_L = \Delta V/\Delta P_L = \frac{(80 - 60)\ ml}{(7 - 3.5)\ cmH_2O}$$

$$= 20\ ml/3.5\ cmH_2O$$

$$= 5.7\ ml/cmH_2O = 0.0057\ liter/cmH_2O$$

That is only about one-sixtieth of the compliance of the adult lung. However, using the average lung volume ($\bar{V}$) during the measurement [(FRC + 50% VC)/2 = (60 + 80)/2 = 70 ml], the

---

* Use whichever form (C_L or E_L) your teachers prefer. Elastance is the better usage, but compliance is more deeply ingrained.

specific compliance is

$$SpC_L = \frac{\Delta V}{\overline{V} \times \Delta P_L} = \frac{0.0057 \text{ liter}}{0.070 \text{ liter} \times cmH_2O} = 0.081/cmH_2O$$

The specific compliance of the baby's lung is not much less than that of the adult lung.

> **Remember:**   When interpreting lung compliance or elastance, due regard should be taken of lung volume.

SURFACE FORCES AND LUNG RECOIL

The adult human lung contains about 300 million tiny anatomic alveoli. This arrangement has the beneficial effect of vastly increasing the surface area for O_2 and CO_2 exchange but has the disadvantage that each anatomic alveolus has a very small radius of curvature (average r in adult human is 110 μm at FRC). This geometric condition plus the fact that there is an interface between air in the alveoli and the tissue gives rise to the complication of **surface tension**. The magnitude and importance of the air-liquid surface tension in the lung and the physiologic mechanisms that have evolved to overcome the problem make a fascinating story.

The significance of the air-liquid surface tension is best demonstrated by determining the complete inflation and deflation pressure-volume curve of the lungs when they are filled with liquid (for example, 0.9% NaCl solution) and by comparing the result with the air P-V loop. This comparison is shown in Figure 5-4. The air P-V loop is the same as that shown in Figure 3-4.

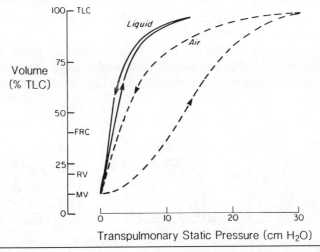

Fig. 5-4.   Complete pressure-volume curves of a normal human lung for the liquid-filled and air-filled states. The curve can begin at either end, but conventionally it begins at minimal volume (MV) and a translung static pressure of zero. The solid line shows the liquid-filled lung. The curve is steep and the inflation and deflation lines are nearly superimposed; that is, there is little hysteresis. Total lung capacity is achieved at a translung pressure of 15 cmH_2O. The pressure-volume curve for the air-filled lung is shown by the dashed line. The deflation curve is displaced to the right of the liquid-state curve; the inflation curve is displaced even further. This means that the pressure-volume curve of the lung is sensitive to the prior condition of the lung, that is, to its volume history.

The pressure-volume curve of the liquid-filled lung is displaced toward lower distending pressure at any given volume. The significance of the shift is that it requires much less pressure to maintain lung volume when the lung is filled with liquid (water) rather than with gas. In some disease conditions (notably respiratory distress syndrome of the newborn) the deflation limb of the air pressure-volume curve is displaced farther to the right (closer to the inflation limb). That means that higher pressures are necessary to hold the lungs inflated.

The difference between the air and liquid P-V loops is not due to tissue elastic forces (collagen, elastin, etc.), since these are not significantly changed by filling the lung with liquid. What has changed is that the alveolar air-liquid interface has been removed by the liquid. One should conclude from this that the pressure necessary to maintain a given lung volume is the sum of the pressures necessary to overcome elastic recoil of tissue elements and of the elastic "skin" (air-liquid interface) at the alveolar surface.

What is Surface Tension?

Within the bulk phase of a liquid, such as water (Fig. 5-5A), there are forces of attraction among the water molecules. On the average these forces are equal in all directions. But at the surface (Fig. 5-5B), the water molecules do not have equal attraction forces in all directions. In the interior of the liquid, the molecules have thermal kinetic energy and occasionally a molecule will achieve sufficient energy to penetrate to the surface or even to escape into the air above. The latter event generates the vapor pressure of the liquid (for example, $P_{H_2O} = 47$ mmHg in the lungs at 37°C). But there are relatively few of these molecules in the gas above the liquid, and they are ineffective in attracting the molecules at the surface. Therefore, the water molecules tend to be pulled toward the interior, away from the surface, which increases the pressure (kinetic energy) in the liquid. When the kinetic energy of the water molecules is raised sufficiently to replace molecules in the surface as rapidly as they are pulled away, an equilibrium is established. The lateral attraction at the surface among the water molecules exerts a force within the plane of the surface, which acts as an elastic **tension** to oppose the energy of bulk phase molecules trying to enter (expand) the surface.

Surface tension has the units of force per unit length. A physical analogy, often used, is to consider the tension generated when one pulls down a window shade (Fig. 5-6A). In a sphere, which for this purpose is analogous to an anatomic alveolus, the surface tension acts in the

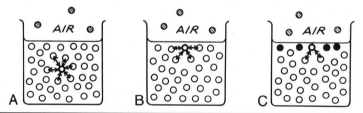

Fig. 5-5. Model to represent the intermolecular forces involved in the generation of surface tension. **(A)** Intermolecular attractive forces among water molecules (open circles) in the interior of the liquid. The resultant (sum) of all directed forces is zero. **(B)** Intermolecular attractive forces on the molecules in the surface showing an imbalance whose resultant tends to pull molecules toward the interior. The sparse molecules in the vapor phase (shaded circles) are insufficient to counterbalance the pull of the water molecules within the bulk phase. **(C)** Surface-active molecules, such as lung surfactant, which is partially hydrophobic (solid circles), displace most of the water molecules from the surface. (From Comroe JH: Physiology of Respiration. 2nd Ed. Year Book Medical Publishers, Chicago, 1974, with permission.)

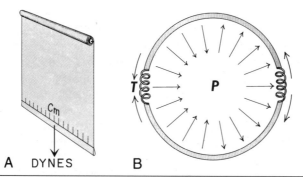

Fig. 5-6. **(A)** Tension in a plane surface (window shade) and in a curved surface (sphere). To pull the shade, one exerts a force (dynes) along the edge (cm). The tension in the fabric of the shade is the force per unit length (dynes/cm). **(B)** For the curved surface, part of the wall tension (T) is directed inward (left half of sphere) but is opposed by the distending pressure (P) (right half of sphere). The tension may be due to structural elements in the wall (rubber balloon) or to the air-liquid surface forces (soap bubble). In the lung's alveoli, both contribute. (From Abramson DI (ed): Blood Vessels and Lymphatics. Academic Press, San Diego, 1962, with permission.)

curved surface to hold the sphere together in opposition to the transmural distending pressure which is trying to force the surface apart (Fig. 5-6B).

The relationship between the tension in the surface and the transmural distending pressure is described by the LaPlace law, the same law that is used to describe mechanical wall tension in the ventricles of the heart and in blood vessels. There are two important differences: (1) in the lung, the tension (T) is in the surface rather than in the tensile strength of the wall structure and (2) for a sphere there are two equal radii of curvature. The LaPlace law for spherical structures, such as alveoli, is

$$P = 2 \times T/r \tag{5-3}$$

where r is the radius of curvature and P is the portion of the translung pressure, P_L, that accounts for the difference between the liquid and air pressure-volume curves at any given volume during inflation or deflation as shown in Figure 5-4.

Soap bubbles are frequently used to describe surface tension. The bubble integrity is maintained by the surface tension of soap molecules acting to counterbalance the distending pressure across the bubble surface.

The surface tension in the alveoli of the lung has the special property of varying as a function of surface area. In Figure 5-4, the inflation limb of the air pressure-volume curve requires a higher transpulmonary pressure at any volume than does the deflation limb. This can only be explained if the surface tension changes with lung inflation and deflation, being greater as the lung surface expands and less as the lung surface contracts. The variable surface tension between inflation and deflation accounts for most of the hysteresis seen in the air pressure-volume curve.

The soap bubble is not a complete analogy for the alveolus because the soap bubble has a constant tension in its surface. The amazing feature of the lung's surface is that specific phospholipid molecules are present in the surface that allow the surface tension to vary in a cyclic manner as alveolar surface area changes during breathing. In ordinary breathing, the variation in surface forces is small, cycling around the equilibrium value of 28 dynes/cm at 37°C. With a large breath, however, as the surface expands, the surface tension rises to 50 dynes/cm. This rising tension opposes expansion of the lung and requires increased transpulmonary pressure (work) to enlarge the lung, but it has the beneficial effect of allowing more molecules of the surface tension-lowering material to enter the air-liquid interface. This in part explains why the previous breathing pattern (volume history) affects the P-V loop and why, for example, static lung compliance is measured on deflation from TLC (Fig. 5-3).

When the lung begins to deflate, the surface molecules are compressed together. This acts to lower surface tension to less than 10 dynes/cm. Consequently, there is a large decrease in transpulmonary pressure before lung volume changes very much, as the deflation limb of the air P-V curve in Figure 5-4 shows. The decreasing surface tension during deflation also acts to stabilize the smallest alveoli, so they do not shrink faster than the largest alveoli.

There are other forces acting at the same time, and the picture is not quite as simple as described. The fact that several alveoli share common surfaces is one such factor. Table 5-1 lists the air-water surface tensions of some common substances.

Let us use the LaPlace equation to compute the surface tension that exists in the air-liquid interface at 50% TLC during deflation from total lung capacity. In Figure 5-4 the pressure difference between the air deflation and liquid deflation curves at 50% VC amounts to about 2 cmH_2O. If the average radius of the anatomic alveoli in the human lung is taken as 120 μm at 50% TLC, then we can compute the surface tension at that volume using Eq. 5-3. The main complication is to be sure that the units are correct. Since tension is in dynes/cm, pressure must be converted from cmH_2O (or mmHg) to dynes/cm^2 and the radius must be converted from micrometers to centimeters.

$$P = 2 \times T/r$$

$$2 \text{ cmH}_2\text{O} \times 980 \text{ dynes/(cm}^2 \times \text{cmH}_2\text{O}) = 2T/(120 \text{ μm} \times 10^{-4} \text{ cm/μm})$$

$$1,960 \text{ dynes/cm}^2 = 2T/(120 \times 10^{-4} \text{ cm})$$

$$T = 12 \text{ dynes/cm}$$

The first term includes the conversion factor for cmH_2O to dynes/cm^2. The second term includes the conversion for micrometers to centimeters.

If surface tension is calculated during inflation at 50% TLC, where the average radius of the alveoli is the same but the pressure difference between air and liquid-filled curves is about 9 cmH_2O (Fig. 5-4), one will find a surface tension value of approximately 53 dynes/cm^2, more than four times as great as during deflation.

There are many substances (surfactants, wetting agents, or detergents) that lower the surface tension of water. Even the proteins and phospholipids in plasma lower the air-liquid surface tension from 70 dynes/cm (pure water) to 50 to 60 dynes/cm (Table 5-1).

Table 5-1. Air-Liquid Surface Tension of Some Common Liquids

Liquid	Surface Tension (dynes/cm)
Water	70
Plasma	50–60
Lung surface-active material	<5–50 (28 at equilibrium)
Detergent solution	30
95% ethanol	22

Some surface tension-lowering molecules are less attracted by the water molecules in the bulk phase because a portion of the molecule is hydrophobic. Therefore, these molecules tend to concentrate at the air-liquid interface (Fig. 5-5C) in preference to the water molecules. They lower the internal kinetic energy necessary to maintain the surface configuration. Consequently, the liquid can exist at a larger volume (surface area) at no increase in trans-surface pressure. The more an agent lowers surface tension, the more the bulk liquid can spread (increase its surface area).

When the surface area of the alveoli decreases during lung deflation, the surfactant molecules at the air-liquid interface become compacted together because they are rather insoluble in water and resist further compression. It is this effect that causes the alveolar surface tension to vary as a function of lung volume.

Lung surfactant consists of a complex phospholipid-protein material, which is produced by the type 2 alveolar lining cells and secreted onto the alveolar surface. The main surface tension-lowering substance in lung surfactant is **dipalmitoyl phosphatidylcholine** (DPPC). This surfactant molecule has two special features: its equilibrium surface tension is less than that of plasma (Table 5-1), and the surface tension changes as a function of the expansion or contraction of the alveolar surface. Surface tension rises (approaching that of plasma, 50 dynes/cm) as the surface is expanded and decreases to less than 10 dynes/cm when the surface is compressed during lung deflation.

Lung surfactant has three physiologic advantages: (1) it reduces the work of breathing, that is, it reduces the muscular effort needed to expand the lungs; (2) it lowers the energy necessary to maintain the lungs at low volume (FRC) and helps to prevent the alveoli from collapsing at the end of each expiration, which would greatly increase the work necessary to reinflate the lung at the next breath (surfactant deficiency is the basic defect in the respiratory distress syndrome that may occur in the lungs of underdeveloped newborns); and (3) it stabilizes alveoli that tend to deflate at different rates. The unit that deflates more rapidly will have a lower surface tension. This slows its rate of volume decrease, allowing a more slowly deflating unit with a higher surface tension to "catch up."

Origin, Composition, Turnover, and Regulation of the Surface-Active Material in the Lung

The surface-active material in the lung is a complex mixture of phospholipids and specific proteins. All its ingredients are necessary for the full expression of its surface tension-lowering properties and for the stability of the air-liquid interface. The main component is dipalmitoyl phosphatidylcholine (DPPC), containing two 16-carbon saturated fatty acid (palmitate) chains. The lipid chains are hydrophobic, whereas the phosphatidylcholine is hydrophilic. The molecules orient themselves at the air-liquid interface with the fatty acid residues arranged so as to project vertically out from the bulk phase. This arrangement is mechanically stable, which is why the lung surface film resists compression during lung deflation and is able to lower surface tension.

The pulmonary surface-active material is secreted by the type 2 alveolar cells (Fig. 2-4A). These cells begin to produce the surface-active material and secrete it in late fetal development (third trimester) as the lung matures and becomes ready for air breathing. As Figure 5-4 implies, the surface-active material is not necessary in the liquid-filled fetal lung, but it is essential for the survival of the air-breathing newborn. Immediately after birth, babies have to change from liquid-filled lungs to air-filled lungs making use of a weak rib cage (see Ch. 2). The first cry of the newborn means its lungs have been successfully inflated with air.

Lung surfactant is continually replaced, as old molecules leave the surface film and new ones enter it. The stability of the alveolar air-liquid interfacial film depends on the sustained metabolism of the type 2 alveolar epithelial cells. Alveolar type 2 cell metabolism and surfactant production are sensitive to pulmonary blood flow. For example, after obstruction of a pulmonary artery by a blood clot, the portion of the lung served by that pulmonary artery does not die, since it has other sources of nutrition. But alveolar type 2 cell metabolism is depressed and less surfactant is produced. The affected lung unit's alveolar surface tension rises and the unit shrinks to a small volume until such time as adequate blood flow is restored.

CHEST WALL DISTENSIBILITY

The functional chest wall includes the rib cage, diaphragm, and abdomen, as described in Chapter 2 (Fig. 2-9). These components work together under central nervous system control to cause the cyclic process of breathing. Diseases affecting the chest wall can be very serious and may be the immediate cause of death (multiple broken ribs causing a collapsible [flail] rib cage, inspiratory muscle paralysis [poliomyelitis]). Understanding the function of the chest wall is vital to a complete understanding of pulmonary mechanics.

Elastic Recoil of the Chest Wall

Before discussing the *active*, coordinated muscle activity that produces normal "negative pressure" breathing (see Ch. 6), I must describe the *passive* elastic recoil of the chest wall.

Consider for a moment the condition of the chest wall relative to that of the lungs at end expiration (FRC). In Figure 5-3 the translung static recoil pressure at FRC was 3.5 cmH_2O. Since in normal breathing the alveolar pressure (P_A) is zero (atmospheric, P_B), the pleural pressure (Ppl) must be -3.5 cmH_2O. Now think about the pressures across the chest wall (diaphragm-abdomen and rib cage), as shown in Figure 5-2. By analogy to the translung pressure, we define a transchest wall static recoil pressure (Pw) as:

$$Pw = Ppl - Pbs$$

where Ppl is pleural pressure, which is also the pressure on the inside of the chest wall, and Pbs is body surface pressure (normally atmospheric pressure, P_B). Thus, at FRC chest wall transorgan pressure is

$$Pw = (-3.5 - 0) \, cmH_2O$$

$$= -3.5 \, cmH_2O$$

Since the sign is negative, the chest wall must be under compression; that is, it is below its unstressed position.

At FRC the lungs are above their minimal volume and the chest wall is below its minimal volume. It is these equal but opposite elastic recoil forces that determine the position of the respiratory system (lungs plus chest wall) at end expiration. If we inject air between the parietal and visceral pleurae (create a pneumothorax) to break the liquid seal that couples the lungs to the chest wall, the lungs will become smaller and the thoracic cavity will become larger. How large will the thoracic cavity get? It will increase its volume until transorgan static recoil pressure equals zero, approximately 1 liter above FRC, according to Figure 5-7.

The **passive** pressure-volume curve of the chest wall is added to that of the lung in Figure

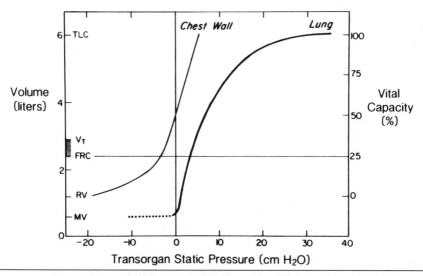

Fig. 5-7. The passive pressure-volume curve of the chest wall added to that of the lung. At FRC the transchest wall pressure is negative (compressive) and is exactly equal and opposite to translung pressure at FRC. Over the range of FRC to total lung capacity, the pressure-volume curve of the chest wall is essentially linear. It becomes alinear at volumes below FRC. When the transchest wall pressure is zero, the resting volume of the thoracic cavity is about 3.5 liters in this example (approximately 50% vital capacity).

5-7. I emphasize the word passive because, unlike the lung, the chest wall also has an active pressure-volume curve, which is completely different, as discussed in Chapter 6.

The pressure-volume curve of the chest wall is located to the left of that of the lung. At FRC, $Pw = -3.5$ cmH$_2$O is equal and opposite to $P_L = +3.5$ cmH$_2$O. At very low volume, below FRC, the chest wall becomes progressively stiffer until at residual volume Pw is about -20 cmH$_2$O. Above FRC, the P-V curve of the chest wall is steep (high compliance) and nearly linear. At TLC Pw is about $+5$ cmH$_2$O.

Even though the chest wall is normally under compression, the compliance of the chest wall (Cw) is still a positive number, since the slope of the P-V curve is positive. Do not be misled by the fact that Pw = -3.5 cmH$_2$O at FRC. Remember, it is only the *change* in Pw that is important.

Let us compute the compliance of the chest wall over the range of FRC to FRC + 50% VC.* At 50% VC, thoracic gas volume is 3.6 liters and Pw is $+0.2$ cmH$_2$O, according to Figure 5-7. Thus

$$Cw = \frac{(3.6 - 2.4) \text{ liters}}{[0.2 - (-3.5)] \text{ cmH}_2\text{O}}$$

$$= \frac{1.2 \text{ liters}}{3.7 \text{ cmH}_2\text{O}}$$

$$= 0.32 \text{ liter/cmH}_2\text{O}$$

---

* There is no hysteresis for the pressure-volume curve of the chest wall; it is the same during inflation as during deflation.

> **Remember:** Chest wall compliance will always be a positive number.

Chest wall compliance (Cw) is about the same as lung compliance (CL). This can be seen in Figure 5-7, where the slopes of the P-V curves of the lung and of the chest wall over the region FRC to 50% VC are nearly parallel.

What else can be read from Figure 5-7? Near TLC, it is not the chest wall that limits thoracic expansion because the compliance of the chest wall remains high; rather, it is the lung that becomes stiff. At the other end, near RV, it is the chest wall that becomes stiff, while the lung remains compliant.

Transdiaphragmatic Pressure

I have not made any distinction between the pressure across the rib cage and the pressure across the diaphragm. At FRC, if Pw is equal everywhere, then the pressure across the diaphragm (Pdi) must be equal to Pw and therefore the abdominal pressure (Pabd) must be equal to the pressure on the body surface (Pbs) (normally PB) and thus equal to 0. To clarify these relationships, refer back to Figure 5-2.

$$Pw = Pdi = Ppl - Pabd$$

$$-3.5 \text{ cmH}_2\text{O} = -3.5 \text{ cmH}_2\text{O} - Pabd$$

$$Pabd = 0$$

In humans this can only be achieved in the supine position with the diaphragm and abdominal muscles completely relaxed, so that abdominal pressure under the diaphragm is equal to atmospheric pressure. At equilibrium, the pressure difference is counterbalanced by passive tension in the diaphragm. Indeed, FRC is lower in the supine position because the diaphragm is pushed into the thoracic cavity by the higher abdominal pressure until the required passive diaphragmatic tension is achieved.

In the standing position, however, Pabd just beneath the diaphragm is the same as pleural pressure (Ppl). At first that may be difficult to believe, but it is true. The transdiaphragm pressure is zero. There is no passive tension in the diaphragm. Thus, the diaphragm moves downward into the abdominal cavity, which explains why FRC increases immediately upon standing.

But somewhere the abdominal pressure must rise to equal body surface pressure. Indeed it does—across the anterior (ventral) abdominal wall. The pressure difference across the abdominal wall equals $-3.5 \text{ cmH}_2\text{O}$ just below the diaphragm. Abdominal pressure rises (1 cmH$_2$O/cm) as one moves down the abdomen. Thus, abdominal pressure rises to equal Pbs about 3.5 cm below the diaphragm. Further down, transabdominal pressure becomes positive, which is why the lower abdomen tends to protrude when the abdominal muscles are relaxed.

> **Remember:** The pressure difference across *all* components of the chest wall must be the same.

Notice in Figure 5-7 that in the normal range of tidal breathing (in fact, up to nearly 50% VC), Pw is negative, which means that no work (P × ΔV) is done on the chest wall to expand it. During deflation, however, when the lungs are doing nearly all the work by delivering elastic recoil energy to expel air, they also work on the chest wall to pull it inward to its FRC position.

Specific Compliance of the Chest Wall

Specific compliance of the chest wall is not usually computed, but this could be done in the same way as for the lung.

ELASTIC RECOIL OF THE TOTAL RESPIRATORY SYSTEM

Normally, the lungs and chest wall move together. The volume changes are identical because the lungs are coupled to the chest wall by molecular cohesion within the liquid layer of the pleural space. The total pressure across the respiratory system (Prs) is the sum of translung (P_L) and transchest wall (Pw) pressures.

$$Prs = P_L + Pw = (P_A - Ppl) + (Ppl - Pbs)$$

$$Prs = P_A - Pbs$$

Remember: Prs only has meaning in terms of lung and chest wall distensibility, when *all* the muscles of breathing, including the abdominal muscles, are completely relaxed (passive pressure-volume curve).

As usual, we begin at FRC (Fig. 5-7), which by definition is the condition of complete relaxation. At that point, Prs = 0 (since P_A = Pbs).

As we progress to different volumes, the passive pressure across the respiratory system must be the sum of the transchest wall pressure and the translung pressure. Thus, at FRC + 1 liter, the transchest wall pressure = 0 (unstressed thoracic volume) and, therefore, Prs is equal to the translung pressure (P_L). This gives us a second point on the P-V curve of the total respiratory system. Now study Figure 5-8, which shows the complete pressure-volume curve for the respiratory system (dashed line), in addition to those of the lung and chest wall. Figure 5-8 is the set of relaxation pressure-volume curves shown in every textbook of respiratory physiology.

The P-V curve for the respiratory system has a lower slope at every point than the corresponding curves for either the lung or the chest wall. This means that the compliance of the respiratory system (Crs) must be less than that of either the lung or the chest wall.

Let us use Figure 5-8 to compute the respiratory system compliance over the range FRC + 50% VC to FRC, that is, during deflation. The computation is as follows:

$$Crs = \Delta V/\Delta Prs = \frac{(3.6 - 2.4) \text{ liters}}{[(P_A - Pbs) - 0] \text{ cmH}_2\text{O}}$$

$$= \frac{1.2 \text{ liters}}{(7.2 - 0) \text{ cmH}_2\text{O}} = 0.17 \text{ liter/cmH}_2\text{O}$$

The compliance of the total respiratory system (Crs) is one-half that of either the lung or the chest wall. But one will not obtain the correct Crs by adding the compliances of the lung and the chest wall directly because distensibilities are considered to be in parallel. It is necessary

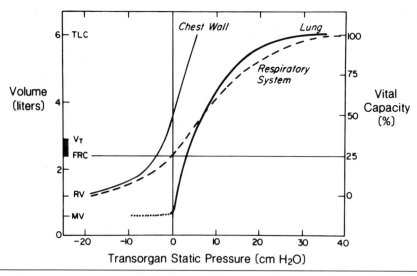

Fig. 5-8. The deflation pressure-volume curve of the respiratory system (dashed line) in addition to those of the chest wall and lung. The slope of the respiratory system line is less than that of either the chest wall or lung. At FRC, the respiratory system must be at equilibrium and the total trans-respiratory system pressure must be zero. At approximately 50% vital capacity, the chest wall is at its unstressed (resting) position; all the pressure needed to distend the respiratory system is expended across the lung.

to add reciprocals: $1/Crs = 1/C_L + 1/Cw$. Compliance is not the best way to consider distensibilities of units *in series*.

Elastance (E), defined as the resistance to distortion of a structure, greatly simplifies the comparison of the whole system to its parts because elastances of two or more series-coupled structures can be added directly; no reciprocals are involved. That is why many pulmonary physiologists prefer to use elastance instead of compliance. The elastance of the respiratory system (Ers) is measured by adding the elastances of the lung (E_L) and chest wall (Ew) together.

$$Ers = E_L + Ew = \frac{1}{0.34} + \frac{1}{0.32} \ cmH_2O/liter$$

$$= (2.94 + 3.12) = 6.1 \ cmH_2O/liter$$

$$Crs = 1/Ers = 1/6.1 = 0.16 \ liter/cmH_2O$$

In disease, there may be profound changes in the distensibility of the various components of the respiratory system, individually or together. For example, the lungs may become very stiff due to fibrotic changes or they may become very flaccid due to destruction of their elastic fibrils (emphysema). The chest wall may be distorted by congenital malformations or by diseases that produce stiffening (kyphoscoliosis, abdominal distension, extreme obesity).

READINGS

Books

1. Bates DV, Macklem PT, Christie RV: Respiratory Function in Disease. 2nd Ed. WB Saunders, Philadelphia, 1971
   Excellent human lung data succinctly summarized.

2. Comroe JH Jr: Premature Science and Immature Lungs. Parts I–III. pp. 140–182. Retro-spectroscope, Von Gehr Press, Menlo Park, CA, 1977
   A delightfully written history of how lung surfactant was discovered and of its relationship to lung disease.
3. Murray JF: The Normal Lung. 2nd Ed. WB Saunders, Philadelphia, 1986
   A useful compilation of information relevant to human lung function. Chapter 4 reviews static lung mechanics, and Chapter 14 is about aging.
4. Weiss L: Histology: Cell and Tissue Biology. 5th Ed. pp. 788–868. Elsevier Biomedical, New York, 1983
   A standard modern textbook of histology; contains a description of the alveolar type 2 cell.

Reviews

5. Clements JA: Surface phenomena in relation to pulmonary function. Physiologist 5:11–28, 1962
   Summary of early work on the physicochemical properties of surfactant.
6. Mead J: Mechanical properties of lungs. Physiol Rev 41:281–330, 1961
   A detailed review of all aspects of lung, but not chest wall, mechanics.
7. Pattle RE: Properties, function and origin of the alveolar lining layer. Nature 175:1125–1126, 1955
   The first report of very low alveolar surface tension in bubbles of edema foam obtained from rabbit lungs.
8. Rahn H, Otis AB, Chadwick LE, Fenn WO: The pressure volume diagram of the thorax and lung. J Appl Physiol 146:161–178, 1946
   The classic description of the deflation pressure-volume curves of the lungs and chest wall.

QUESTIONS*

Drill

1. Calculate the missing values and state the significance of the data in each subquestion. Data are given in cmH_2O/liter for elastance and liters/cmH_2O for compliance.
   a. $C_L = 0.3$; $Cw = 0.1$; $Crs = ?$
   b. $Crs = 0.04$; $Cw = 0.05$; $C_L = ?$
   c. $Ers = 10$; $E_L = 5$; $Ew = ?$
   d. $Ers = ?$; $C_L = 0.05$; $Cw = 0.1$
   e. $C_L = ?$; $Ew = 5$; $Ers = 7$

Problems

2. (a) At a depth of 100 m (328 feet), what is the pressure at the airway opening necessary to maintain the normal FRC of a skin diver? (b) What is the transdiaphragm-abdominal wall pressure at normal FRC? (c) Suppose the pressure at the airway opening suddenly dropped to zero. Describe (in words) some of the immediate sequelae affecting air-containing cavities such as the lungs and chest wall.

3. A person has a lung compliance of 0.15 liters/cmH_2O over the range 50% VC to FRC (average volume during the measurement is 1.7 liters). State how you would determine whether the static mechanical properties of the lungs are normal. How might the reduced compliance be explained?

4. In clinical pulmonary edema due to lung injury by a toxic substance, plasma proteins may enter the alveoli and inactivate the surfactant material. This fixes alveolar surface tension at a constant value of 50 dynes/cm. (a) On the copy of Figure 5-4 below, draw the deflation limb of the air pressure-volume curve, assuming the normal TLC point is not displaced. (b) Draw the inflation limb of the air pressure-volume curve. (c) Is the pressure-volume hysteresis more or less than normal? Why? (d) What changes occur in the liquid-filled pressure-volume curve?

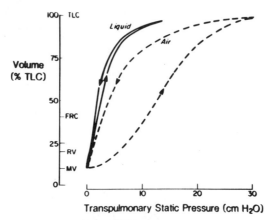

5. When evaluating problems in lung mechanics, it is usually helpful to make a simple model and add the appropriate conditions, parameters, and variables. The figure below suffices for most situations.
   In the "old days" (1940s to 1950s), when poliomyelitis epidemics were common, thousands

---

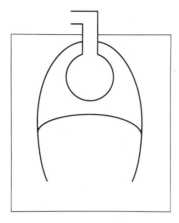

of patients with paralyzed respiratory muscles were sustained in "iron lungs." The principle of the iron lung is simple: passively ventilate the lungs and thorax by changing the pressure around the body (Pbs). Suppose we are able to measure all necessary parameters and variables in a paralyzed subject in an iron lung. Assume that chest wall and lung compliances are linear and equal to 0.2 liter/cmH$_2$O over the range of minimal volume to 70% VC, and minimal volume = 1 liter, FRC = 2 liters, and 50% VC = 3 liters. (a) What is Crs over the range FRC to 50% VC? (b) What is Ppl at FRC? (c) When the iron lung pressure = −10 cmH$_2$O and the breathing apparatus is static (Pao − P$_A$ = 0), what is lung volume? (d) For the conditions in (c), what is transdiaphragm-abdominal wall pressure? (e) If, from the condition in (c), the airway opening is temporarily occluded by a pressure-measuring device and iron lung pressure is returned to zero, what is P$_A$? (f) For the condition described in (e), what is Ppl?

6. Assume for simplicity that the shape of the diaphragm is a portion of a sphere with a 15-cm radius of curvature. In a supine person at FRC, the abdominal pressure just under the diaphragm equals P$_B$ and pleural pressure equals −4 cmH$_2$O. The passive tension in the diaphragm (dynes/cm) is about:

    a. 40   b. 7,000   c. 22,000   d. 29,000   e. 59,000

7. Aging affects the elastance of the lung. The static translung pressure at 60% TLC varies as a function of age, as shown in the figure below. The translung pressure at age 56 is

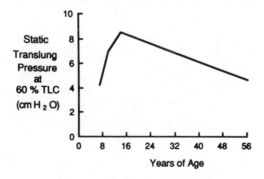

one-half that at age 16. (a) What is the most likely cause of such a change? (b) If chest wall elastance decreased with age in a parallel fashion to lung elastance, how would that affect your answer in (a)?

Use the normal deflation pressure-volume curve of the lung and the numbered points shown below to answer Questions 8 and 9.

8. Which point represents the FRC of a person with markedly reduced static lung recoil, such as may occur with destruction of lung parenchyma in chronic obstructive pulmonary disease (emphysema)?

    a. 1   b. 2   c. 3   d. 4   e. 5

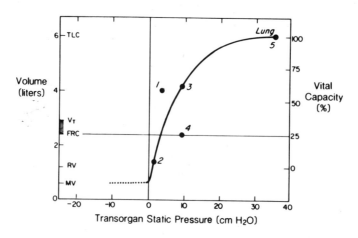

9. Which point probably represents the FRC of a hospitalized teenager with severe hyper-reactivity of the airways (asthma) with overinflated lungs due to expiratory airway obstruction but without any lung tissue destruction?

    a. 1   b. 2   c. 3   d. 4   e. 5

10. The P-V curve for the air-filled lung shown below is a copy of Figure 3-4. Locate the point at normal FRC when breathing at normal V_T for a long time (20 minutes). Explain why you located the point there.

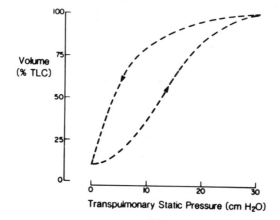

Mechanical Properties in Breathing: Dynamics

THE BOTTOM LINE

Dynamic Lung Compliance

The dynamic compliance of the lung is about 0.2 liter/cmH$_2$O, which is less than the static compliance, due mainly to a rise in air-liquid surface tension toward its equilibrium value during tidal breathing. An occasional large sighing breath restores the surfactant and increases compliance.

Dynamic Chest Wall Compliance

Dynamic chest wall compliance is the same as its static compliance.

Active Pressure-Volume Curve of the Chest Wall

The active pressure-volume curve of the chest wall is the mirror image of the lung pressure-volume curve. The difference is explained by the contraction of the muscles of breathing. One cannot compute the compliance of the chest wall during active breathing.

Resistance to Airflow

During breathing, the pressure difference across the lung includes both elastic and resistive components. The translung pressure due to static lung elastic recoil, P$_A$ − Ppl, must be added to the pressure due to airflow resistance, Pao − P$_A$, so that P$_L$ = Pao − Ppl. Alveolar pressure equals ambient pressure only at end inspiration and end expiration (points of no airflow).

Measurement of Airway Resistance

Airway resistance (Raw) equals (Pao − P$_A$)/V̇. As in blood vessels, the main factor regulating airflow resistance is the radius raised to the fourth power, r^4. Turbulence, which occurs even in quiet breathing, adds an additional pressure drop. In normal

(Continues).

(Continued).
humans, the total driving pressure ΔP due to airflow resistance is given by $\Delta P = 2.4 \times \dot{V} + 0.03\dot{V}^2$. The last term, which accounts for turbulence, increases rapidly as airflow rate increases. Breath sounds are due to turbulence in the upper airways. During tidal breathing, peak airflow is about 0.5 liter/sec. An important *physical factor* affecting airway resistance is the transmural pressure, especially of the larger intrathoracic airways (bronchi), because the walls of these vessels are distensible and collapsible. In normal breathing, the transmural pressure is always positive (distending), but in a forced expiratory maneuver pleural pressure may rise above large airway pressure and cause airway narrowing. This is called **dynamic compression** and limits peak expiratory flow velocity. It is effort independent. The *flow-volume relationship* is another way to represent breathing dynamics. It clearly shows expiratory flow limitation during a forced vital capacity maneuver.

Neurohumoral Regulation of Airway Resistance
Airway resistance is regulated via the autonomic nervous system. The vagus nerve (parasympathetic) is the main motor nerve, whereas sympathetic (adrenergic) nerve stimulation inhibits airway smooth muscle contraction. $P_{A_{CO_2}}$ has local effects. A number of biologic amines (histamine, acetylcholine, thromboxane, leukotrienes, substance P) cause airway constriction. β-Adrenergic agonists and atropine lead to dilation.

Work and Power of Breathing
The work of breathing for one breath at rest is small (0.25 joule), and the power requirement is 0.05 watt (0.05 joule/sec). Normally, the oxygen cost of quiet tidal breathing is <2% of oxygen consumption. In pulmonary disease, the power requirement may be increased to such an extent that respiratory muscle fatigue develops and respiratory failure occurs (increased $P_{A_{CO_2}}$).

While the static properties of the lungs and thorax are important to the understanding of lung and thoracic distensibility, the concept of statics requires the assumption of an equilibrium, a condition not likely to be achieved in life, because breathing at the normal resting rate of 12 breaths per minute allows only 2 seconds for inspiration and 3 seconds for expiration. Indeed, the special maneuver used to measure static translung (elastic recoil) pressure (Fig. 5-1), namely, a large inspiration to total lung capacity, followed by very slow deflation to the desired translung pressure or volume, should be sufficient to warn one that normal breathing may not give the same result.

DYNAMIC LUNG COMPLIANCE

As we breathe normally, we do not go to TLC but cycle over the range FRC to FRC + V_T. Figure 6-1 shows the normal dynamic tidal volume loop added to the pressure-volume curve from Figure 5-4. The tidal volume loop is located approximately in the center of the static P-V loop.

In Figure 6-1 at FRC during quiet breathing, the translung static pressure is approximately 5 cmH$_2$O, not 3.5 cmH$_2$O as in Figure 5-4. A normal 0.5-liter tidal volume increases lung volume to approximately 50% of TLC, at which point the translung pressure is 7.5 cmH$_2$O.

The tidal inspiration and expiration curves show only a little hysteresis, and that is due mainly to frictional energy losses (airflow resistance), not to changes in surface tension, which are very small because of the slight change in alveolar surface area. The average compliance of the lung

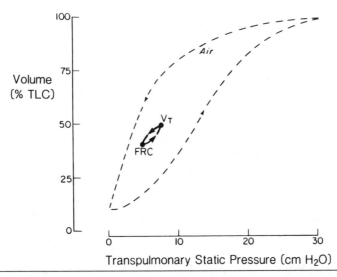

Fig. 6-1.   The normal dynamic pressure-volume loop during tidal breathing added to the normal static air pressure-volume curve. Dynamic compliance is calculated as the slope of the straight line ($\Delta V/\Delta P$) drawn between the points of no flow, namely, FRC and FRC + V_T. Dynamic compliance is less than static compliance even in normal individuals.

during tidal ventilation (or at any ventilation up to vital capacity) can be calculated as the slope of the line joining the end-inspiratory and end-expiratory points (no flow). The compliance calculated this way during breathing is called the **dynamic** compliance (dynC_L):

$$dynC_L = \frac{\Delta V}{\Delta P} = \frac{V_{FRC+VT} - V_{FRC}}{P_{L_{FRC+VT}} - P_{L_{FRC}}}$$

$$= \frac{(2.9 - 2.4) \text{ liter}}{(7.5 - 5.0) \text{ cmH}_2\text{O}} = \frac{0.5 \text{ liter}}{2.5 \text{ cmH}_2\text{O}}$$

$$= 0.2 \text{ liter/cmH}_2\text{O}$$

It is obvious from Figure 6-1 that the average dynamic compliance during breathing is less than the static compliance measured from the deflation limb of the pressure-volume curve. Lung compliance (elastance) is sensitive to the previous state of the lung (volume history). In Appendix 2, I used a dynamic compliance of 0.2 liter/cmH$_2$O for the resting condition but used static compliance (0.34 liter/cmH$_2$O) for exercise, in which tidal volume is much larger (one-half vital capacity).

Why is dynamic compliance less than static compliance? It is because the small change in alveolar surface area associated with tidal breathing is inadequate to bring new surfactant molecules into the air-liquid interface as old molecules are depleted. Thus, a relative deficiency of surfactant develops, and surface tension rises toward its equilibrium value (28 dynes/cm at 37°C). In other words, the recoil of the lung (elastance) increases with time as surface tension rises. A single large lung inflation (sigh or yawn) suffices to restore the normal surfactant layer. This is a normal event, which occurs every few minutes in healthy people. In addition, with all our other ventilatory activities (coughing, sneezing, talking, etc.), tidal volume is not constant. If one continued constant tidal breathing indefinitely, the lungs would become stiffer and increasingly difficult to ventilate, and some alveoli would collapse (microatelectasis). Fortunately, the gradually stiffening lung is detected by neural receptors (deflation receptors) in the lungs and in the chest wall. When activated, these receptors drive the central breathing controller in the brain (Fig. 1-2) to increase V_T to restore the normal, steady-state condition.

DYNAMIC CHEST WALL COMPLIANCE

Since surface tension does not affect the thoracic cage directly, the dynamic compliance of the chest wall is no different from its static compliance. Clearly, however, if the translung (or transpulmonary) pressure (P_L) at FRC during tidal breathing is 5 cmH$_2$O, then pleural pressure must be -5 cmH$_2$O. That is incompatible with the FRC as shown in Figure 5-7. But that figure shows only the *static* lung P-V curve. One must use the *dynamic* tidal volume curve from Figure 6-1. What happens is that FRC decreases until the transchest wall pressure (Pw) equals -5 cmH$_2$O, which is sufficient to balance the new translung pressure. Fortunately, the slope of the chest wall P-V curve decreases rapidly at that volume, so FRC only decreases a little.

> **Remember:**   At FRC the lungs and chest wall are recoiling equally but in opposite directions. The pressure difference across the respiratory system (Prs) must equal zero.

THE ACTIVE PRESSURE-VOLUME CURVE OF THE CHEST WALL

There is one further complication that must be mentioned briefly. The chest wall has an active pressure-volume curve. When we contract our muscles of breathing, the transchest wall pressure (Pw) becomes more negative (not positive) as the lung is expanded. In fact, the active pressure-volume curve of the chest wall during normal breathing is the *mirror image* of the passive pressure-volume curve of the lung, as shown in Figure 6-2. It must be so because alveolar pressure and body surface pressure both equal zero, if there is no airflow. Thus, the pressure-volume curve of the whole respiratory system is a vertical line at Prs = 0 in Figure 6-2; that is, the respiratory system has infinite compliance (zero elastance) during active normal breathing.

The commonsense explanation of this apparent contradiction, of course, lies in the contraction of the muscles of breathing. Chest wall compliance is not considered as a factor in active breathing, and one must remember that compliance of the chest wall or the respiratory system cannot be computed under that condition.

RESISTANCE TO AIRFLOW

In Figure 6-1 the tidal breathing pressure-volume curve forms a small loop, not a straight line. That means that some of the work (pressure times change in volume) used to expand the lungs is not recovered during expiration. Whenever there is movement, inertia (acceleration of mass), and flow (velocity), resistance must be considered. Resistance causes frictional losses that are unrecoverable. Fortunately, the inertia of the respiratory system is very low, so we will ignore it. But airflow resistance cannot be ignored.

During breathing, the total pressure difference across the lung (P_L) is

$$P_L = P_{compliance} + P_{resistance} = (P_A - Ppl) + (Pao - P_A)$$
$$= Pao - Ppl$$

(6-1)

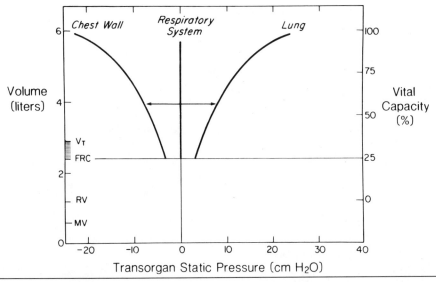

Fig. 6-2. The pressure-volume curve of the chest wall and respiratory system during active breathing is completely different from the passive curve (Fig. 5-8). The chest wall curve is the mirror image of the lung curve, which is always passive. At any point between FRC and near TLC, the static alveolar pressure is equal to body surface pressure. Thus, the curve for the respiratory system is a vertical line at Prs = 0, which makes the respiratory system appear to be infinitely distensible (compliant). This is not true, however, because the active tension in the muscles of breathing has not been included.

where Pao is the pressure at the airway opening (nose or mouth). When there is no airflow, Pao = P_A, which is why dynamic compliance must be computed only at end inspiration and end expiration. During airflow, Pao − P_A ≠ 0. The difference may be positive or negative depending on whether air is flowing into or out of the lung.

Physical Factors Determining Resistance to Airflow in Rigid Tubes

Resistance in the airways (Raw) is determined by the same factors that govern the flow of liquid through blood vessels, since air is a fluid of low viscosity. By analogy to the equation for pulmonary vascular resistance (Eq. 3-6), we can compute airway resistance as driving pressure (the pressure difference between airway opening and alveoli) divided by flow

$$Raw = \frac{Pao - P_A}{\dot{V}} \tag{6-2}$$

When airflow is laminar, we can describe resistance using Poiseuille's equation

$$Raw = \frac{8}{\pi} \times \eta \times \frac{1}{r^4} \tag{6-3}$$

I have arranged the factors in the order I believe is easiest to remember; namely, a constant $(8/\pi)$, viscosity (η), and geometry (length/radius^4).

Resistance is directly proportional to the viscosity, η, and airway length, l. Resistance is inversely proportional to the fourth power of the airway radius, r. In normal breathing, air viscosity does not vary and the length of the airway is almost constant. The main factor affecting airway resistance is the radius of the tubes, as for the vascular system. The term r^4 means that small changes in radius greatly affect airway resistance.

There is just one small difference between airflow and blood flow. Even in quiet breathing airflow is *turbulent* (chaotic) in the upper airways (nose, mouth, glottis, trachea, cartilaginous bronchi), which increases the resistance to airflow. Thus, the driving pressure for airflow (ΔP) is more than is predicted from the Poiseuille equation and Eq. 6-2

$$\Delta P = \text{Pao} - \text{P}_A = 2.4 \times \dot{V} + 0.03 \times \dot{V}^2 \qquad (6\text{-}4)$$

where the first term describes the pressure drop due to laminar flow and the second term describes the pressure drop due to turbulence (square of the velocity), which is greatest in the large upper airways. Turbulence increases as airflow rate ($\dot{V}$) increases. The factor 2.4 in the laminar flow term is normal expiratory airway resistance, and the factor 0.03 in the second term means that turbulence causes little extra pressure until $\dot{V}^2$ becomes large.

The clearest evidence for turbulence in breathing is the sounds one hears over the chest during breathing. Laminar flow is silent.

Airflow resistances in series are additive. Pulmonary physiologists and chest physicians usually limit the separation of longitudinal resistance distribution to the upper airways (nasopharynx and large airways [bronchi of >2 mm diameter]) and small airways (<2 mm diameter). Normally, 70 to 80% of total airway resistance (Raw) is in the large airways. In clinical pulmonary function testing, airway resistance refers to the resistance measured while breathing through the mouth. It includes resistance in the mouth, throat (glottis), and cartilaginous and membranous airways.

$$\text{Raw} = \text{R}_{\text{large airways}} + \text{R}_{\text{small airways}}$$

Small airway resistance is low because flow is laminar and its velocity is very low. You will recall from Chapter 2 that the airways branch in a manner described as irregular dichotomy. The "child" branches have a total cross section larger than the "parent" airway, and the "child/parent" ratio increases rapidly in the smallest airways beyond the terminal bronchioles, where the radius of the successive branches is nearly constant. Also, the small airways, although narrow (respiratory bronchioles and alveolar ducts are about 0.25 mm in radius), are exceedingly numerous. Resistances of tubes in parallel are added reciprocally

$$\frac{1}{R} = \frac{1}{R_1} + \frac{1}{R_2} + \cdots + \frac{1}{R_n}$$

where n represents the number of parallel airways of a given radius. For example, the huge number ($n = 30,000$) of terminal bronchioles makes their equivalent resistance very low even though r is only 0.03 cm (300 μm).

In disease conditions, the longitudinal distribution of airway resistance may vary markedly. For example, in a disease known as bronchiolitis (inflamed bronchioles) in infants, swelling (edema) of the mucosa of the bronchioles may drastically reduce their radii. A reduction by one-half increases their contribution to resistance 16-fold because of the fourth power factor ($2^4 = 16$) in Poiseuille's equation (Eq. 6-3). Thus, even if normal small airway resistance is only 20% of total resistance, that portion is increased to

$$\text{Raw} = 80\% + 16 \times (20\%) = 400\%$$

Total airway resistance (Raw) is quadrupled.

MEASUREMENT OF AIRWAY RESISTANCE

The partitioning of longitudinal resistance between large and small airways is beyond the scope of this book. From now on, we will only consider total airway resistance (Raw) as described by Eq. 6-2.

To do this, one must measure two variables: alveolar pressure (PA) and airflow velocity ($\dot{V}$). There are a number of ways to measure airflow continuously. The modern procedure is to use a device known as a pneumotachograph, which measures the very small pressure difference required for flow across a low fixed resistance. The main problem in calculating airway resistance is to measure the alveolar pressure, which is the downstream pressure during inspiration and the upstream pressure during expiration. Since alveolar pressure is not the same as ambient pressure during airflow, methods had to be devised to estimate alveolar pressure.

One widely used method to estimate PA is to briefly occlude the airway opening. At the instant after airflow stops, Pao = PA. Do not be concerned about the procedure, just believe that PA during airflow can be measured.*

Figure 6-3 is a graph of volume, flow, and relevant pressures during one normal tidal breathing cycle. There are three points of no airflow—at the beginning of inspiration ($t = 0$), at the end of inspiration ($t = 2$ sec), and at the end of expiration ($t = 5$ sec) (same as the beginning of inspiration). At these three points, alveolar pressure equals atmospheric pressure. It is between these points of no airflow that physiologists compute dynamic compliance.

In terms of airflow resistance, the important features of Figure 6-3 are that airflow reaches a peak velocity of $+0.5$ liter/sec during inspiration and of -0.5 liter/sec during expiration (the minus sign means flow out of the lung) and that alveolar pressure decreases below the pressure at the airway opening by 0.8 cmH$_2$O at peak airflow during inspiration and exceeds the pressure at the airway opening by 1.2 cmH$_2$O at peak airflow during expiration. A little later, I will explain why the driving pressure is less during inspiration.

The total pressure difference from ambient to pleural space during airflow is the pressure difference due to lung distensibility (dynamic compliance) plus the pressure difference due to airflow resistance. The sum of these pressures gives PL in Eq. 6-1. The complex solid line on the segment of the graph for pleural pressure in Figure 6-3 was obtained by assuming a linear change in PL generated by constant dynamic compliance (dashed line) and adding to it the resistive pressure difference (Pao − PA) from the alveolar pressure curve above.

Common sense tells us that PL must be increased during airflow into the lung and be reduced during airflow out of the lung, and that is exactly what is shown by the solid pleural pressure line in Figure 6-3.

Using Eq. 6-2, we can compute airway resistance at any point during the breathing cycle by dividing alveolar pressure by airflow velocity ($\dot{V}$). In Figure 6-3, if we do that at peak velocity during inspiration, we obtain the following:

$$\text{Raw, I} = \frac{\Delta P}{\dot{V}} = \frac{\text{Pao} - \text{PA}}{\dot{V}} = \frac{[0 - (-0.8)] \text{ cmH}_2\text{O}}{0.5 \text{ liter/sec}}$$

$$= \frac{1.6 \text{ cmH}_2\text{O} \times \text{sec}}{\text{liter}}$$

---

* The method has some additional complications, including delayed relaxation of elastic and collagen tissue fibrils and surface stresses, which slowly change alveolar pressure, but the PA − Pao as measured by the airway occlusion technique is the true airway resistive driving pressure.

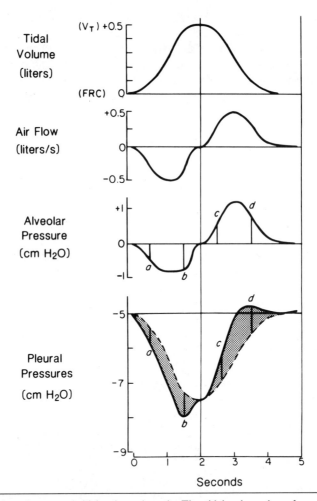

Fig. 6-3.   Dynamics of a normal tidal volume breath. The tidal volume loop from Figure 6-1 is spread out over 5 seconds (12 breaths/min). The inspiratory time, 2 seconds, is shorter than the expiratory time, 3 seconds. In part, this is because airflow resistance is higher during expiration, as indicated by the fact that the maximal alveolar pressure deflection is only 0.8 cmH$_2$O during inspiration but is 1.2 cmH$_2$O during expiration, even though peak airflow is 0.5 liter/sec in each phase. The dashed line in the pleural pressure graph (bottom) represents the pressure necessary to overcome lung elastance. It is essentially the mirror image of the tidal volume curve (top). The alveolar pressure curve (second from bottom) is in phase with the airflow curve (third from bottom). When the alveolar pressure swing due to airflow is added to the elastic recoil pressure, one obtains the complex curve shown by the heavy solid line in the bottom graph. It may not be obvious to the eye, when adding rapidly changing pressures, how the curve should look. Therefore, line segments a, b, c, and d show four examples in which the resistive pressure has been added to the elastic pressure. The shaded area during inspiration is less than the area during expiration because the work to overcome airflow resistance is less.

Likewise, during expiration

$$\text{Raw, E} = \frac{\Delta P}{\dot{V}} = \frac{(0 - 1.2) \text{ cmH}_2\text{O}}{-0.5 \text{ liter/sec}}$$

$$= \frac{2.4 \text{ cmH}_2\text{O} \times \text{sec}}{\text{liter}}$$

These are in the normal range for adult humans, namely, 1.5 to 2.5 cmH$_2$O × sec/liter (Appendix 2). The signs of the airflow and the alveolar pressure difference are always the same, so resistance is a positive number.

Other Factors in Lung Resistance to Movement

In addition to airway resistance, there is tissue resistance to movement (inertia), which is normally dissipated over a few seconds (stress relaxation), and to a phenomenon known as *pendelluft* ("swinging air," like the pendulum on a clock), which is due to air moving back and forth among terminal respiratory units that are inflating and deflating at slightly different rates because of different time constants (R × C), which are discussed in Chapter 8.

Normally, these extra "resistive" effects are small (<20% of Raw) but in disease states they may become large. If one uses the total resistive driving pressure to compute resistance, the result is called **total pulmonary resistance** (RT). For the remainder of this chapter, I will ignore lung tissue resistance.

Resistance to airflow is affected by lung volume. In Chapter 3, I mentioned that dead space volume (VD) increased as lung volume increased. Since the dead space volume is altered principally by a change in airway radius, there is an inverse relationship between dead space volume and airway resistance. Airway resistance decreases as lung volume increases toward total lung capacity and increases as lung volume decreases toward residual volume.

Physical Factors Influencing Airway Resistance

In rigid cylindrical tubes, resistance during laminar flow is fixed because the physical dimensions of the tube never change, regardless of the transmural pressure difference across the tube walls. But if the tube is distensible and collapsible, then the transmural pressure may have important nonlinear effects. This concept should not be new; it is identical to that which applies to blood vessels (as taught in cardiovascular physiology). This concept reoccurs in Chapter 7 on the pulmonary circulation.

Figure 6-4 represents flow in a nonrigid tube. In Figure 6-4A, the pressure in the tube always exceeds the external pressure. Therefore, the transmural pressure (Ptm) is positive (Ptm = P$_{\text{inside}}$ − P$_{\text{external}}$). As the tube expands, flow resistance decreases. Thus, flow is proportional not only to the driving pressure along the tube but also to the actual pressure inside the tube. In Figure 6-4B, the external pressure is raised above the outflow or downstream pressure. Thus, as flow resistance dissipates the driving pressure, the pressure inside the tube falls. When it falls below the external pressure, the transmural pressure becomes negative (compressive), and the tube begins to narrow. As Ptm becomes more negative, the tube is compressed more and more until a new stable condition is reached in which the collapsed zone (always at the outflow end of the uniform tube) limits the flow rate. The regulation of flow in this manner is called *dynamic compression*, which is a variant of the "Starling resistor."* Under

---

* Ernest Starling, the early twentieth century English physiologist (law of the heart; law of the intestine; Starling's hypothesis), popularized the use of a collapsible tube resistor in his heart-lung preparation. Perhaps the simplest everyday application of the collapsible tube principle is the blood pressure cuff, which by external compression collapses a suitable artery.

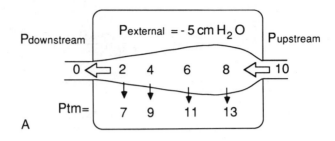

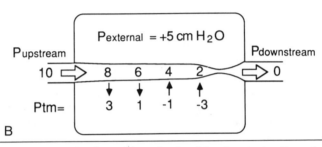

Fig. 6-4. Pressure and diameter of a distensible and collapsible tube passing through a closed chamber in which the external pressure on the tube can vary. **(A)** Flow is from right to left and $P_{external} = -5$ cmH$_2$O. The tube is distended due to the positive (distending) transmural pressure (Ptm). **(B)** Flow is from left to right and $P_{external} = +5$ cmH$_2$O. The transmural pressure decreases until it becomes negative (compression). The tube collapses near the outflow end of the chamber.

such conditions, airflow is independent of the total driving pressure (Pao − P$_A$). The real airways are more complicated than the model in Figure 6-4 because they are not uniformly distensible and collapsible. Nevertheless, the principle of dynamic compression holds.

Transmural Pressure Across the Airways
Transmural pressure across the airways varies at different airway levels. In the neck, the external pressure on the trachea is atmospheric pressure, whereas inside the thorax (mediastinum) the pressure outside the trachea and main stem bronchi is pleural pressure. Inside the lung, the transmural pressure of the cartilaginous airways is a pressure proportional to pleural pressure, but for the bronchioles, which are attached directly to the respiratory tissue, there is no transmural pressure difference. Recall that this is one of the important functional distinctions between bronchi and bronchioles (see Ch. 2). Bronchiolar radius is a function of lung volume because of the radial tension of lung connective tissue fibers on the airways.

During inspiration, as pleural pressure decreases and lung volume increases, all the airways expand. The main phases of a normal inspiration are diagrammed in Figure 6-5 (left-hand column). During airflow, transpulmonary pressure (P$_L$) is equal to the sum of the dynamic elastic recoil pressure and the pressure difference between the airway opening and the alveoli, which is dependent on airflow resistance. By studying the models in Figure 6-5, which show FRC, early inspiration, the midpoint of inspiration, and end inspiration, it can be seen that the transmural pressure across the intrathoracic airways is always positive.

Similar phases during expiration are also shown in Figure 6-5 (right-hand column). Pleural pressure rises to increase alveolar pressure above the pressure at the airway opening. However,

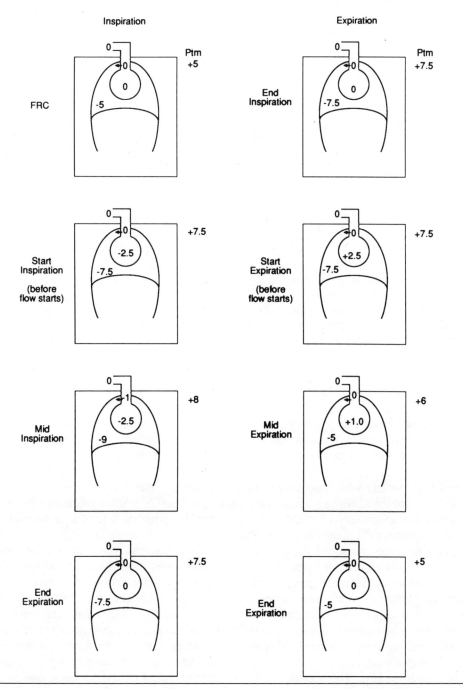

Fig. 6-5. Series of respiratory system models demonstrating changes in airway transmural pressure (Ptm) during tidal volume breathing under normal resting conditions. Ptm is shown at each stage of the breathing cycle. Ptm increases during inspiration (left-hand column) and decreases during expiration (right-hand column). Since pleural pressure never rises above ambient pressure (Pao), Ptm is always positive (distending). There is no airway collapse during expiration.

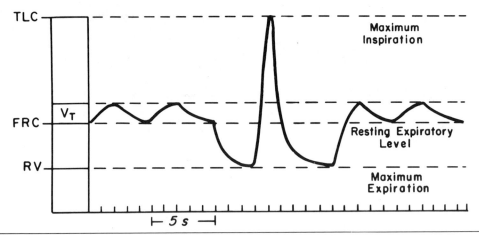

Fig. 6-6.   Spirogram (volume versus time) of a forced vital capacity maneuver. Compare this figure with the spirogram in Figure 5-3. After expiration to RV, there is a rapid inspiration to TLC. The time required is less than 1.5 seconds. When the forced expiration begins, 80% of the vital capacity is expelled in the first second and all of it is expelled in 3 seconds. If the normal vital capacity is 4.8 liters and is achieved in 1.5 seconds, then the average inspiratory flow rate is 3.2 liters/sec. During expiration, the mean airflow is only 1.6 liters/sec, which gives some idea of the dynamic compression of the airways and the increase in expiratory airflow resistance that occurs when pleural pressure becomes positive relative to airway pressure.

the pleural pressure never exceeds the pressure at the airway opening in normal quiet breathing. Therefore, although transmural pressure decreases, it is never negative (compressive). The airways narrow during expiration, which explains why airway resistance is higher during expiration. The small airways are less sensitive to the phases of breathing because in normal tidal breathing, the change in lung volume is small ($<20\%$), so the radii of the small airways remain nearly constant.

Now let us consider what happens when a normal person takes a very large inspiration from FRC to TLC and then breathes out as hard and fast as possible (maximum expiratory flow) by contracting the abdominal and chest wall muscles.* A spirogram tracing of a **forced vital capacity maneuver** is shown in Figure 6-6.

During inspiration, as shown in Figure 6-7 (left-hand column), the transmural distending pressure is always positive. In early expiration (Fig. 6-7, right-hand column), however, pleural pressure rises to a high level to generate the large driving pressure necessary for forced airflow. This raises pleural pressure above atmospheric pressure (pressure at the airway opening). Thus, as airflow begins, there is compression of the intrathoracic airways. This further increases flow velocity at the site of narrowing, which reduces the lateral pressure, according to the Bernoulli principle (venturi effect). This limits expiratory airflow. The dynamic compression reaches a stable condition, such that no matter how hard one tries, one cannot increase the rate of expiratory flow. The reason is that any further rise in pleural pressure causes more airway compression, which opposes the increase in flow. This generates a maximum expiratory flow rate that is *independent of effort*. One cannot generate a flow rate independent of effort

---

* The diaphragm cannot assist expiration. It is purely an inspiratory muscle. During a forced expiration, the anterior abdominal wall muscles are active, in addition to the intercostal muscles.

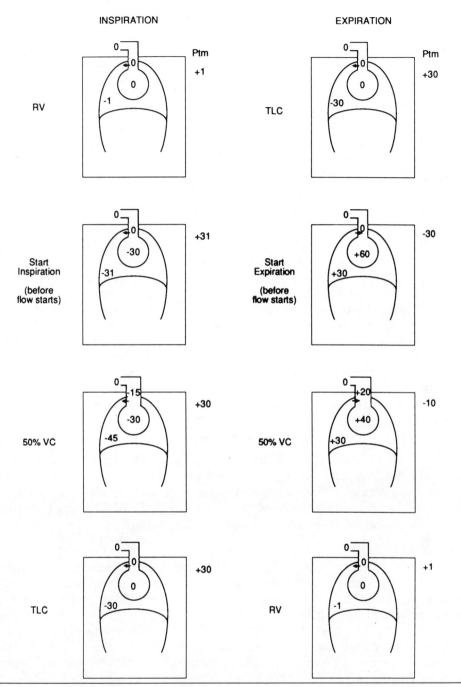

INSPIRATION

EXPIRATION

Fig. 6-7. Series of respiratory system models to demonstrate transmural pressure (Ptm) across the main bronchi during a forced (maximal effort) vital capacity maneuver in a normal individual. The forced vital capacity begins at residual volume (RV), where Ptm is approximately 1 cmH$_2$O (left-hand column). Ptm is large and positive during inspiration. The airways are passively dilated. During forced expiration (read right-hand column from top down), pleural pressure becomes positive, and soon after airflow begins, Ptm becomes negative (compression).

during inspiration, since the airways are distended and not compressed. The only limitation to the velocity of inspiratory airflow is the length-tension characteristics of the muscles of breathing.

Coughing

Coughing is a naturally occurring example of expiratory dynamic airway compression. Coughing involves a rapid inspiration, followed by closure of the glottis. One then rapidly raises pleural and alveolar pressures by contraction of the abdominal and internal intercostal muscles. The glottis is partially opened. There is a sudden fall in tracheal pressure to atmospheric pressure, causing rapid acceleration of gas out of the lung. The strongly compressive transmural pressure, coupled with the decreased lateral pressure in the airways, causes the main stem bronchi to collapse at their weakest point. This further increases local flow velocity. The high flow velocity moves irritating debris from the upper airways, particularly the glottis, trachea, and main stem bronchi.

Chronic Obstructive Pulmonary Disease

People with the degenerative lung disease called emphysema (chronic obstructive pulmonary disease) have lost lung elastic recoil. The transpulmonary pressure at any lung volume is reduced, so that pleural pressure at the end of a normal inspiration is closer to atmospheric pressure than in a normal individual. In addition, the airways are often flaccid, particularly the main bronchi and trachea. During expiration, to generate sufficient airflow in a reasonable period of time so that minute alveolar ventilation is adequate, the individual increases expiratory airflow. The elevated pleural pressure may compress the large airways, thus adding to the expiratory resistance. Emphysematous patients learn to inspire quickly and breathe out slowly to avoid airway collapse. In addition, some purse their lips, thereby generating expiratory flow limitation at the mouth, which maintains a positive distending pressure across the airways. As chronic obstructive pulmonary disease becomes more severe, the afflicted patient can generate less and less maximal expiratory flow.

Airway Hyperirritability

A person with hyperirritable airway disease (asthma) has a different problem. In asthma, the airways are narrowed by smooth muscle contraction, mucosal edema, and excessive secretions. Thus, both inspiratory and expiratory flow resistances increase. However, the patient with asthma breathes at an increased FRC and has normal lung elastance. This acts to distend the airways during inspiration and limits compression during expiration.

Flow-Volume Relationship

If we take the spirometer tracings of tidal and forced inspiratory and expiratory flow shown in Figure 6-6 and make them into closed loops by connecting the end of maximum expiration back to the beginning of inspiration, and then plot flow velocity against the lung volume at each point along the breathing loop, we generate a **flow-volume curve**. Figure 6-8 shows some flow-volume curves. In Figure 6-8A, the small loop (FRC) is the flow-volume curve for a normal tidal breath. It is reminiscent of the tidal breathing loop in Figure 6-1, but here airflow velocity (not translung pressure) has been plotted against volume. The peak inspiratory and expiratory flows achieved during tidal breathing are about 0.5 liter/sec, as already indicated.

Figure 6-8A also shows a complete *maximal* flow-volume curve (large loop). Inspiratory flow is not limited except by effort, that is, how hard one tries. But the expiratory flow curve is the maximal flow that can be achieved no matter how much effort is made. The expiratory flow limitation allows one to assess dynamic airway compression. Figure 6-8B shows several normal flow-volume loops made at different lung volumes or at different expiratory flow velocities. Notice that all the loops eventually achieve the same expiratory slope.

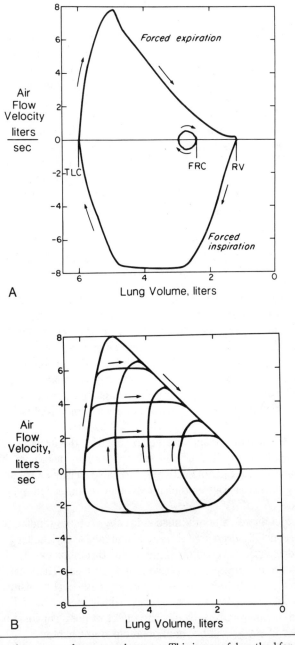

A

B

Fig. 6-8. (**A**) Flow-volume curve for a normal person. This is a useful method for showing the relationship between lung volume (x-axis) and airflow velocity (y-axis). During tidal breathing (small loop labeled FRC) the velocity of airflow in inspiration and expiration reaches 0.5 liter/sec. During the forced vital capacity maneuver (large loop), inspiratory flow velocity reaches almost 8 liters/sec. During expiration, airflow velocity rises rapidly to a maximum before lung volume has changed much. Then airflow velocity decreases steadily as volume decreases to RV. Peak inspiratory flow may exceed peak expiratory flow and is maintained over a larger change in lung volume, since the airways are distended, not compressed. (**B**) Stylized set of flow-volume curves, which show that no matter at what volume the forced expiratory maneuver begins, expiratory flow cannot exceed the maximum value for that volume. The expiratory portion of the flow-volume curve is **effort independent** because of dynamic airway compression occurring as pleural pressure becomes positive relative to airway pressure.

One reason that inspiration cannot produce high flow velocity is that inspiratory effort decreases as the thorax enlarges. In other words, the strongest inspiratory effort occurs before the diaphragm and chest wall muscles have expanded the thoracic cavity. Even though the force available decreases, inspiratory flow tends to remain constant until near total lung capacity, at which point flow falls rapidly to zero.

During expiration the curve is entirely different. Contracting the powerful anterior abdominal muscles and the intercostal muscles generates a high flow velocity near TLC. Velocity decreases rapidly (approximately linearly) as volume decreases, but not because of decreasing muscular effort. Once the linear portion of the expiratory flow-volume curve is reached, it is **effort independent**. No matter how hard the subject tries, the maximum flow cannot be exceeded at the given volume. Dynamic compression of the airways (Starling resistor) limits expiratory flow, and this limitation increases at lower lung volumes. ˙

NEUROHUMORAL REGULATION OF AIRWAY RESISTANCE

The vagus nerve (parasympathetic, cholinergic) is the motor nerve to the smooth muscle of all the cartilaginous airways and possibly to the membranous bronchioles and alveolar ducts. Stimulation of the efferent vagal fibers, either reflexly or directly, leads to airway constriction, a decrease in anatomic dead space volume (V_D), and an increase in airway resistance (Raw).

Stimulation of the sympathetic (adrenergic) nerves has the opposite effect. In humans, sympathetic nerves to the lungs are believed to innervate only vascular smooth muscle, not airway smooth muscle. But diffusion of the sympathetic postganglionic neurotransmitter norepinephrine to nearby parasympathetic ganglia or directly to the airway smooth muscle inhibits airway constriction.

Some agents act reflexly via the vagus nerve to constrict the airways and to induce cough. Inhalation of smoke, dust, cold air, and irritant substances may also have this effect. Exercise-induced asthma is common among people with hyperirritable airways. One suggested mechanism is increased osmolality within airway epithelial cells due to increased evaporative losses from the airway-lining liquid.

Some substances affect airway smooth muscle directly. Agents tending to cause airway constriction in this manner include *decreased* $P_{A_{CO_2}}$, histamine, acetylcholine, some adrenergic α-receptor agonists,* adrenergic β-receptor antagonists, thromboxane A_2, leukotrienes C_4 and D_4, and substance P (one of a group of bioactive neuropeptides). Histaminelike compounds are sometimes used in provocative tests on patients who may have hypersensitive airways (asthma). Agents or effects tending to cause airway dilatation include *increased* $P_{A_{CO_2}}$, adrenergic β-receptor agonists, and atropine (which blocks the effect of postganglionic parasympathetic impulses). Only the effect of $P_{A_{CO_2}}$ will be mentioned again in Chapter 8.

In the normal lung, there is continuous modulation of airway muscle tone, presumably to provide a balance between airway resistance (Raw) and anatomic dead space (V_D) to maintain minimal work for each breath.

---

* The explanation of the apparent contradiction of the previous statement about adrenergic nerve stimulation is that direct action of mediators on cells with suitable receptors cannot automatically be equated with effects via selective nerve stimulation. Also, the local concentration may determine whether an adrenergic agent has mainly α or mainly β effects.

WORK AND POWER OF BREATHING

The work involved in taking a single breath has been defined as

$$W = P \times \Delta V$$

Work is measured in joules (pressure times volume) and **power** (the rate of doing work) is measured in watts (joules per second). Clearly, if tidal volume increases, more work is needed to inflate the lung and, if minute ventilation increases (increased volume flow per unit time), power utilization increases. The work of breathing and the power requirement of breathing are commonly used interchangeably, although work should be restricted to a single breathing cycle, whereas power should be used when time is a factor.

The work of breathing is commonly divided into two portions, namely, the work of moving the lungs and the work of moving the chest wall. Many diseases affect the work and power requirement of breathing.

The work of moving the chest wall cannot be assessed during active breathing for the same reason that the compliance of the chest wall cannot be measured: there is no simple way to assess the mechanical work done by the muscles of breathing on themselves. However, the ventilation of a person who is paralyzed either by disease or through a neuromuscular blocking drug can be maintained by a mechanical device. Under these conditions, the lungs, thorax, and gas are moved passively by the ventilator, so that the total work of breathing can be determined. From such measurements, the total work of a single breath at normal tidal volume is about 0.25 joule, of which one-half is expended in moving the lung.* The power requirement of breathing is approximately 50 mW [0.25 joules/breath × (1 breath/5 sec) = 0.05 joules/sec = 0.05 W].

In thinking about work and power, it may be difficult to obtain a sense of what the units mean. To get some idea of how little power is used in breathing, a dim 7-W night-light consumes about 150 times as much power as resting minute ventilation. On the other hand, riding a bicycle up a moderately steep hill may require 100 W of power (100 joules/sec).

As Figure 6-9 shows, one can equate the work done on the lung (only) during a single breath with the area bounded by FRC and FRC + V_T and the pressure axis. During inspiration (Fig. 6-9A), work is done to move the lung, whereas during expiration (Fig. 6-9B), work is done by the potential energy stored in the elastic recoil of the lung. The difference between the work (areas) in Figures 6-9A and B is due to the work necessary to overcome frictional (resistive) losses during inspiration. During expiration, there is actually more potential energy available to do work than is necessary to overcome resistance. This is shown in Figure 6-9C. Since in the steady state there can be no energy left over, the extra energy is used to pull the chest wall back to its resting configuration. Remember that during tidal breathing the chest wall is compressed below its unstressed volume and therefore loses potential energy during inspiration. In addition, some energy loss goes into the velocity of air leaving the airway opening.

During exercise, the work of each breath increases more rapidly than does tidal volume because airflow is more rapid, which increases turbulence. A 10-fold increase in airflow rate increases the turbulence factor by $\dot{V}$, namely, 100-fold.

There is a maneuver called the *maximum voluntary ventilation* during which an average person, trying to ventilate as much as possible, may move 160 liters/min. Reasonable values are 4 liters/breath × 40 breaths/min. The resistive driving pressure across the respiratory

---

* The work calculation is based on a tidal volume of 0.5 liter and a respiratory system compliance (Crs) of 0.1 liter/cmH$_2$O (1 joule = 10 liters × cmH$_2$O).

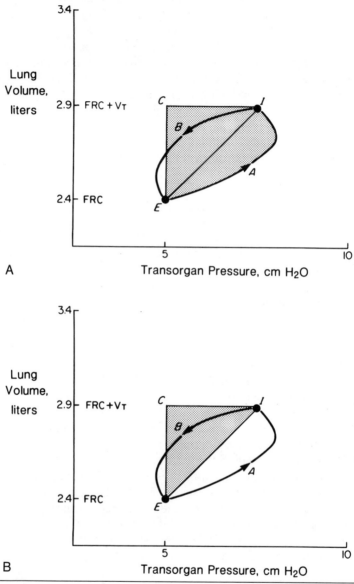

Fig. 6-9. Work of breathing done on the lungs (not the whole respiratory system) is shown for a normal tidal volume (this is an enlargement of the tidal volume loop of Figure 6-1). **(A)** Shaded area EAIC represents the total pressure-volume work needed to inflate the lungs. **(B)** Shaded area EIC represents the elastic potential energy (recoil force) stored in the lung at end inspiration. Sufficient energy must be stored during inspiration to complete expiration to FRC. The lost work, represented by the unshaded inspiratory portion of the loop, EAI, was used to overcome airway and tissue resistances and was dissipated as heat (friction) or breath sounds. (*Figure continues.*)

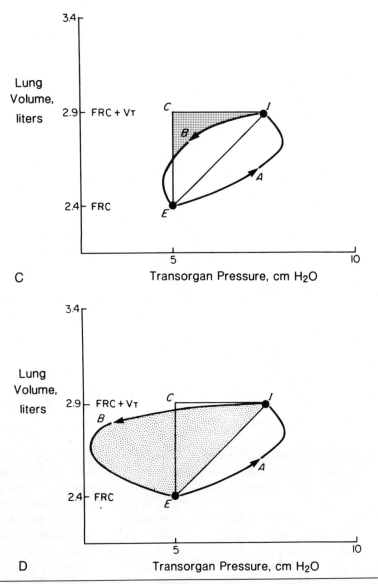

Fig. 6-9 (*Continued*). (**C**) Shaded area represents the excess work available during expiration over and above what is needed to overcome airflow resistance. It is the energy used to pull the chest wall back to its FRC position and to impart velocity to the expiratory gas as it leaves the airway opening. (**D**) Forced expiration coming after a normal inspiration. The shaded area EIB represents the total expiratory work done on the lungs. Obviously, there was not enough potential energy stored in the triangle EIC to permit such a rapid expiration. The expiratory muscles (abdominal and intercostal) had to be used to increase velocity for the forced exhalation. The extra work during expiration was required to overcome the increased resistive work and to add kinetic energy to the expired gas.

system may reach 20 cmH_2O. The power requirement is 5 W, almost enough to power that night-light.

During resting tidal breathing, the power requirement is so small that the oxygen cost of quiet breathing ($\dot{V}_{O_2}$ of the respiratory muscles) cannot be reliably measured. The increase in oxygen consumption associated with forced ventilation, however, has been measured and extrapolation made to the normal resting condition. The normal O_2 cost of breathing (O_2 consumption of the muscles of breathing) is 1 to 2% of resting oxygen consumption (3 to 5 ml O_2/min).

The mechanical efficiency of breathing is defined as

$$\text{Efficiency} = \frac{P \times \Delta V}{O_2 \text{ cost of breathing}} \tag{6-5}$$

The efficiency of the breathing apparatus is low (<10%) compared with that of skeletal muscle, the efficiency of which is about 15 to 20%.

In patients with diseases that increase lung elastance (reduced compliance) or increase airway resistance, the work of breathing may be markedly increased. Ordinarily, there is a large safety factor for the muscles of breathing, so that they are adequately supplied with oxygen and metabolic substrates to do their work indefinitely (aerobic metabolism). But muscle fatigue can occur when the elastic or resistive load is too great for the available blood supply.

Under such conditions *respiratory fatigue* occurs. This means the muscles of breathing are unable to ventilate the lungs adequately to supply the body's oxygen requirements. Thus, Pa_{CO_2} rises. Respiratory muscle fatigue can be corrected by reducing the work load (for example, by dilating the airways in a patient with asthma) or by mechanically assisting ventilation (for example, in a patient with emphysema complicated by bronchitis).

Although the normal oxygen cost of breathing is less than 2% of resting oxygen consumption, during voluntary hyperventilation up to 30% of oxygen consumption (0.30×250 ml O_2/min = 75 ml O_2/min) may be used just to move the lungs and chest wall. Obviously, in patients who are already expending more O_2 than normal to move air at rest, the oxygen cost of breathing may limit their exercise capability.

Although there is sufficient potential energy stored in the lungs and thorax during inspiration to restore the breathing apparatus to its FRC position (by the definition of the steady-state condition), if one makes a forced expiration, as in a forced vital capacity test, then the muscles of breathing are used to accelerate expiratory airflow and the work of expiration is increased (Fig. 6-9D). Active expiration also occurs in exercise because air must be moved quickly.

If the work of inspiration is increased owing to increased resistance to airflow, as in asthma, the potential energy stored in the lungs and chest wall is not increased, since the extra work was dissipated as frictional (heat) loss during inspiration. Since expiratory resistance is also increased, there may not be sufficient elastic potential energy to move air fast enough for the lungs to reach their original FRC position *within the expiratory time* (T_E) *available*. If T_E is not sufficient for the lung to reach its normal FRC position, that is, if expiratory airflow continues right up to the beginning of the next inspiration, alveolar pressure will be greater than atmospheric pressure (pressure at the airway opening, Pao) at the end of expiration. This is referred to by pulmonary physiologists as "intrinsic" PEEP, meaning a built-in form of *positive end-expiratory pressure*, not caused by an external device. Consequently, FRC will increase until sufficient elastic energy is stored by the lungs to achieve a new steady state. Intrinsic PEEP is another way of saying that the potential energy stored in the breathing apparatus is insufficient to return the lungs to their normal FRC in the time available. The timing of the respiratory cycle will be discussed in more detail in Chapter 11.

> **Remember:** Breathing is a dynamic process, and therefore time is an important variable.

One of the difficulties associated with increased work of breathing in pulmonary disease is that as breathing becomes more labored (requires more muscular effort), the low efficiency of the breathing apparatus causes an exorbitant increase in the oxygen cost of breathing. If the entire increase in oxygen consumption is required just to meet the demands of the breathing apparatus, then no additional oxygen is available for other metabolic requirements. This can be extremely limiting to patients with severe lung disease, such as those with advanced emphysema or infants with marked airway narrowing (bronchiolitis or severe asthma).

The concept of the minimal work of breathing as the set point in normal breathing has been used to explain the normal tidal volume and frequency of breathing (12 breaths per minute) as well as the normal airway resistance (2 cmH$_2$O × sec/liter) relative to the volume of the dead space (150 ml). From the point of view of elastance, it would be better to have a high frequency of breathing and a small tidal volume. In that case, the lungs and thorax would scarcely have to move at all. This is the principle of *high-frequency ventilation*, which has achieved some popularity in recent years. On the other hand, frictional losses in airflow increase rapidly with frequency, since the velocity of airflow (turbulence) is markedly increased. Thus, the concept arose that the controller in the brain selects an airflow velocity, a frequency, and a tidal volume that requires the least amount of breathing power. Although the concept of minimal power of breathing is reasonable, the power requirement of breathing is normally little affected by substantial changes in tidal volume or frequency.

It is not clear whether there is a control mechanism to sense power utilization. In disease, the tendency is to breathe more rapidly and shallowly when lung elastance is increased and to breathe more slowly and deeply when airflow resistance is increased. These two factors, resistance (R) and compliance (C) affect breathing in opposite ways. Therefore, their product, R × C (the time constant), is another important variable. Since the time constant concept is more applicable to the distribution of the ventilation, further discussion will be delayed until Chapter 8.

READINGS

Books

1. Forgars P: Lung Sounds. Bailliere Tindall, London, 1978
   Chapter 1 on acoustics of airway sounds and Chapter 4 on the physiology of dynamic compression are recommended.
2. Forster RE, Dubois AB, Briscoe WA, Fisher AB: The Lung. 3rd Ed. Year Book Medical Publishers, Chicago, 1984
   Chapter 4 on mechanics of breathing covers mainly dynamic properties. It is easy to read and well illustrated. The several clinical methods for measuring lung function are clearly described. In the appendix, the work of breathing is well described.
3. Nunn JF: Applied Respiratory Physiology. 3rd Ed. Butterworths, London, 1987
   The best respiratory physiology textbook available, although weighted heavily toward anesthesiology and too advanced for beginners. Chapter 3 on airflow resistance contains everything except dynamic compliance, which is in Chapter 2 on statics. Work of breathing is covered in Chapter 5.

Reviews

4. Dayman H: Mechanics of air flow in health and emphysema. J Clin Invest 30:1175–1190, 1951
   One of the first descriptions, with radiographic evidence, of large airway compression during forced expiration.
5. Derenne JPH, Macklem PT, Roussos CS: The respiratory muscles: mechanics, control and pathophysiology. Parts I, II, III. Am Rev Respir Dis 48:119–133, 373–390, 581–601, 1978
   Up-to-date review of the physiology, pathophysiology, and clinical importance of the diaphragm and other muscles of breathing.
6. Fry DL, Hyatt RE: Pulmonary mechanics: a unified analysis of the relationship between pressure, volume and gas flow in the lungs of normal and diseased human subjects. Am J Med 29:672–689, 1960
   The classic description of the flow-volume loop.
7. Knowlton FP, Starling EH: The influence of variations in temperature and blood pressure on the performance of the isolated mammalian heart. J Physiol 44:206–219, 1912
   Contains the original description of what is now called the Starling resistor.
8. Macklem PT, Mead J: Resistance of central and peripheral airways measured by a retrograde catheter. J Appl Physiol 22:395–401, 1962
   The proof that airway resistance is greater in the larger airways, exactly opposite to what had been believed for many years.
9. Otis AB: The work of breathing. Physiol Rev 34:449–458, 1954
   Detailed review.

QUESTIONS*

Drill

1. Calculate the missing variable and state the phase of breathing.

	Raw, cmH$_2$O × sec/liter	Pao, cmH$_2$O	P$_A$, cmH$_2$O	Flow, liters/sec
a.	?	20	5	4.0
b.	6	0	20	?
c.	?	0	−20	8
d.	1.8	0	?	7
e.	5.0	?	+10	4

2. Calculate total resistance for the airways given the following partial resistances.
   a. R_{large} = 1.5 cmH$_2$O × sec/liter; R_{small} = 0.7 cmH$_2$O × sec/liter
   b. Parallel airways: R1 = 1.8, R2 = 1.0, R3 = 0.6, R4 = 3.5 cmH$_2$O × sec/liter.
   c. For the trachea and main stem bronchi, R = 1.5; for the left lung, R = 3.5, for the right lung, R = 1.5 cmH$_2$O × sec/liter.

Problems

3. What is the average dynamic lung compliance for the normal lung during a vital capacity (RV-TLC) maneuver?
4. a. Immediately after a large sighing breath, show the position of the *next* tidal P-V loop on the copy of Figure 6-1 below.
   b. Describe what happens to the tidal P-V loop after constant tidal volume breathing for several minutes.

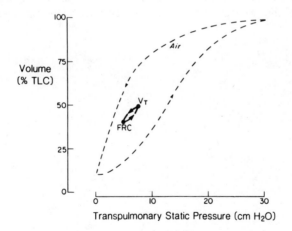

5. a. Calculate dynamic lung compliance at 1 second after the beginning of inspiration in Figure 6-3.
   b. Calculate dynamic lung elastance at 1 second after the onset of expiration.

---

* Answers begin on page 211.

6. Using the copy of Figure 6-9A below, draw the pressure-volume loop during a rapid *inspiration* to pleural pressure $= -10$ cmH$_2$O followed by a relaxed passive expiration. Explain how the work of breathing is distributed during this maneuver.

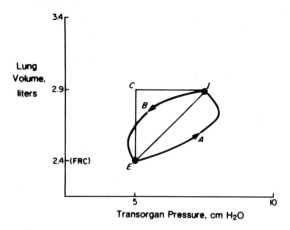

Lung Volume, liters

Transorgan Pressure, cm H$_2$O

7. a. What is the total respiratory system work of breathing done on a paralyzed man in an iron lung for a breath equal to 50% VC from FRC, assuming average Crs $= 0.1$ liter/cmH$_2$O?
   b. What is the power requirement for ventilating this patient's respiratory system, if the frequency of breathing is set at 20 breaths per minute?
8. If P$_L$ at FRC $= 5$ cmH$_2$O during normal breathing, what is FRC? Explain how you obtained your answer.
9. If Ppl $= +5$ cmH$_2$O at normal FRC, what are two explanations? (*Hint:* Consider *static* and *dynamic* events.)
10. a. At a peak inspiratory airflow of 5.0 liters/sec, what is the driving pressure for flow?
    b. What fraction of the driving pressure is needed to overcome turbulence?

7

Pulmonary and Bronchial Circulations

THE BOTTOM LINE

Pulmonary blood flow ($\dot{Q}$) is as important as $\dot{V}_A$ in determining the overall efficiency of gas exchange according to the ventilation/perfusion ratio, $\dot{V}_A/\dot{Q}$.

Pressure and Resistance

In normal humans, the cardiac output flows through the lung at pressures much lower than those in the systemic circulation. Resting normal pulmonary vascular resistance $[(Ppa - Pla)/\dot{Q} = (19 - 11)/5 = (1.6 \, cmH_2O \times min)/liter]$ is only about one-fifteenth that of the systemic circulation, in part because the pulmonary circulation is nearly maximally dilated. Comparing *pressure-flow curves* is an excellent way to assess changes in pulmonary hemodynamics under various conditions.

Pulmonary Blood Flow

Blood passing from the systemic venous system to the systemic arterial system without being fully oxygenated (venous admixture, right-to-left shunt) decreases systemic arterial oxygen tension (Pa_{O_2}), and concentration (Ca_{O_2}). In congenital heart disease, blood may flow from the systemic arterial system to the venous system (left-to-right shunt). Under these conditions, pulmonary blood flow is increased but the systemic arterial oxygen tension and concentration and systemic blood flow are normal. The *distribution* of pulmonary blood flow is sensitive to gravity over the height of the air-filled lung because the pulmonary arterial and left atrial pressures are normally low, the vessels are distensible or collapsible, and interstitial and alveolar pressures are not determined by gravity. This gives rise to three major flow conditions: in zone 1, alveolar > arterial > venous pressure, so there is no flow; in zone 2, arterial > alveolar > venous pressure, so flow is regulated by compression of microvessels at the venous outflow from the alveolar walls (Starling resistor effect); in zone 3, arterial > venous > alveolar pressure, so flow is dependent on driving pressure, vascular geometry, and smooth muscle tone.

(Continues).

(*Continued*).

Although normally *passive (gravity-dependent) regulation* of pulmonary blood flow distribution predominates, in some circumstances *active regulation* may become very important. The main regulator is *alveolar oxygen tension* ($P_{A_{O_2}}$). Alveolar hypoxia leads to an immediate and sustained local increase in vascular resistance by causing the small pulmonary arteries to constrict. When more than 20% of lung mass is affected, pulmonary arterial pressure rises, as in high-altitude pulmonary hypertension. *Thromboxane A_2* and *prostacyclin* (PGI_2), metabolites of arachidonic acid, are a powerful constrictor and a powerful dilator, respectively. Their blood concentrations may increase dramatically, especially during acute lung vascular disturbances.

Bronchial Circulation

The bronchial circulation nourishes the walls of the airways and blood vessels, warms and humidifies incoming air, and supplies substrate to airway glands, mucosa, and smooth muscle. The bronchial supply maintains tissue viability when pulmonary arterial vessels are obstructed by an embolus.

Pulmonary blood flow ($\dot{Q}$) is the denominator of the ventilation-perfusion ratio, $\dot{V}_A/\dot{Q}$, and is equal in importance with breathing in determining the overall efficiency of gas exchange. Historically, the pulmonary circulation was called the "lesser circulation." Certainly, it is not "lesser" in terms of blood flow, since more blood flows through the lungs than any other organ. The term lesser circulation derives from the fact that the walls of the pulmonary arteries are not well endowed with elastic fibers and smooth muscle and are therefore much thinner than the walls of the systemic arteries. One can deduce that pulmonary arterial pressure is less than systemic arterial pressure. The major anatomic features of the pulmonary circulation are described in Chapter 2.

The right ventricle pumps the mixed venous blood through the pulmonary arterial distribution system and then through the alveolar wall capillaries (where O_2 is added and CO_2 is removed) and on to the left atrium. The main stumbling block for students of hemodynamics is to understand how *all* of the cardiac output flows through the pulmonary circulation at a much lower pressure than through the systemic circulation. The difference is due in part to the enormous number of resistance vessels (small muscular pulmonary arteries) and in part to the dilated condition of the resistance vessels. At rest, most systemic arterioles and precapillary sphincters are partially constricted. Thus, in the *systemic* circulation about 75% of total resistance is located in the arterioles. Probably the major quantitative difference in the *pulmonary* circulation is that the arterioles, both by their enormous number and by their low basal smooth muscle tone, contribute much less resistance.

If all systemic vessels were maximally vasodilated, the hemodynamics of the systemic circulation would be similar to those of the pulmonary circulation. Such a situation actually occurs in some kinds of shock (for example, low systemic arterial pressure due to widespread vasodilation).

Remember: The pulmonary circulation is normally dilated, and the systemic circulation is normally constricted.

The small muscular arteries and arterioles of the pulmonary circulation have much less smooth muscle than do those of the systemic circulation. That is clearly part of the reason for the lower resistance in the pulmonary circuit.* The importance of having low resistance in the pulmonary circulation should be obvious. Since the total cardiac output must flow through the lung, it is useful not to expend much metabolic energy (power) to move that blood.

In certain conditions—both physiologic (living at high altitude, where the inspired air has a low oxygen partial pressure) and pathologic (primary pulmonary hypertension)—the lung's arterioles may become as well muscularized as those of the systemic circulation, and the pressure in the pulmonary artery may approach that in the aorta. The right ventricle hypertrophies (forming a thicker free wall). Right heart failure due to excessive power demand may ensue. This is a serious clinical problem and difficult to treat.

The alveolar wall capillary network is the main exchange system of the pulmonary circulation. In this, it functions identically to the capillaries of the systemic circulation. Some O_2 and CO_2 may diffuse through the thin walls of vessels other than capillaries, but in everyday life nearly all the O_2 and CO_2 exchange occurs in the alveolar wall capillaries.

The pulmonary capillary bed is a remarkable structure. At rest, it contains about 75 ml of blood, spread out in a vast array of thin-walled interconnecting vessels. During exercise, the capillary blood volume increases, approaching the maximum anatomic capillary volume, which in adults is about 200 ml. The average thickness of the capillary walls is only 0.1 μm, which helps to optimize oxygen diffusion between the alveolar gas and the hemoglobin in the red blood cells. The total capillary surface area for gas exchange is about 70 m^2 (40 times body surface area).

Remember: Lung capillary blood volume is approximately equal to the stroke volume of the right ventricle under most conditions.

At a heart rate of 75 beats/min, the erythrocytes entering the pulmonary capillaries remain there for one 0.75-second cardiac cycle, which is more than adequate for O_2 and CO_2 equilibration between alveolar gas and blood (see discussion of diffusion in Ch. 9).

The total blood volume of the pulmonary circulation (main pulmonary artery to left atrium) is 500 ml, which is 10% of the total circulating blood volume (5,000 ml). In life, the lung is 40% blood by weight. Nearly one-half of the shadows seen in a radiograph of the lung are blood (Fig. 2-1). The well-trained radiologist can tell a great deal about the pulmonary circulation by a careful examination of the plain chest radiograph.

The vascular volume, except for the amount in the capillaries, is distributed approximately equally between the arterial and venous vessels. The large pulmonary vascular volume serves as a capacitance reservoir (buffer) for the left atrium. If venous return to the right ventricle suddenly changes, diastolic filling of the left ventricle does not change for two or three cardiac cycles. During normal breathing, the right and left ventricles are out of phase. As pleural pressure falls during inspiration, the right ventricle receives more blood because the pressure gradient for flow into the heart (venous return) is increased, whereas the left ventricle ejects less blood

---

* In the fetus, the pulmonary arterioles are well muscularized and tightly constricted, so that nearly all of the right ventricular output is shunted to the systemic circulation through the *foramen ovale* and the *ductus arteriosis*. The pressures in the cavities of the right and left ventricles are essentially equal. After birth, when the pulmonary vascular bed dilates because of expansion of the lung and the onset of air breathing (alveolar oxygen tension is one of the main factors regulating pulmonary vascular resistance), the right ventricle slowly regresses relative to the left ventricle. In the normal adult, the right ventricle is a mere appendage of the left ventricle and the pulmonary arterioles have little muscle.

because the left ventricle is in a lower pressure chamber (thorax) so the systemic arteries are at a relatively higher pressure (increased afterload). During expiration the opposite occurs.

PRESSURE AND RESISTANCE

Figure 7-1 shows normal pressures in the human pulmonary circulation compared with those in the systemic circulation. The data are for an adult at rest lying supine (minimal gravitational effect). The pressures are given in millimeters of mercury (mmHg) to compare the systemic and pulmonary circulations. However, pulmonary physiologists usually refer to pulmonary vascular pressure in centimeters of water (cmH_2O). Table 7-1 lists the normal pulmonary vascular pressures. The pressure in the pulmonary artery is about one-fifth that in the aorta. Left atrial pressure is higher than right atrial pressure.

Let us use the data in Table 7-1 to calculate pulmonary vascular resistance (PVR) at the

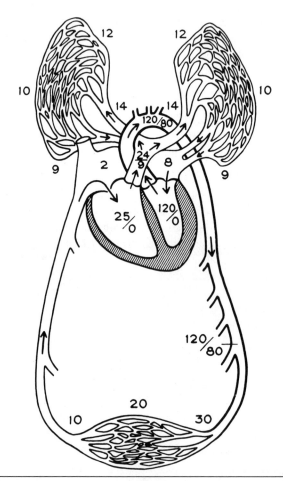

Fig. 7-1.   Pressures in the pulmonary and systemic circulations in a normal, resting, supine human adult. Pressures are shown in mmHg. (From Comroe JH: Textbook of Respiratory Physiology. 2nd Ed. Year Book Medical Publishers, Chicago, 1974, with permission.)

Table 7-1. Pressures in the Pulmonary Circulation of
Normal, Resting, Supine Adult Humans

	mmHg	cmH$_2$O
Pulmonary artery[a]		
Systolic/diastolic	24/9	33/11
Mean	14	19
Arterioles		
Mean	12	16
Capillaries		
Mean	10.5	14
Venules		
Mean	9	12
Left atrium		
Mean	8	11

[a] The pulmonary arterial and left atrial pressures are measured at cardiac catheterization—the former directly, the latter by wedging the arterial catheter. The capillary pressure is computed by the standard equation P$_{cap}$ = Pla + Rv × (Ppa − Pla), where Rv is the fraction of resistance downstream from the midpoint of the capillary, normally taken as 0.4.

normal resting cardiac output ($\dot{Q}$) of 5 liters/min and at mean pulmonary arterial pressure (Ppa) of 19 cmH$_2$O and mean left atrial pressure (Pla) of 11 cmH$_2$O.

$$\text{PVR} = \frac{\Delta P}{\dot{Q}} = \frac{Ppa - Pla}{\dot{Q}} = \frac{(19 - 11) \text{ cmH}_2\text{O}}{5 \text{ liters/min}}$$

$$= \frac{8}{5} = \frac{1.6 \text{ cmH}_2\text{O} \times \text{min}}{\text{liter}}$$

Pulmonary vascular resistance is one-fifteenth that in the systemic vascular bed. In the pulmonary circulation, the complete driving pressure (Ppa − Pla) must be used when computing resistance. Right atrial pressure can usually be omitted when computing systemic vascular resistance, but left atrial pressure cannot be omitted in computing pulmonary vascular resistance.

Pressure-Flow Curves

One way to achieve an overall view of pulmonary hemodynamics is to examine the change in driving pressure as cardiac output varies. These are called **pressure-flow** curves (see Ch. 3). Four representative curves in different physiologic conditions are shown schematically in Figure 7-2. Vascular resistance (driving pressure divided by flow) is represented on a pressure-flow curve by the slope of a line from the origin to any particular point on a curve. The shapes of the pressure-flow curves are due to the large distensibility (high compliance) of the pulmonary vessels. On curve 1 (normal), the resistance during exercise (E) is less than that at rest (R). Alveolar hypoxia (line 2) causes vasoconstriction, and therefore, there is a greater driving pressure (and consequently resistance) at any given flow (for example, at rest, HR). During exercise while hypoxic, the resistance still may decrease, as shown by point HE, where the resistance is fortuitously the same as that for a person at rest breathing air.

PRESSURE-FLOW CURVES

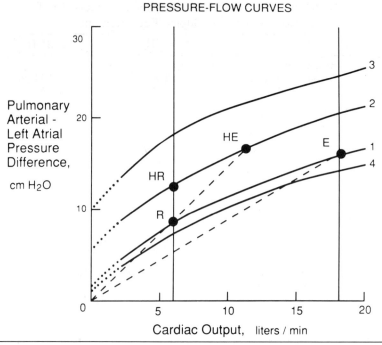

Fig. 7-2.   Representative pressure-flow curves that might be obtained in the human pulmonary circulation. Line 1 is normal. Point R is the normal resting point, and point E is maximum steady-state exercise. The data are from Appendix 2. The slopes of the dashed lines from the origin to the points on the curve represent pulmonary vascular resistance ($\Delta P/\dot{Q}$). Curves 2 and 3 lie above line 1, meaning there is increased resistance at any given flow, for example, point HR. Notice the positive y-axis intercepts of these curves; that is, flow stops even though the driving pressure is not zero. The reason why flow stops cannot be ascertained from the graph alone. Curve 2 represents hypoxic pulmonary vasoconstriction, and curve 3 represents continuous positive pressure breathing (15 cmH_2O). Curve 4 is slightly below the normal line, indicating a decreased resistance at any given flow when a normal person breathes 100% oxygen.

Continuous positive pressure breathing (line 3) may also increase resistance at a given flow because the increased alveolar pressure tends to compress the microvessels in the alveolar walls, thereby increasing their resistance. Curve 4 (for breathing 100% oxygen) shows only slight vasodilation, indicating that at the normal $P_{A_{O_2}}$ of 100 mmHg there is little hypoxic vasoconstriction. Each of the pressure-flow lines will be discussed further in the appropriate section.

PULMONARY BLOOD FLOW

In Chapter 3, I used the Fick equation (Eq. 3-5) to compute cardiac output from the resting oxygen consumption ($\dot{V}_{O_2}$) and the oxygen concentration difference across the lung [($\bar{v}$ − a)ΔC_{O_2}]. Although the Fick equation is still the primary reference for measuring cardiac output, there are several faster methods in common use, all based on what is known as the *indicator dilution principle*. In the 1980s, the thermodilution (caloric) method has come to supersede all others. The thermodilution method is another application of the volume of dilution principle (see Ch. 3). It is so widely used in cardiac catheterization laboratories, intensive care units, and recovery rooms that beginning students should know something about it.

In the thermal indicator dilution method, a suitable quantity (C × V) of cold blood or 5% dextrose solution is injected rapidly into the right atrium, and the temperature of pulmonary arterial blood is recorded continuously until it returns to normal. The time-temperature tracing (Fig. 7-3) depends on the volume rate of blood flow, since it is into that volume that all the tracer has been diluted. The flow can be determined if one can measure the mean concentration of tracer (as indicated by the mean temperature, $\overline{T}$) and the time (a–f) during which the tracer passed the temperature detector. Both values can be obtained from the time-temperature tracing if the recirculation of the indicator is taken into account or eliminated. One major advantage of the thermal dilution method for measuring cardiac output is that recirculation is minimal because the body is a huge heat sink.

These days the procedure and the calculations are automated and easy to carry out. The only limitation to wider application of the method is the need to have a pulmonary arterial (or alternately a systemic arterial) catheter equipped with a sensitive heat probe (thermistor) to detect the small temperature changes.

Shunts Between the Right and Left Heart

Right-to-Left Shunt
An important functional test of the adequacy of the pulmonary circulation is to determine what fraction of the cardiac output *effectively* flows through pulmonary capillaries (exchanges with "ideal" alveolar gas) and what fraction bypasses the lungs to enter the systemic arteries unox-

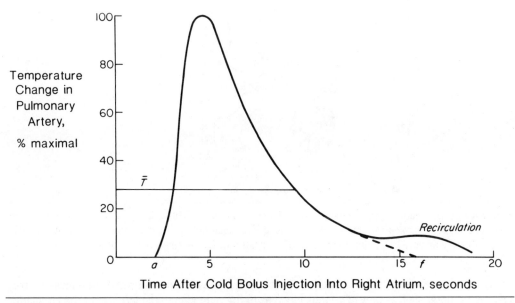

Fig. 7-3. The time-temperature change as measured in the pulmonary artery after a bolus injection of cold blood intravenously. After a brief delay until the bolus reaches the detector (a), the temperature change rises to a peak and then declines exponentially to zero (f), although the latter is masked by the small recirculation of the cold blood. Using methods that eliminate the recirculation component, the mean temperature ($\overline{T}$) and the time (a–f) during passage of the tracer can be obtained and used to determine the cardiac output.

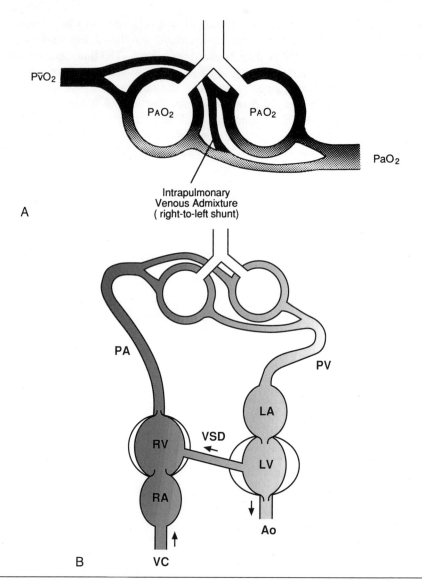

$P\bar{v}O_2$

PAO_2 PAO_2

PaO_2

Intrapulmonary
Venous Admixture
(right-to-left shunt)

A

PA

PV

LA

RV   VSD   LV

RA

Ao

B   VC

Fig. 7-4.   Diagramatic representation of (**A**) venous admixture (right-to-left shunt) and (**B**) left-to-right shunt (interventricular septal defect). Abbreviations: VC, vena cava; RA, right atrium; RV, right ventricle; PA, pulmonary artery; PV, pulmonary vein; LA, left atrium; LV, left ventricle; Ao, aorta.

ygenated (venous admixture, "shuntlike effect") (Fig. 7-4A). **Venous admixture** includes true anatomic shunts, such as flow of venous blood from the right side to the left side of the circulation (as in cyanotic congenital heart disease) or intrapulmonary flow through portions of the lung that do not receive adequate ventilation.

A small amount of venous admixture is normal because some venous blood enters the left ventricle by way of the bronchopulmonary venous anastomoses and the intracardiac thebesian veins. This amounts to 1 to 2% of the cardiac output normally, but in some diseases bronchial anastomotic blood flow may rise to 10 to 20% of cardiac output. In certain congenital anomalies the right-to-left anatomic shunt may account for 50% of cardiac output.

The way to quantify venous admixture is to use the Fick equation for oxygen uptake and to partition cardiac output into two independent streams (effective blood flow to normal lung and shuntlike flow), which mix in the left ventricle. Thus, one must measure $\dot{V}_{O_2}$, $C\bar{v}_{O_2}$, and Ca_{O_2} to calculate cardiac output (see the sample calculation in Ch. 3, p. 37). The next step is to partition cardiac output into the two independent streams. Unfortunately, the oxygen concentrations of systemic arterial and mixed venous blood are not linear functions of P_{O_2} (see Fig. 1-2 or Fig. 9-1).

Let us proceed, as in Chapter 4, first with a simple example and then with more complex ones. Some of the calculations may seem complicated, but if each part is worked separately, the equations are straightforward and make common sense.

Example 1: Mixing Plasma
Calculate the P_{O_2} of a mixture of 1 liter of plasma at $P_{O_2} = 100$ mmHg and 0.25 liter of plasma at $P_{O_2} = 40$ mmHg. To do this, one must apply the volume of dilution equation (mixing equation) that was presented as Eq. 4-1 as follows:

$$(V_1 \times C_1) + (V_2 \times C_2) = (V_1 + V_2) \times \bar{C} \tag{7-1}$$

The O_2 concentration is calculated by using the O_2 solubility coefficient (α), which equals 0.03 ml O_2/(liter × mmHg), assuming that its physical solubility in plasma is the same as in whole blood (see the section on blood gas concentration and Eq. 3-3 in Ch. 3 to refresh your memory). Equation 7-1 becomes

$$(1 \times 100 \times 0.03) + (0.25 \times 40 \times 0.03) = (1 + 0.25) \times \bar{C}_{O_2}*$$

$$\bar{C}_{O_2} = \frac{(3.0 + 0.3)}{1.25} = 2.64 \text{ ml } O_2/\text{liter}$$

By Eq. 3-3, the O_2 partial pressure of the mixture is

$$P_{O_2} = \frac{\bar{C}_{O_2}}{\alpha} = \frac{2.64 \text{ ml } O_2/\text{liter}}{0.03 \text{ ml } O_2/(\text{mmHg} \times \text{liter})} = 88 \text{ mmHg}$$

The result makes common sense. There is four times as much plasma at the higher P_{O_2}, therefore, the average P_{O_2} of the mixture should be closer to 100 than to 40 mmHg.

Example 2: Mixing Blood
Calculate the systemic arterial oxygen tension (Pa_{O_2}) in a person with a normal cardiac output ($\dot{Q}_T$) of 5 liters/min but with 20% of it (1 liter) bypassing the lung. The subject's resting oxygen consumption is 250 ml O_2/min (normal). The mixed venous P_{O_2} ($P\bar{v}_{O_2}$) is 35 mmHg (a little lower than normal). The hemoglobin concentration of the blood is 150 g/liter (normal), and the HbO_2 equilibrium curve shown in Figures 1-2 or 9-1 applies.

Because of the alinear HbO_2 equilibrium curve, one must work with the *concentration* of oxygen in whole blood, not its P_{O_2}. We obtain Ca_{O_2} by adding the oxygen bound to hemoglobin (O_2 capacity × S_{O_2}/100) to that in physical solution. Normal O_2 capacity is 1.34 ml O_2/g Hb × 150 g Hb/liter = 201 ml O_2/liter (see Ch. 3, p. 35). In Figures 1-2 or 9-1, the $S_{O_2} = 97.5\%$ or 0.975 (as a fraction) at $P_{O_2} = 100$ mmHg and 70% or 0.70 at $P_{O_2} = 35$ mmHg. Now write down the mixing equation (Eq. 7-1), as in the previous example

---

* Since α is a common term, you could use P_{O_2} instead of $\bar{C}_{O_2}$, but that will not work in the next examples. It is better to do it this way.

$$Ca_{O_2} = \frac{(201 \times 0.975 + 100 \times 0.03) \times 4 + (201 \times 0.70 + 35 \times 0.03) \times 1}{5}$$

$$= \frac{(196 + 3.0) \times 4 + (141 + 1) \times 1}{5} = \frac{796 + 142}{5} = \frac{938}{5}$$

$$= 188 \text{ ml } O_2/\text{liter}$$

Before continuing, be sure you know what each number means. For example, the expression in the first parentheses shows the bound O_2 (201×0.975) added to the dissolved O_2 (100×0.03) and the whole multiplied by 4 liters of normal pulmonary blood flow. The expression in the second parentheses is the shunt flow, of which there is 1 liter (20% shunt). When all the oxygen is added together and divided by the cardiac output (5 liters/min), the systemic arterial concentration is obtained.

One may think that the amount in physical solution is too trivial to consider but, as will be seen in example 3, it sometimes has a substantial effect on the result.

To calculate the P_{O_2} of the systemic arterial blood, apportion the oxygen concentration into the amount in solution and the amount bound to hemoglobin *with the constraint that the P_{O_2} be the same for both*. Since the HbO_2 equilibrium curve has no simple equation, P_{O_2} must be obtained by numerical approximation.

As a first approximation, use Figure 1-2 to estimate the P_{O_2} corresponding to $S_{O_2} = 188/201 = 93.5\%$. By ignoring the amount of physical solution, one obtains the upper limit of P_{O_2}. The P_{O_2} is approximately 60 mmHg. Now compute the oxygen in solution at that P_{O_2}

$$C_{O_2}, \text{ dissolved} = \frac{60 \text{ mmHg} \times 0.03 \text{ ml } O_2}{\text{mmHg} \times \text{liter}} = 1.8 \text{ ml } O_2/\text{liter}$$

Subtract the amount in physical solution from the total oxygen content and obtain $188 - 2 = 186$ ml O_2/liter. Use this for a second approximation to obtain the lower limit of S_{O_2} and P_{O_2}.

In the second approximation, $S_{O_2} = 186/201 = 92.5\%$ and $P_{O_2} = 55$ mmHg. P_{O_2} changes more than S_{O_2} because the slope of the HbO_2 equilibrium is relatively flat over its upper portion. Finally, compute the dissolved O_2 at $P_{O_2} = 55$ mmHg and obtain a value of 1.6 ml O_2/liter.

The correct P_{O_2} must lie between 55 and 60 mmHg and the S_{O_2} between 92.5 and 93.5%. Since the HbO_2 equilibrium curve can be considered straight over such a narrow range, take the mean P_{O_2} as 58 mmHg and S_{O_2} as 93%. Because of its curved shape, the HbO_2 equilibrium curve will *always* make the P_{O_2} of a blood mixture less than that for equal volumes of plasma in which O_2 is only in physical solution, provided the P_{O_2} is less than necessary for 100% S_{O_2} (about 200 mmHg).

Now there's an idea. Suppose one could do the test in a manner such that the Pa_{O_2} was >200 mmHg. Then the O_2 bound to hemoglobin could be ignored, thereby avoiding the problem of the odd shape of the HbO_2 equilibrium curve. The wily pulmonary physiologist accomplishes this by having the subject breathe 100% O_2 for several minutes on the reasonable assumption that all areas of the lung, no matter how poorly ventilated, will eventually achieve an FA_{O_2} of 94% (5.6% CO_2), except for those regions that are completely unventilated ($\dot{V}A/\dot{Q} = 0$) or are true anatomic shunts.

Example 3: Shunt Calculation while Breathing 100% O_2
Compute the Pa_{O_2} while the person with a 20% shunt in example 2 is breathing 100% oxygen, $P\bar{v}_{O_2} = 43$ mmHg (a little higher than normal), and $PA_{O_2} = 600$ mmHg. Write down the volume of dilution equation as before with the additional information that for $P_{O_2} = 200$ mmHg, the S_{O_2} is about 100% (O_2 capacity). Use Figure 1-2 to estimate the oxygen saturation as 78% at $P\bar{v}_{O_2}$ of 43 mmHg.

Table 7-2. Summary of Venous Admixture Examples

	$P_{A_{O_2}}$ (mmHg)	$\dot{Q}s$ (fraction)	$P\bar{v}_{O_2}$ (mmHg)	Pa_{O_2} (mmHg)	$(A - a)\Delta P_{O_2}$ (mmHg)
Plasma	100	0.20	40	88	12
Blood ($F_{I_{O_2}} = 0.21$)	100	0.20	35	58	42
Blood ($F_{I_{O_2}} = 1.0$)	600	0.20	43	188	412

$$Ca_{O_2} = \frac{(201 \times 1.0 + 600 \times 0.03) \times 4 + (201 \times 0.78 + 43 \times 0.03) \times 1}{5}$$

$$= \frac{(201 + 18) \times 4 + (157 + 1.3) \times 1}{5}$$

$$= \frac{876 + 158}{5} = 207 \text{ ml } O_2/\text{liter}$$

Here the dissolved O_2 concentration of the blood flowing through normal lung (second term in first parentheses) is substantial—18 ml O_2/liter. This is nearly 10% of that bound to hemoglobin and has a large effect on the computation (as can be verified by trying the calculation without it). In the expression in the second parentheses, the amount of dissolved O_2 is small because the P_{O_2} is low. Finally, from the total Ca_{O_2} subtract the O_2 capacity to obtain the content of dissolved oxygen as 6 ml/liter. The P_{O_2} necessary to keep 6 ml O_2/liter in solution is 6/0.03 = 188 mmHg. The example shows how much easier the computation is when the resultant mixture is fully saturated.

In Table 7-2, the three examples are summarized together with the alveolar − arterial P_{O_2} difference, $(A - a)\Delta P_{O_2}$. This variable is markedly different among the three examples. In example 3, it is enormous. The mixed venous P_{O_2} varies because the cardiac output is kept constant at 5 liters/min and the oxygen consumption is normal (250 ml/min). Therefore, the systemic arterial to mixed venous oxygen concentration difference had to be 50 ml/liter by the Fick equation (see Ch. 3). The variation of $P\bar{v}_{O_2}$ is small compared with the Pa_{O_2} variations because of the shape of the hemoglobin-oxygen equilibrium curve. Near the normal mixed venous P_{O_2} of 40 mmHg, the curve is steep. Small changes in P_{O_2} have large effects on saturation.

Remember: Right-to-left shunts always reduce systemic arterial oxygen tension and concentration. Breathing 100% O_2 accentuates the $(A - a)\Delta P_{O_2}$ and usually makes the venous admixture calculation easier.

Example 4: Quick Estimate of Venous Admixture
There is a rapid method for estimating the shunt fraction in a subject breathing 100% oxygen. In example 3, the $(A - a)\Delta P_{O_2}$ was 400 mmHg for a 20% shunt. The clever physiologist estimates the shunt will be 1% of cardiac output for each 20 mmHg difference between alveolar and arterial oxygen tensions. It is a useful rule of thumb but, of course, requires several assumptions, namely, that the HbO_2 equilibrium curve, the oxygen capacity of the blood, and the $\dot{V}_{O_2}$ are all normal.

If you think of venous admixture as a stream of blood being pumped around and around the body without delivering any O_2 or picking up any CO_2, then it is clear that venous admixture reduces the efficiency of blood flow. Thus, venous admixture is the blood flow equivalent of wasted ventilation.

Left-to-Right Shunt

Of particular interest to the pulmonary physiologist is that a left-to-right shunt does not affect systemic arterial oxygen tension (Pa_{O_2}). Suppose a patient has a 20% left-to-right shunt through an interventricular septal defect. The patient otherwise has normal physiology with Pa_{O_2} = 100 mmHg, $\dot{V}_{O_2}$ = 250 ml/min, and a normal $(\bar{v} - a)\Delta C_{O_2}$, so the blood flow to the systemic tissues must be normal at 5 liters/min. Thus, a left-to-right shunt is always *in addition to* the systemic flow; that is, pulmonary blood flow exceeds systemic blood flow. In this example, pulmonary blood flow (6.25 liters/min) exceeds the systemic flow (5 liters/min) by 1.25 liters/min ($\dot{Q}s/\dot{Q}T$ = 1.25/6.25 = 20%).

As pulmonary physiologists, we are interested in understanding and quantifying the effect of the left-to-right shunt on the mixed venous O_2 concentration and P_{O_2}. To do this we must reconsider what we mean by the mixed venous oxygen tension, $P\bar{v}_{O_2}$.

Until now, I have used pulmonary arterial blood as representative of $P\bar{v}_{O_2}$, and so it is normally. But with a left-to-right shunt, pulmonary arterial P_{O_2} is not the same as the P_{O_2} of all the systemic venous blood returning to the heart via the inferior and superior vena cavae and the coronary sinus.*

The characteristic finding at cardiac catheterization in a person with a left-to-right intrathoracic shunt is a step *increase* in the oxygen concentration of blood somewhere on the right side of the heart. When one knows which chamber has the increase, one knows the anatomy of the shunt and can estimate its size from the shunt flow. This is vital information for the cardiac surgeon to have before attempting to repair the defect. In our example, the patient has an opening between the left and right ventricles; therefore, the oxygen concentration and P_{O_2} are increased in the right ventricle compared with the right atrium. Examine Figure 7-4B. Although the anatomy is distorted, the scheme shows the abnormal connection between the ventricles. The mean systemic venous P_{O_2} equals 40 mmHg; S_{O_2} = 75% (normal). To calculate the O_2 concentration of blood in the pulmonary artery (Cpa_{O_2}), set up the mixing equation

$$Cpa_{O_2} = \frac{(201 \times 0.975 + 100 \times 0.03) \times 1.25 + (201 \times 0.75 + 40 \times 0.03) \times 5}{6.25}$$

$$= \frac{(196 + 3) \times 1.25 + (151 + 1) \times 5}{6.25}$$

$$= \frac{249 + 760}{6.25} = 161 \text{ ml } O_2/\text{liter}$$

This time the shunt appears first. The mean concentration of blood in the pulmonary artery is 161 ml O_2/liter. From the HbO_2 curve (Fig. 1-2) and interpolating between P_{O_2} = 40 and 50 mmHg, the pulmonary arterial (mixed venous) oxygen saturation ($S\bar{v}_{O_2}$) is 79%, with $P\bar{v}_{O_2}$ = 44 mmHg.

Remember: With a left-to-right intrathoracic shunt: (1) the pulmonary blood flow exceeds the systemic blood flow; (2) the systemic arterial oxygen concentration and P_{O_2} are normal; (3) somewhere within the right side of the heart (right atrium, ventricle, or pulmonary artery) P_{O_2} increases.

---

* Some physiologists refer to the mean systemic venous oxygen tension as a "virtual" oxygen tension, "virtual" meaning that it can't be directly measured because there is incomplete mixing of the venous streams before they reach the right ventricle.

Right-to-left shunts (venous admixture) occur rather commonly in pulmonary diseases and in some forms of congenital heart disease, such as the tetralogy of Fallot, as well as when pulmonary vascular resistance rises (pulmonary hypertension) in a child with a patent ductus arteriosus. Left-to-right shunts are not common and are usually due to congenital heart disease (atrial septal defect, ventricular septal defect, patent ductus arteriosus). Left-to-right shunts do not occur in pulmonary disease.

Distribution of Blood Flow

The normal pressures in the aorta (120/80 mmHg) refer to pressures at the level of the heart (Fig. 7-1). In the upright position pressure varies by 0.74 mmHg/cm body height. In a standing adult human who is 175 cm tall, systemic arterial pressure is 130 mmHg higher in the feet than in the head. Systemic venous pressure varies in the same manner.

The effects of gravity are *relatively* greater in the pulmonary circulation because the pressures in the pulmonary artery and left atrium are much lower than systemic vascular pressures. In the chest radiographs in Figure 2-1, the lung at FRC is 24 cm high. The average pressures shown in Table 7-1 are only valid at the level of the heart (left atrium). What are the pressures up and down the lung from that point? At FRC the bottom of the lung is about 12 cm below the left atrium. That means that for each centimeter *below the left atrium* the pulmonary arterial pressure increases by 1 cmH_2O. At the bottom of the lung in the costodiaphragmatic recess, pulmonary arterial pressure is $19 + 12 = 31$ cmH_2O and left atrial pressure is $11 + 12 = 23$ cmH_2O. Both the arterial and venous pressures are increased equally, so the driving pressure (Ppa − Pla) across each level of lung remains constant at 8 cmH_2O.

The opposite effect occurs as one goes up the lung—one must subtract 1 cmH_2O/cm height. At FRC mean pulmonary arterial pressure at the top of the lung will be $19 - 12 = 7$ cmH_2O. During systole the pressure will be higher and during diastole it will be lower. Late in diastole, when the pulmonary arterial pressure is at its lowest value, the pressure in the pulmonary artery at the top of the lung may drop to zero or below. The *effective* left atrial pressure equals zero at 11 cm above the reference level. Above that level, the effective venous outflow pressure is less than alveolar (atmospheric) pressure.

The pressure pattern is important because changing pulmonary arterial pressure affects the distribution of blood flow over the height of the lung. Figure 7-5 is a cartoon showing the analogous effect of height on water flow in an apartment house if the water pressure is not adequate to maintain high inflow pressure throughout the building.

Effect of Gravity on Distensible Tubes

If a horizontal rigid tube, open at one end to atmospheric pressure, is filled with water, as shown in Figure 7-6A, pressure at every point in the tube is atmospheric. This is equivalent to a human lying in the horizontal position. If the tube is turned into the vertical position (Fig. 7-6B), the pressure at the top will still be atmospheric but the pressure in the water increases by 1 cmH_2O per centimeter down the tube owing to the weight of the column of water (density, 1 g/ml). At the bottom of the tube, the pressure is 15 cmH_2O higher than atmospheric. This is equivalent to a human in the standing position in whom pulmonary arterial pressure over the height of the lung differs by the weight of a column of blood equal to lung height.

Next we examine a rigid, water-filled U-tube (each limb of equal length), as shown in Figure 7-6C. The pressure in each limb is atmospheric at the open top and increases at the rate of 1 cmH_2O per centimeter down the tube. There is no flow because the driving pressure is zero at each level in each arm of the tube. Since the U-tube is rigid, it can be rotated around the horizontal axis through the open ends without any effect, as shown in Figure 7-6D, except that now atmospheric pressure is at the bottom and the pressure at the top is $- 15$ cmH_2O, since the direction of gravity is downward.

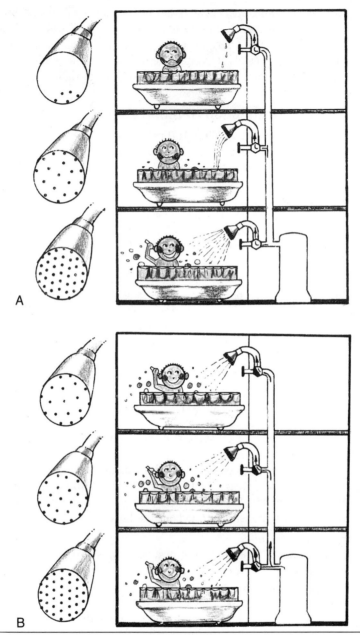

Fig. 7-5. Effect of gravity on regional pulmonary perfusion is represented by three showers on different floors of an apartment house. **(A)** When all showers are on, there is less flow as one goes upstairs because the pressure in the reservoir tank is insufficient to maintain adequate pressure at the top of the building. This represents the normal pulmonary arterial pressure and regional lung blood flow distribution. **(B)** If the pressure in the reservoir is increased, flow is more evenly distributed over the height of the building, although pressure and flow are still less at the top. This represents the pulmonary circulation during exercise or during global hypoxic pulmonary vasoconstriction (high altitude). (From Wagner WW: Capillary recruitment in the pulmonary circulation. Chest 93:855–885, 1987, with permission.)

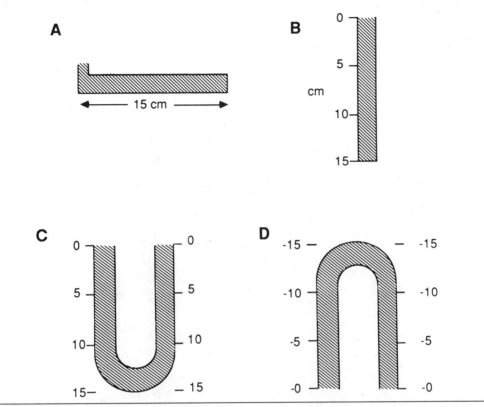

Fig. 7-6.   (A) In a horizontal rigid tube pressure is equal at all points. (B) In a vertical rigid tube transmural pressure increases down the tube owing to the weight (density) of the liquid filling the tube. For water (blood) the pressure increases by 1 cmH_2O/cm height. (C) In a right U-tube the transmural pressure increases down the tube. The increase is the same in each arm of the tube, so there is no flow. (D) The orientation of the tube has no effect.

If we combine the horizontal tube in Figure 7-6A and the two U-tubes in Figure 7-6C and D, everything said up to now still applies (Fig. 7-7A). Pressure at the top of the structure is -15 cmH_2O and that at the bottom is $+15$ cmH_2O relative to zero at the middle horizontal tube. The pressure difference between the top and the bottom is 30 cmH_2O. There is no flow because there is no driving pressure, since the inflow and outflow pressures are equal.

The results are not influenced by the manner in which the y-axis is labeled because all the pressures are relative. Thus, the pressure in the middle is labeled 20 cmH_2O, so that the pressure at the top is $20 - 15 = 5$ cmH_2O and at the bottom is $20 + 15 = 35$ cmH_2O.

Now consider the same system but with liquid flowing, as shown in Figure 7-7B. Relative to the horizontal tube (MID), the pressure in the inflow reservoir is 19 cmH_2O and that in the outflow reservoir is 11 cmH_2O. There is a driving pressure for flow across the structure which is exactly equal to the inflow minus the outflow pressure, namely, $19 - 11 = 8$ cmH_2O. The anatomy of the structure in between is irrelevant in terms of flow, *as long as all the tubes are rigid*. Thus, flow will occur equally through the top, middle, and bottom sections, since each path has the same resistance to flow.

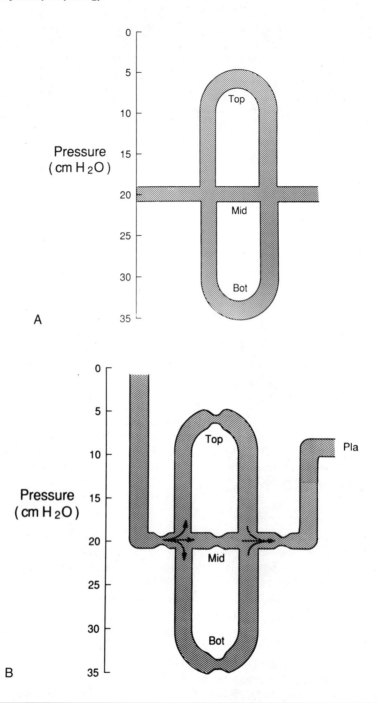

Fig. 7-7. **(A)** Any combination of tubes, as in the complex manifold shown, does not alter the pressure relationships. **(B)** Flow has no effect on the rigid tube structure. The system is 30 cm high with MID at 20 cm. The inflow pressure is 19 cmH$_2$O and the outflow pressure is 11 cmH$_2$O. The driving pressure, 8 cmH$_2$O, is the same across each arm of the manifold. The labeling of the y-axis is irrelevant since all pressures are relative. The constrictions at various points represent resistances to flow.

The final step is to go from a rigid system to a distensible one and to add *variable* resistances for the arteries (Ra), capillaries (Rc), and veins (Rv), as shown in Figure 7-8. In the real pulmonary circulation all the vessels are *distensible*. Each vessel tends to dilate when its transmural pressure increases, just as the airways do during inspiration (Fig. 6-4A). Although the higher pressures toward the bottom do not change the driving pressure, they do change the transmural distending pressure.

One consequence is that the higher transmural pressure toward the bottom of the lung model distends the tubes and, according to Poiseuille's equation (Eq. 6-3), decreases the resistance to liquid flow. Thus, flow is greater toward the bottom of the lung because the resistance is less, not because the driving pressure is greater.

Another consequence is that the pressure in the microvessels near the bottom of the lung is higher, which increases the hydrostatic pressure for liquid filtration according to the Starling equation for capillary liquid exchange. In patients with congestive heart failure (high left atrial pressure), interstitial edema liquid tends to accumulate first at the bottom of the lung.

Using the model in Figure 7-8 to represent the pulmonary circulation, it is possible to explain the distribution of blood flow over the height of the lung. Before doing so, however, a few more words are needed about the difference between *alveolar* and *extra-alveolar* vessels (see Ch. 2).

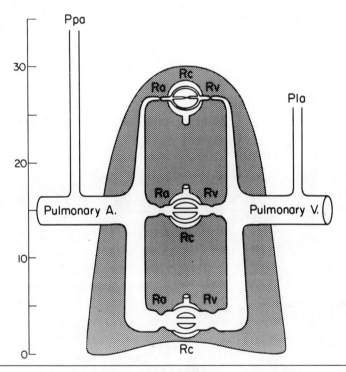

Fig. 7-8. The distensible pulmonary vascular bed differs from the rigid system by allowing transmural pressure to affect the radii of the various tubes. Although the driving pressure (Ppa − Pla) is the same at all levels, flow is no longer uniform because resistance increases as one goes up the lung owing to narrowing of vessels as transmural pressure decreases. Since alveolar pressure surrounding the capillaries is normally the same throughout the lung, the vascular pressures are decreasing relative to alveolar pressure as one moves up the lung. Ra, Rc, and Rv are arterial, capillary, and venous resistances, respectively.

In Figure 7-8, the extra-alveolar vessels are represented by the main arterial and venous tubes, whereas the alveolar vessels are mainly the alveolar wall capillaries, shown within the alveoli. The pressure outside the alveolar vessels is alveolar gas pressure (P_A), which is ordinarily atmospheric (relative zero). The pressure outside the extra-alveolar vessels, however, is below alveolar pressure and is similar to pleural pressure (Ppl) (-5 cmH$_2$O at FRC). When the lung expands and pleural pressure falls, the pressure outside the extra-alveolar vessels decreases relative to alveolar (atmospheric) pressure. This causes the extra-alveolar vessels to enlarge during inspiration (increased pulmonary blood volume).

On the other hand, alveolar pressure does not vary much with breathing except for the small cyclic variations caused by airway resistance (see Ch. 6). Near the top of the lung, where the effective venous pressure falls below alveolar pressure, the transmural pressure across the small veins becomes negative; that is, it becomes a compressive pressure at the outflow from the alveolar wall network. As the blood vessels are compressed, vascular resistance increases. This is another example of a Starling resistor.

The uneven distribution of blood flow on a gravitational basis is divided into three zones depending on the relative values of pulmonary arterial, venous, and alveolar pressures. The effect of each set on zonal conditions on blood flow distribution is sketched in Figure 7-9 and listed in Table 7-3.

In zone 1, flow is zero because pulmonary arterial pressure is less than alveolar pressure. In zone 3, flow is high and changes only because of the increasing transmural distending pressure, as one moves down the lung. Zone 2 is the one that usually gives students headaches. But now

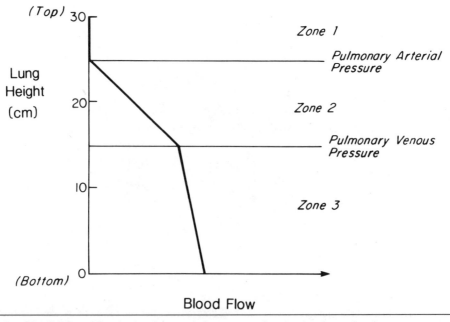

Fig. 7-9. Distribution of flow in the three main lung zones. In zone 1, where alveolar pressure exceeds both venous and arterial pressures, there is no flow. In zone 2, where pulmonary arterial pressure exceeds alveolar pressure, flow is regulated by alveolar pressure compressing the outflow from the alveolar capillaries (Starling resistor). In zone 3, the driving pressure is constant because arterial and venous pressures exceed alveolar pressure. Note that flow continues to increase going down zone 3 owing to the passive distension of the vessels by the increasing transmural pressure. Compare with Figure 7-8.

Table 7-3.   Pressure-Flow Conditions in the Three Lung Zones

Zone	Relative Pressures	Flow
1	Alveolar > arterial > venous	0
2	Arterial > alveolar > venous	Increases as one moves down the lung, Pla → PA
3	Arterial > venous > alveolar	Increases as one moves down the lung owing to increased distension of resistance vessels

that you know about Starling resistors and dynamic compression of the airways (see Fig. 6-4 and associated text), transferring the concept to the pulmonary circulation should be straight-forward.

Throughout zone 2, the alveolar pressure exceeds the venous outflow pressure (effective left atrial pressure). The transmural pressure of these vessels is negative (Pla − PA < 0). The vessels exposed to alveolar pressure are compressed at the outflow end of the alveolar compartment. It may help to review Figure 6-4B and imagine that it is a capillary instead of a bronchus. At the top of zone 2 (at the border between zones 1 and 2), flow ceases as PA begins to exceed Ppa (entering zone 1). In the opposite direction, flow increases going down zone 2 because the compressive transmural pressure is decreasing as the effective left atrial pressure rises toward PA. At the lowest part of zone 2 (at the border between zones 2 and 3), PA = Pla, and flow becomes independent of alveolar pressure (entering zone 3).

Although all three zones can exist in the human lung, normally pulmonary arterial pressure is high enough so that zone 1 does not occur (except briefly late in diastole), and even zone 2 is limited to the upper third of the lung because left atrial pressure is normally well above alveolar pressure.

From the clinical point of view, however, during mechanical ventilation, alveolar pressure is artificially increased because positive pressure is applied to the airway opening. This increases the amount of lung in zone 2 (alveolar pressure rises relative to pulmonary venous pressure), which increases resistance to blood flow. Thus, in pressure-flow curve 3 in Figure 7-2, the line is shifted upward and the extrapolated intercept shows a substantial driving pressure when flow is zero. At that point the entire lung must be in zone 1 (PA > Ppa > Pla).

When pulmonary vascular pressures are increased, the distribution of blood flow over the height of the lung is more uniform. Thus, in heavy exercise blood flow distribution is nearly even, as the cartoon in Figure 7-5B suggests.

Regulation of Pulmonary Blood Flow

Longitudinal Distribution of Resistance
The resistance to blood flow in the pulmonary arteries and arterioles is much less than that in the systemic circulation. Recent measurements by the technique known as micropuncture have revealed that in the normal range of tidal breathing the alveolar wall capillaries contribute 35 to 40% of the total resistance; the arteries about 50%; and the veins 10 to 15%. Recall that in the systemic circulation the arterioles contributed 75% of the resistance and the venous circulation about 20%. The resistance to blood flow in the capillaries was considered trivial (<5%).

What is trivial in the systemic capillaries, namely, a pressure fall of several centimeters of water, is a substantial quantity in the pulmonary circulation. In Table 7-1 the average pressure difference across the lung (Ppa − Pla) is 19 − 11 = 8 cmH$_2$O. An approximately 3 cmH$_2$O pressure drop occurs in the alveolar wall capillaries. This depends on the dimensions and dis-

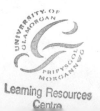

tensibility of the alveolar wall capillary network since there is no active regulation of capillary dimensions. The fraction of resistance within the alveolar wall vessels is sensitive to lung volume (less at low volume), to blood flow rate (less at high flow), and to the vascular distending pressure (greater at low pressure).

Passive Regulation

Although passive regulation has been amply discussed in relation to the vascular transmural pressures in the three lung zones, it is important to mention the passive mechanical effects of changes in pulmonary blood flow in exercise. When humans perform submaximal sustained exercise, cardiac output may rise threefold above the resting level. This increase in blood flow is accommodated by the pulmonary circulation without an equivalent rise in the pulmonary vascular driving pressure. This is due to **recruitment** and **distension** of microvessels caused by the increasing transmural pressure in the very small vessels (arterioles, capillaries, and venules). As already noted, in humans during exercise the volume of blood in the pulmonary capillaries may double; therefore, the contribution of the capillaries to resistance decreases substantially. At a threefold increase in flow, the driving pressure across the lungs may increase only about 50%, which means that the calculated pulmonary vascular resistance must have decreased by 50%.

Active Regulation

One may argue that there is no need for active regulation of pulmonary blood flow in the adult because all the cardiac output must flow through the lung, and it is better to maintain low vascular resistance to keep the power requirement of the right ventricle as low as possible. In many organs the resistance vessels have the property of constricting when the transmural pressure rises, which opposes passive dilation resulting from the increased transmural distending pressure. When transmural pressure decreases, the smooth muscle responds by relaxing. This is called **autoregulation**. The mechanism is a local property of the vascular wall. Within limits, this maintains fairly constant flow. The lung does not exhibit autoregulation, which is good because otherwise it would be more difficult to increase cardiac output in exercise.

Although the passive effects of pressure on the distensible pulmonary vascular bed are prominent, active regulation does occur under physiologic and pathologic conditions. There is adequate smooth muscle associated with the small muscular pulmonary arteries, arterioles, and veins to substantially alter pulmonary vascular resistance. The smooth muscle may hypertrophy remarkably in pathologic conditions.

A number of naturally occurring substances will selectively affect the vasomotor tone of pulmonary arterial or venous vessels. Some are normally constrictors (decreased P_{AO_2}; thromboxane A_2; α-adrenergic catecholamines; histamine; angiotensin; several prostaglandins; neuropeptides; leukotrienes; serotonin; a newly discovered endothelial cell peptide, endothelin; and increased P_{CO_2}) and some are normally dilators (increased P_{AO_2}; β-adrenergic catecholamines; prostacyclin; endothelium-derived relaxing factor; acetylcholine when vascular tone is increased; bradykinin; and dopamine).

Alveolar Oxygen Tension

The factor of overriding importance governing minute-to-minute active regulation of the pulmonary circulation is the alveolar oxygen tension (P_{AO_2}). The partial pressure of oxygen in the air spaces is far more important than the oxygen tension within the mixed venous blood, which does not change much (Table 7-2). The reason P_{AO_2} is so important is that the small muscular pulmonary arteries and veins are surrounded by the alveolar gas of the terminal respiratory units they subserve (see Ch. 2). Ordinarily, the P_{AO_2} is high (100 mmHg), so the smooth muscle cells of microvessels in or near the alveolar walls are bathed in the highest oxygen tensions of any organ. Oxygen diffuses through the thin alveolar wall tissues into the smooth muscle cells.

There is a marked difference between the response of pulmonary vascular smooth muscle and that of the systemic circulation to low P_{O_2}. In the lung, low alveolar oxygen tension causes local constriction of the nearby arterioles, whereas in the systemic circulation low oxygen tension tends to relax the local resistance vessels, which permits passive dilation to occur. Why the response in the lung is opposite to that in the systemic circulation is not known, but it appears to be a direct effect of oxygen tension on the vascular smooth muscle cells.

As alveolar oxygen tension falls, the adjacent arterioles constrict. This decreases local blood flow and shifts it to other regions. Very small changes in local vascular resistance can cause marked shifts of blood flow without any significant effect on overall pulmonary vascular resistance, provided the volume of lung involved is not too large (say, 20% of the total lung mass).

On the other hand, a global reduction in alveolar oxygen tension, such as occurs at high altitude or in a person breathing low-oxygen mixtures, leads to a rise in pulmonary vascular resistance. Pulmonary vascular resistance in acute alveolar hypoxia may be more than twice the normal level. This is a sustained effect in humans and in most mammals. The effect of alveolar oxygen tension on pulmonary vascular resistance is chiefly on the arterioles and small muscular arteries. In many types of lung pathology, hypoxic vasoconstriction plays a major compensatory role. On the other hand, if a disease process (such as lobar pneumonia) blocks local hypoxic vasoconstriction, Pa_{O_2} may fall (increased shunt fraction). Thus, an important clinical test of the vasoconstrictor component of pulmonary hypertension is to determine the effect of oxygen inhalation on pulmonary vascular resistance. Pressure-flow curve 4 in Figure 7-2 shows the slight dilating effect of oxygen breathing in a normal person. This means that little hypoxic vasoconstriction occurs normally.

Remember: Alveolar oxygen tension regulates the pulmonary circulation locally. Increased Pa_{O_2} dilates and decreased Pa_{O_2} constricts the small arteries.

Thromboxane and Prostacyclin
The most important of the vasoconstrictors is **thromboxane A_2** (a product of arachidonic acid metabolism*), which is produced within the pulmonary circulation in several types of acute lung injury. Many cells, including leukocytes, macrophages, and endothelial cells, are capable of producing and releasing thromboxane. Thromboxane A_2 is one of the most powerful known constrictors of pulmonary arterial and venous smooth muscle. As with oxygen, the effect is mainly localized to the region where the thromboxane is released, although recirculation and diffusion through the lung interstitium sometimes spread its effect to airways and other vessels. Thromboxane constricts both arteries and veins.

Prostacyclin (prostaglandin I_2), another product of arachidonic acid metabolism, is a potent vasodilator. Endothelial cells are probably the chief source of this substance. Some physiologists hypothesize that a balance between thromboxane and prostacyclin production regulates normal pulmonary vascular tone. But there is little production of either thromboxane or prostacyclin normally. The normal smooth muscle tone of the pulmonary vascular bed is low.

---

* Arachidonic acid is a component of cell membranes and therefore ubiquitous in the body. It is readily metabolized by well-known intracellular pathways into several potent vasoactive compounds that diffuse into the surrounding media.

Remember: Thromboxane is a potent smooth muscle stimulant and is frequently detected in conditions in which pulmonary vasoconstriction occurs. It acts locally.

BRONCHIAL CIRCULATION

The bronchial arteries supply water and other nutrients to the mucosal cells and glands and to the airways, down to and including the terminal bronchioles. They also nourish the pleurae, interlobular septal supporting tissues, and pulmonary arteries and veins. Under normal conditions the bronchial circulation does not supply the terminal respiratory unit (alveoli, alveolar ducts, or respiratory bronchioles), which receives its nutrition via the alveolar wall capillaries.

The pressure in the main bronchial arteries is nearly the same as that in the aorta, so that regardless of body position there is a high driving pressure. Although bronchial blood flow is <1% of cardiac output, it is appropriate for the portion of the lungs it serves. Bronchial vascular resistance is much higher than that of the pulmonary circulation.

About one-half of bronchial blood flow returns to the right side of the heart via the bronchial veins. The remainder flows through small bronchopulmonary anastomoses (<100 μm diameter) into the pulmonary veins, thus contributing to the normal venous admixture (right-to-left shunt). In certain inflammatory diseases of the airways (bronchitis, bronchiectasis, bronchogenic carcinoma), the bronchial circulation expands dramatically and may contribute as much as 10 to 20% to the venous admixture.

When the pulmonary circulation is obstructed (due to thrombosis or embolism), the bronchial arteries dilate, enlarge, and develop connections with precapillary vessels of the pulmonary circulation. When this occurs, the blood flowing through the alveolar capillaries is systemic blood, which takes up little oxygen from the alveolar gas but can still give up carbon dioxide. Thus, the bronchial circulation keeps the lung alive when the pulmonary blood flow is shut off.

The bronchial circulation participates in conditioning the inspired air, especially under circumstances in which air bypasses the upper air passages (breathing through the mouth during exercise or in a patient with a tracheostomy [surgical opening of the trachea in the neck]). The bronchial circulation also supplies heat to warm the incoming air. Indeed, it is essentially impossible for air to be moved fast enough to reach the alveoli without having been completely warmed and humidified in air passages. Thus, there is no evaporation from the alveolar surfaces.

The bronchial circulation is the only angiogenic portion of the lung's circulation in the adult. Only in the fetus and newborn does the pulmonary circulation grow. In adult life, all new blood vessel growth in the lung comes from the bronchial circulation. Thus, all scars and tumors are supplied by bronchial vessels, even if, in the case of tumors, the original cancer cells arrived in the lung through the pulmonary circulation.

READINGS

Books

1. Forster RE II, Dubois AB, Briscow WA, Fisher AB: The Lung: Physiologic Basis of Pulmonary Function Tests. 3rd Ed. Year Book Medical Publishers, Chicago, 1986
   Chapter 6 is an excellent review of the pulmonary circulation and describes methods, including indicator dilution, for measuring flow. Also see the appendix.
2. Grover RF, Wagner WW Jr, McMurtry I, Reeves JT: Pulmonary circulation. pp. 103–136.

In Handbook of Physiology. Vol. III. The Cardiovascular System. American Physiological Society, Bethesda, MD, 1984
An extensive review particularly strong on the modern view about hypoxic pulmonary vasoconstriction. Includes a very extensive reference list.

3. Harris P, Heath D: The Human Pulmonary Circulation. 2nd Ed. Churchill Livingstone, Edinburgh, 1978
A thorough standard reference but heavy emphasis on pathology.

4. Nunn JF: Applied Respiratory Physiology. 3rd Ed. Butterworths, London, 1987
Chapter 6 thoroughly and clearly describes the indicator dilution method and lung zones. Venous admixture is described in a separate section.

Reviews

5. Deffenbach ME, Charan NB, Lakshminarayan S, Butler J: The bronchial circulation: small, but a vital attribute of the lung. Am Rev Respir Dis 135:463–481, 1987
The definitive up-to-date review of this underappreciated part of basic lung circulatory physiology.

6. Hyman AL, Spannhake EW, Kadowitz PJ: Prostaglandins and the lung. Am Rev Respir Dis 117:111–136, 1978
A thorough examination of the actions of numerous arachidonic acid metabolites on the pulmonary circulation.

7. McGregor M: Pulsus paradoxicus. N Engl J Med 301:480–482, 1979
An excellent brief review of how pleural pressure affects filling and emptying of the right and left hearts.

8. Mitzner W: Resistance of the pulmonary circulation. Clin Chest Med 4:127–137, 1983
A well-written discussion of pressure-flow curves under zone 2 conditions. The author is careful to distinguish between total pulmonary vascular resistance and what he refers to as *incremental resistance*. I do not think beginning physiology students should be concerned about such subtleties, but if you are fascinated by pulmonary hemodynamics, you will want to read this review.

Original Research

9. Bhattacharya J, Staub NC: Direct measurement of microvascular pressures in the isolated perfused dog lung. Science 210:327–328, 1980
The first direct micropuncture data on the longitudinal profile of lung microvascular pressure.

10. West JB, Dollery CT, Naimach A: Distribution of blood flow in isolated lung: relation to vascular and alveolar pressures. J Appl Physiol 19:713–724, 1964
The classic demonstration of lung blood flow zones in relation to vascular and alveolar pressure.

QUESTIONS*

Drill

1. Calculate the missing variable and explain the lung zone condition.

	PVR, cmH₂O × min/liter	Ppa, cmH₂O	PA, cmH₂O	Pla, cmH₂O	Q̇, liters/min
a.	?	40	0	20	10
b.	?	36	15	8	7
c.	4	22	0	12	?
d.	1	?	10	10	15
e.	?	12	?	6	0
f.	12	70	?	10	5

2. Calculate the total resistance across the pulmonary circulation, given the following partial resistances (cmH₂O × min/liter).
   a. Ra = 0.5; Rc = 0.4; Rv = 0.1
   b. Ra = 1.0; Rc, top = 1.0; Rc, mid = 0.75; Rc, bottom = 0.5; Rv = 0.2 (Top, mid, and bottom refer to three levels of the parallel capillaries shown in Fig. 7-8.)

Problems

3. Use the copy of Figure 7-2 below to calculate pulmonary vascular resistance at 3 and 10 liters/min for all four curves.

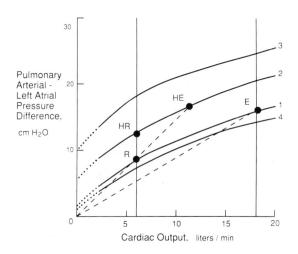

4. a. Given that bronchial blood flow equals 1% of cardiac output, calculate bronchial vascular resistance using whatever normal resting parameters from Appendix 2 are needed. b. Explain why bronchial vascular resistance is so high compared with overall systemic resistance.
5. If one injects 10 ml of blood at 0°C into the right atrium, what would cardiac output be if the mean pulmonary arterial temperature during passage of the bolus decreased 0.25°C and the time of tracer passage was 15 seconds. Normal pulmonary arterial temperature is 37.5°C in humans.

---

* Answers begin on page 211.

6. In a lung containing all three blood flow zones, flow in zone 2 is 50% of flow in zone 3. For a total cardiac output of 6.6 liters/min, what are the mean resistances in zones 1, 2, and 3, respectively, if Ppa = 24 and Pla = 7 cmH$_2$O? What is total resistance?

7. A patient enters the intensive care unit with her entire left lung (45% total lung mass) consolidated (unventilated) due to pneumococcal lobar pneumonia. She is observed to have bluish lips, fingernail beds, and skin (cyanosis), even though she is feverish (40°C) and the room is warm. Subsequent measurements reveal that her Pa$_{O_2}$ is 65 mmHg, even though she is breathing 100% O$_2$, $\dot{V}_{O_2}$ is 380 ml/min, and cardiac output is 7 liters/min.

   a. What is her venous admixture in liters per minute, assuming that any unstated parameters are normal? b. What can you infer about the factors regulating her pulmonary circulation?

   Using the pressure-flow graph of the normal human pulmonary vascular bed shown below, answer questions 8 and 9.

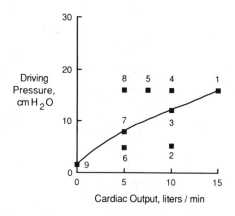

8. Which point best represents the lowest resistance?
   a. 1   b. 2   c. 4   d. 6   e. 9

9. Which pairs of points have the same resistance?
   a. 1 and 3   b. 6 and 8   c. 4 and 8   d. 4 and 7   e. 6 and 9

10. An unconscious patient is in the intensive care unit with his upper body at a 60-degree elevation, as represented by the figure below. He is breathing spontaneously but has an

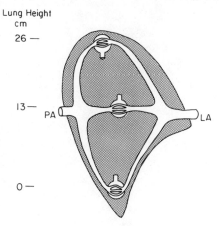

endotracheal tube in place. The tube has two channels so that each lung can breathe separately. The left lung is breathing against 10 cmH$_2$O continuous positive airway pressure; that is, Pao and P$_A$ = 10 cmH$_2$O whenever there is no airflow.

Which of the following statements is most nearly correct?

a. Mean pulmonary arterial pressure is probably increased above normal.
b. Mean pulmonary arterial pressure is probably decreased below normal.
c. Left atrial pressure is probably decreased below normal.
d. All of the right lung is in zone 2.
e. All of the left lung is in zone 1.

8

Matching Ventilation to Perfusion

THE BOTTOM LINE

Ventilation and Perfusion

The overall distribution of ventilation/perfusion, $\dot{V}_A/\dot{Q}$, is obtained by dividing the alveolar ventilation equation (Eq. 4-4) by the Fick blood flow equation (Eq. 3-5) to obtain

$$\frac{\dot{V}_A}{\dot{Q}} = \frac{0.863 \times R \times (Ca_{O_2} - C\bar{v}_{O_2})}{Pa_{CO_2}}$$

Thus, three independent variables determine the $\dot{V}_A/\dot{Q}$ ratio. For the whole lung, normal resting $\dot{V}_A/\dot{Q}$ is 0.84. The distribution of ventilation/perfusion ratios among terminal respiratory units, however, is not uniform, even in the normal lung, and may show marked deviations from normalcy in disease. The limiting $\dot{V}_A/\dot{Q}$ ratios are *wasted ventilation* ($\dot{V}_A/\dot{Q} = \infty$) and *venous admixture* ($\dot{V}_A/\dot{Q} = 0$). Other $\dot{V}_A/\dot{Q}$ distributions between these extremes are often shown on the O_2-CO_2 diagram.

Distribution of Ventilation

Ventilation is distributed nonuniformly in the lung on both a regional (gravitational) and a local (nongravitational) basis. Regional distribution predominates in the normal upright human. There is a twofold variation over the height of the lung (greater at the bottom) due to the regional variation of FRC (lung is more expanded toward the top). Local factors affecting ventilation distribution to each terminal respiratory unit are its resistance (R) and compliance (C), whose product, $R \times C$, equals τ, the time constant. The time constant determines the rate at which the unit will be ventilated. Furthermore, the unit's compliance determines its maximum ventilation relative to its starting (FRC) volume.

Distribution of Perfusion

Blood flow is distributed nonuniformly in the lung on both a regional (gravitational) and a local (nongravitational) basis. Regional distribution predominates in the normal upright

(Continues).

(*Continued*).

human. There is a fivefold variation over the height of the lung (greater at the bottom) that is due to the effect of gravity on the distensible vessels. The main local factor affecting perfusion distribution is the alveolar oxygen tension (P_{AO_2}). Hypoxic vasoconstriction is very effective provided the amount of lung tissue affected is small (<20% of lung mass).

Overall $\dot{V}A/\dot{Q}$ Distribution

In the normal upright human, the $\dot{V}A/\dot{Q}$ varies regionally from 0.7 at the bottom to 3 or higher at the top. Local $\dot{V}A/\dot{Q}$ imbalance due to variation of time constants among terminal respiratory units is not significant in the normal lung but becomes important in disease. Although the precise quantification of the $\dot{V}A/\dot{Q}$ distribution is beyond the scope of this text, nevertheless one can assess the overall effect on arterial oxygenation by determining the alveolar-arterial oxygen tension difference (A − a)ΔP_{O_2}. Normally, this difference is 10 to 15 mmHg, with wasted ventilation and venous admixture accounting for one-third and regional variation of $\dot{V}A/\dot{Q}$ accounting for two-thirds. In disease the (A − a)ΔP_{O_2} is often markedly increased, principally because of nonuniform $\dot{V}A/\dot{Q}$ distribution. Although ventilation/perfusion mismatching is usually described by its effect on arterial oxygen tension, P_{aCO_2} is also affected, although to a much lesser degree.

VENTILATION AND PERFUSION

The concept of matching gas flow (ventilation) and blood flow (perfusion) for successful oxygen and carbon dioxide exchange is simple, but the details and quantification can be extremely difficult. One example was presented in Chapter 7, where the P_{aO_2} due to venous admixture was calculated. Inequalities of the distribution of ventilation/perfusion ratios are the most common explanation for impairment of O_2 and CO_2 exchange. This chapter deals with the principal causes of ventilation/perfusion mismatching both under normal and pathologic conditions.

In the ideal lung, inspiration draws air at constant composition uniformly into each of the terminal respiratory units, so that each receives a fair share in relation to its FRC (constant fractional alveolar ventilation). In the ideal lung, the right ventricle distributes mixed venous blood to the alveolar wall capillaries flowing through each terminal respiratory unit so that each receives its fair share of pulmonary blood flow in relation to its ventilation. In the ideal lung, the blood leaving each terminal respiratory unit has the same P_{O_2} and P_{CO_2}. The main criteria for ideal matching of ventilation to perfusion are (1) no wasted alveolar ventilation and (2) no wasted blood flow. Ideally, the ventilation/perfusion ratio, $\dot{V}A/\dot{Q}$, is uniformly distributed.*

Since resting normal alveolar ventilation ($\dot{V}A$) is 4.2 liters/min and since normal resting pulmonary blood flow ($\dot{Q}$) is 5 liters/min, the normal $\dot{V}A/\dot{Q}$ = 4.2/5.0 = 0.84. Since it is a ratio, there are no units. There is no magic about these numbers, except that they give the normal P_{aO_2} of 100 mmHg and P_{aCO_2} of 40 mmHg at R = 0.80. If the alveolar ventilation equation (Eq. 4-4) is divided by the Fick equation for pulmonary blood flow using oxygen (Eq. 3-5) while keeping in mind the definition of R (Eq. 3-4), the whole lung ventilation/perfusion ratio will be obtained:

$$\frac{\dot{V}A}{\dot{Q}} = \frac{0.863 \times R \times (Ca_{O_2} - C\bar{v}_{O_2})}{P_{aCO_2}} \tag{8-1}$$

---

* Nearly everyone pronounces the abbreviation as "vee-aye-cue" or "vee-cue," instead of saying "ventilation/perfusion ratio."

In exercise $\dot{V}A/\dot{Q}$ rises. For example, during maximum steady-state exercise, $\dot{V}_{O_2} = 1,500$ ml/min (six times resting), $\dot{V}A = 26$ liters/min, and $\dot{Q} = 15$ liters/min, so $\dot{V}A/\dot{Q} = 1.7$. But $Pa_{O_2} = 100$ mmHg and $Pa_{CO_2} = 40$ mmHg because the $(\bar{v} - a)$ and ΔC_{CO_2} have increased, as described in Chapter 3. Thus, to interpret the $\dot{V}A/\dot{Q}$ ratio correctly one needs to know R (respiratory exchange ratio) and $\dot{V}_{O_2}$, as well as ventilation and blood flow.

In the real lung, neither ventilation nor blood flow is uniformly distributed, even in a healthy normal young adult. In patients with cardiopulmonary disease, the most frequent cause of systemic arterial hypoxemia is not hypoventilation or venous admixture (right-to-left shunt) but uneven alveolar ventilation in relation to alveolar blood flow.

We generally speak of ventilation/perfusion mismatching in terms of its effect on the alveolar-arterial P_{O_2} difference $(A - a)\Delta P_{O_2}$. There is a parallel but much smaller effect on CO_2 tension, which is generally ignored because the main cause of CO_2 retention is hypoventilation (see Ch. 4).

The two extreme instances of ventilation/perfusion mismatching are *wasted ventilation* (see Ch. 4) and *venous admixture* (see Ch. 6).

Wasted Ventilation

Wasted ventilation is shown schematically in Figure 8-1 (bottom). Such a situation may occur clinically when a large blood clot (pulmonary embolism) obstructs a pulmonary artery branch. In Figure 8-1, lung A has its blood flow cut off. It is assumed that no compensatory changes in ventilation or blood flow occur and that before the obstruction one-half of total pulmonary blood flow and one-half of alveolar ventilation went to each lung. Immediately after the occlusion, all the blood flow is diverted to lung B but one-half of ventilation still goes to lung A. Clearly, the ventilation to lung A is wasted because it is ineffective in oxygenating any of the mixed venous blood. Thus, this extra wasted ventilation greatly increases the physiologic dead space, and since it is located anatomically in the terminal respiratory units, it is called **alveolar dead space**. The overall efficiency of lung ventilation is decreased (see Eq. 6-8), since more than one-half the power used in breathing moves air that serves no useful purpose.

The ventilation/perfusion ratio of lung A is infinite because the denominator (blood flow) equals zero (2.1/0). But what is the ventilation/perfusion ratio of lung B in Figure 8-1 (bottom)? Clearly, it cannot be the normal value of 0.84. Lung B is receiving its normal portion of alveolar ventilation but *all* of the cardiac output. Its ventilation/perfusion ratio is 2.1/5.0 = 0.42. I will return to this problem near the end of this chapter, when I discuss compensatory changes that occur. However, something must change to bring the $\dot{V}A/\dot{Q}$ back toward its normal value, or else Pa_{CO_2} will be increased and Pa_{O_2} will be decreased. If that statement makes no sense, please review the section on alveolar ventilation in Chapter 4 before proceeding.

Venous Admixture

Venous admixture is shown schematically in Figure 8-1 (top), where lung A has no ventilation but still has its normal blood flow. Clearly, hypoxemia will result because there is now an absolute shunt of 50% of cardiac output. For lung A the $\dot{V}A/\dot{Q} = 0/2.5 = 0$. In other words, a right-to-left shunt is equivalent to saying the ventilation/perfusion ratio is 0. On the other hand, ventilation of lung B has doubled relative to its blood flow. For lung B the $\dot{V}A/\dot{Q} = 4.2/2.5 = 1.68$. This is clearly hyperventilation, as described in Chapter 4. Thus, the arterial P_{CO_2} will be decreased. The oxygen tension of blood in the pulmonary veins (Ppv_{O_2}) will rise, but due to the flat slope of the HbO_2 equilibrium curve at P_{O_2} values near 100 mmHg, the ventilated lung B is not able to compensate for the low P_{O_2} of the shunt through lung A, so Pa_{O_2} will be decreased.

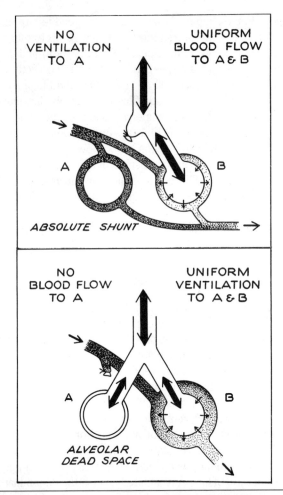

Fig. 8-1. Extremes of uneven ventilation or perfusion. (Top) One lung unit receives no ventilation but has normal blood flow; its $\dot{V}A/\dot{Q} = 0$. (Bottom) One lung unit receives normal ventilation but has no blood flow; $\dot{V}A/\dot{Q} = \infty$. (Modified from Comroe J: Physiology of Respiration. 2nd Ed. Year Book Medical Publishers, Chicago, 1974, with permission.)

Other Ventilation/Perfusion Distributions

If alveolar dead space ($\dot{V}A/\dot{Q} = \infty$) and right-to-left shunt ($\dot{V}A/\dot{Q} = 0$) represent the extremes of ventilation/perfusion mismatching, then all other possible ventilation/perfusion ratios must lie between these values. Figure 8-2 shows two examples. In the top panel, ventilation to lung B is reduced but is not zero; in the bottom panel, blood flow to lung B is reduced but is not zero. You can, however, imagine the units as if each were composed of two parts (concept of independent streams)—normal and shunt (top, inset) or normal and alveolar dead space (bottom, inset).

Even in the normal lung the $\dot{V}A/\dot{Q}$ distribution is not perfect, although on the average, the value of 0.84 is correct. Some lung units are overventilated and some are underventilated, thus forming a distribution around the mean. Figure 8-3A shows the distribution of $\dot{V}A/\dot{Q}$ in a normal human adult. The average normal value of 0.84 is shown as the thin vertical line. The y-axis is labeled in absolute units of ventilation or perfusion (liters per minute). The $\dot{V}A$ or $\dot{Q}$ value is read at each ventilation/perfusion ratio between 0 and 2 on the linear x-axis. This range is adequate to cover nearly all ventilation/perfusion ratios in the normal lung, but in disease there may be significant portions of lung with $\dot{V}A/\dot{Q}$ values above these limits. Thus, it has become customary to use a logarithmic x-axis, as shown in Figure 8-3B. I showed the linear x-axis first to demonstrate clearly that in the normal lung, the $\dot{V}A/\dot{Q}$ distribution is skewed; that is, there is more overventilation than overperfusion, something not readily seen on the more symmetrical logarithmic plot.

An elegant way of measuring the $\dot{V}A/\dot{Q}$ distribution in the lung is called the **multiple inert gas procedure**, in which six inert gases of differing gas-to-blood solubility ratios are infused intravenously until a steady state of gas elimination and infusion is established. From the infused ($P\bar{v}$) and expired ($PA = Pa$) partial pressures of each gas, a computer determines the most likely pattern of $\dot{V}A/\dot{Q}$ distribution that accounts for the data. Figure 8-3 shows the result of one such study.

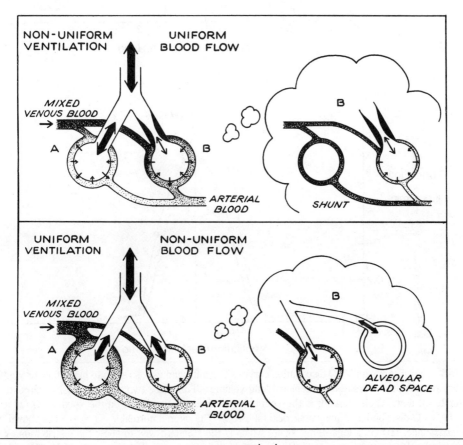

Fig. 8-2.   Examples of intermediate types of mismatched $\dot{V}A/\dot{Q}$. (Top) One lung unit (B) is underventilated owing to increased airway resistance. (Bottom) One lung unit (A) is underperfused owing to increased vascular resistance. One can imagine (balloons) that the affected lung is composed of two parts: one normal and one a shunt (top) or one normal and one alveolar dead space (bottom). (Modified from Comroe J: Physiology of Respiration. 2nd Ed. Year Book Medical Publishers, Chicago, 1974, with permission.)

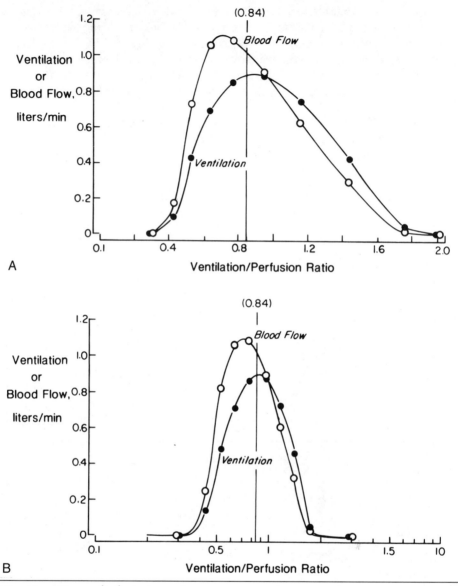

Fig. 8-3.   Normal human $\dot{V}A/\dot{Q}$ distribution curves. The left-hand y-axis refers to blood flow or ventilation (in liters per minute, corrected for regional lung volume). There are two curves, one for ventilation and one for blood flow. Their quotient is the ventilation/perfusion ratio shown on the x-axis. **(A)** On a linear scale the $\dot{V}A/\dot{Q}$ distribution is unsymmetrical (skewed). The overall normal $\dot{V}A/\dot{Q} = 0.84$ is shown by the thin vertical line. **(B)** On a logarithmic scale, which is the standard way to show the distribution, $\dot{V}A/\dot{Q}$ is symmetrically distributed (log normal distribution). In addition, a much wider range of $\dot{V}A/\dot{Q}$ can be conveniently shown, as is often necessary in disease. (Unpublished data courtesy of P. Wagner and J. West, University of California, San Diego.)

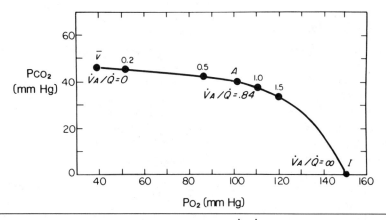

Fig. 8-4.   The O_2-CO_2 diagram indicating the extremes of $\dot{V}A/\dot{Q}$ as well as some intermediate points. Point I represents the inspired gas ($\dot{V}A/\dot{Q} = \infty$) and point $\bar{v}$ represents venous admixture ($\dot{V}A/\dot{Q} = 0$). Ideal $\dot{V}A/\dot{Q}$ is shown at point A.

O_2-CO_2 Diagram

Another way to look at the $\dot{V}A/\dot{Q}$ distribution is shown in Figure 8-4, which is a modification of the O_2-CO_2 diagram shown in Figure 4-4. The point marked A represents the normal Pa_{CO_2} and Pa_{O_2} for an ideal $\dot{V}A/\dot{Q} = 0.84$. All $\dot{V}A/\dot{Q}$ ratios greater than the normal value (overventilation) lie to the right of A. The extreme value of dead space (wasted) ventilation is the inspired point (I). To the left of the normal point A are all $\dot{V}A/\dot{Q}$ ratios less than 0.84 (overperfused). The mixed venous point $\bar{v}$ represents $\dot{V}A/\dot{Q} = 0$ (venous admixture).

In Figure 8-4, I have also added points for some representative $\dot{V}A/\dot{Q}$ ratios. Notice that the $\dot{V}A/\dot{Q}$ values are not arranged linearly along the line. Examine the shape of the O_2-CO_2 curve carefully. As the $\dot{V}A/\dot{Q}$ increases (moves to the right), P_{CO_2} falls more and more rapidly toward zero (inspired gas). At low $\dot{V}A/\dot{Q}$ values, however, the oxygen tension falls steeply but the P_{CO_2} cannot rise above that of mixed venous blood.

> **Remember:**   Any deviation of $\dot{V}A/\dot{Q}$ from ideal impairs the efficiency of O_2 and CO_2 transfer; that is, it increases the (A − a) gas tension differences, especially that for oxygen.

DISTRIBUTION OF VENTILATION

The normal lung is not uniformly ventilated. Regional nonuniform ventilation is mainly due to gravitational effects, such as from top to bottom in the upright human lung. Local nonuniform ventilation among terminal respiratory units is due to variable airway resistance (R) or compliance (C) and is described by the time constant ($\tau = R \times C$).

Regional Ventilation Distribution

In Chapter 2 the point was made that the lungs are not well supported by the trachea nor do they rest upon the diaphragm. They are suspended by their own weight, each level of lung being supported by the level above it. Ultimately, the force maintaining lung support is transmitted through the pleural liquid layer between the lung and the chest wall. Consequently, as one moves *up the lung* (see Fig. 2-1) the mass of lung that must be supported below each level increases. This means that the weight of the lung pulling down or away from the chest wall increases. Thus, pleural pressure decreases. If pleural pressure is decreased, then static translung pressure ($PL = PA - Ppl$) must be increased.

The result is that at all lung volumes below TLC the lung is expanded more near the top. Indeed, the relative alveolar volume follows the *dynamic* compliance curve of the lung. Figure 8-5A shows the end-expiratory volume of alveoli over the height of the lung. Lung height is shown along the x-axis with the bottom of the lung to the left. The alveoli at the bottom are at residual volume, while those at the top are above 60% TLC, even though the lung as a whole is at FRC (open circle). The PL for each 20% of lung volume is shown on the right-hand y-axis, which is not linear because lung compliance is not a linear function of lung volume (Fig. 8-5B). It is important to know the difference between regional terminal respiratory unit end-expiratory volume (regional FRC) and overall lung FRC.

Figure 8-5B shows the dynamic pressure-volume curve for the lung. The slope for the compliance curve for the alveoli at lower FRC (bottom of lung) is greater than the slope of the alveoli at higher FRC (top of lung). This means that at slow inspiration rates (<1.5 liters/sec, as in normal breathing) the lower lung is easier to ventilate (smaller time constant). Thus, two factors tend to increase ventilation toward the bottom of the lung relative to the top; namely, the lower end-expiratory volume (FRC) and the higher dynamic compliance.

The distribution of ventilation over the height of the lung varies about twofold (Fig. 8-5C). The regional distribution of ventilation is a major factor in determining the composition of alveolar gas when measured during expiration, since the better-ventilated alveoli tend to empty first. This is the basis of an important, commonly used pulmonary function test, known as the **single-breath nitrogen test**, for the uniformity of ventilation distribution.

Local Ventilation Distribution

Nongravitational uneven distribution of ventilation is due to variation in the time constants ($\tau = R \times C$). In Figure 8-6, three pairs of lung units show how the time constant concept works. A larger time constant means slower ventilation. Thus, a unit with increased resistance, increased compliance, or both will take longer to fill, all else being constant.

Since breathing is a dynamic process, time is important even at rest. At the normal breathing rate of 12 breaths per minute, inspiratory time (TI) is 2 seconds and expiratory time (TE) is 3 seconds, which may not be long enough for every terminal respiratory unit to achieve a new steady state. In diseases such as chronic obstructive pulmonary disease (emphysema), some lung units may fill and empty very slowly. When chest physicians refer to "fast" and "slow" alveoli, they are referring to the time constants of those units.

The local ventilation distribution depends on breathing frequency. In normal adult humans, the dynamic compliance is not much affected by a wide range of breathing rates, but in disease there may be dramatic frequency dependence.

Figure 8-6A shows two normal terminal respiratory units that have equal $R \times C$ and thus have equal time constants (τ). These units fill equally and synchronously in 2 seconds (normal inspiratory time), as shown in the inset graph. Figure 8-6B shows two units, one of which has twice the airway resistance of the other. This unit will eventually fill as much as its mate, given enough time, but during a normal 2-second inspiration, it fills less completely (that is, its ventilation will be reduced). Figure 8-6C shows two units, one of which has a reduced compliance. This unit fills less completely but faster than its mate because its time constant is reduced.

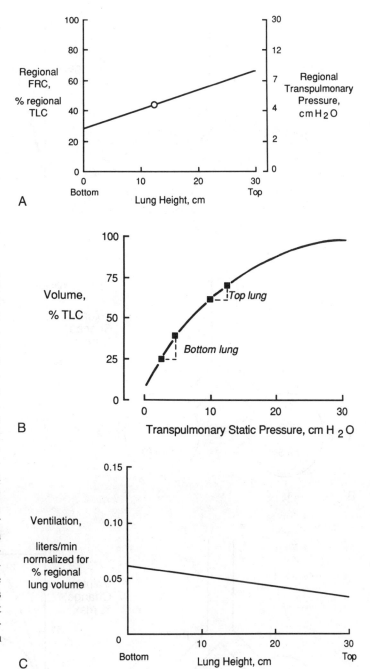

Fig. 8-5. Regional distribution of lung volume. **(A)** Regional FRC normalized to percentage of regional TLC (left-hand y-axis). This corrects for the uneven distribution of lung shape. The FRC increases as one moves up the lung because the static translung pressure (PL) (right-hand y-axis) also increases. The PL scale is not linear since lung volume is not a linear function of PL (Fig. 5-3). For example, PL at the bottom is 3.0 cmH$_2$O (28% of TLC) compared with 8.0 cmH$_2$O at the top (65% of TLC). The average FRC (45% of TLC at PL of 4.5 cmH$_2$O) occurs at a point 12.5 cm up from the base of the lung. **(B)** Increasing transpulmonary pressure (inspiration) affects regional expansion because of the position of different regions of the lung on the dynamic compliance curve. Units near the bottom of the lung are close to residual volume (RV) and have a higher compliance (steeper slope on the dynamic compliance curve) than those near the top, which are already at 65% of TLC. Thus, during inspiration more fresh air goes to the units of the bottom of the lung, as their time constant is lower. **(C)** The distribution of ventilation from the bottom to the top of the lung is shown for the normal upright human lung. Ventilation distribution shows a twofold variation over the height of the lung.

These are three examples of many to illustrate the complex effects of resistance and compliance variations on local ventilation distribution.

Interestingly, airway resistance of lung units is affected by the local ventilation because PA$_{CO_2}$ affects airway smooth muscle tone. This effect compensates for under- or overventilation. Decreasing PA$_{CO_2}$ increases local airway resistance.

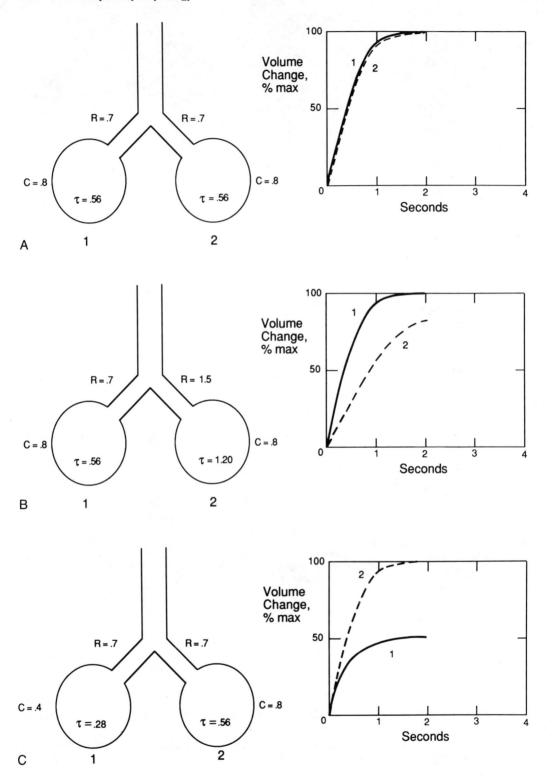

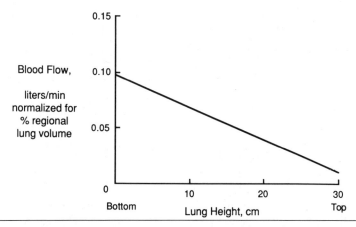

Fig. 8-7.   Distribution of blood flow over the height of the lung in a normal upright human. Blood flow distribution varies more than does ventilation distribution (cf. Fig. 8-5C).

DISTRIBUTION OF PERFUSION

Regional Perfusion Distribution

Chapter 7 described the distribution of blood flow on a regional basis from top to bottom of the lung, explaining it in terms of the effect of gravity on the transmural distending pressure of the blood vessels and the relative arterial, venous, and alveolar pressures (lung zones). Figure 8-7 confirms that in the normal lung the blood flow distribution varies from top to bottom. For simplicity the distribution is shown as linear, which is reasonably correct. Quantitatively, the normal distribution of blood flow shows a greater (fivefold) variation between the bottom and the top of the lung than does ventilation (twofold variation).

Local Perfusion Distribution

An important nongravitational distribution of blood flow to terminal respiratory units occurs. Here the main regulating factor is the alveolar oxygen tension ($P_{A_{O_2}}$), which affects the arterial resistance to a particular unit by the hypoxic vasoconstrictor mechanism. This is a useful compensatory mechanism to decrease blood flow to underventilated alveoli.

The effectiveness of the hypoxic vasoconstrictor phenomenon depends on the fraction of lung involved. If only a small volume (<20% of lung mass) is vasoconstricted because of alveolar hypoxia, the effect on the overall pulmonary hemodynamics is trivial; that is, pulmonary arterial

←
_____

Fig. 8-6.   Examples of local regulation of ventilation due to variation of resistance (R) or compliance (C) of individual lung units. Although normally regional distribution of ventilation predominates, in lung disease the local distribution may be of overriding importance. **(A)** The normal lung is represented as two units, which have equal R and C; the time constant (τ) of each unit is 0.56 second. These units fill equally and reach 97% of final equilibrium in 2 seconds, the normal inspiratory time, as shown in the graph. **(B)** One unit has doubled resistance, so its time constant is doubled. That unit fills more slowly and reaches only 80% equilibrium during a normal breath. The unit is underventilated. **(C)** One unit has reduced compliance (it is stiff), which acts to reduce its time constant. This unit fills faster than the normal unit but only receives one-half of the ventilation. It is also underventilated.

pressure is not increased. This is a critical point about the physiologic usefulness of local regulation of blood flow distribution, which allows adjustment of local perfusion to local ventilation.

When a large fraction of the lung (>20%) is involved, then hypoxic vasoconstriction causes increased pulmonary arterial pressure because total pulmonary vascular resistance is increased. The extreme case is global alveolar hypoxia, in which pulmonary arterial pressure may be doubled. This actually improves the $\dot{V}_A/\dot{Q}$ distribution because the rise in pulmonary arterial pressure tends to even out the normal gravitational maldistribution of blood flow (see Fig. 7-6).

OVERALL $\dot{V}_A/\dot{Q}$ DISTRIBUTION

Regional $\dot{V}_A/\dot{Q}$

To determine the regional distribution of ventilation relative to perfusion, we combine the ventilation and blood flow distribution of Figures 8-5C and 8-7. This is shown in Figure 8-8A for a normal human lung at FRC. At the bottom, blood flow exceeds ventilation; at the top, ventilation exceeds blood flow. The only location in the lung where the $\dot{V}_A/\dot{Q}$ = 0.84 (the average value for the normal whole lung) is approximately halfway up the lung. To obtain the distribution of $\dot{V}_A/\dot{Q}$ over the height of the lung, divide the number for ventilation by the number for blood flow, as read from the left-hand y-axis. For example, at the bottom of the lung, the ventilation is 0.07 liter/min compared with a blood flow of 0.1 liter/min. Therefore the $\dot{V}_A/\dot{Q}$ of that portion of the lung is 0.07/0.1 = 0.7.

The curved line with the solid squares in Figure 8-8A represents the distribution of $\dot{V}_A/\dot{Q}$ for nine regions of the normal human lung. Over the lower two-thirds of the lung the $\dot{V}_A/\dot{Q}$ ratio does not vary much. It is only near the top, where blood flow falls to low levels (high in zone 2 approaching zone 1) that the ratio rises steeply. This partially explains why the $\dot{V}_A/\dot{Q}$ distribution on a linear scale (Fig. 8-3A) is skewed.

To complete the description of the $\dot{V}_A/\dot{Q}$ distribution, examine Figure 8-8B, which is the O_2-CO_2 diagram again but this time with the $\dot{V}_A/\dot{Q}$ points associated with each of the nine regions in Figure 8-8A. With the aid of the O_2-CO_2 diagram, one can read the $P_{A_{O_2}}$ and $P_{A_{CO_2}}$ corresponding to each $\dot{V}_A/\dot{Q}$ ratio. Toward the bottom of the lung, where the ventilation/perfusion ratios are below the normal value of 0.84, the $P_{A_{CO_2}}$ is slightly increased, while the $P_{A_{O_2}}$ is markedly decreased. Toward the top of the lung, where the ventilation/perfusion ratios are increased, the $P_{A_{CO_2}}$ falls rapidly toward zero, while $P_{A_{O_2}}$ rises toward that of inspired gas.

Local $\dot{V}_A/\dot{Q}$

Unfortunately, there is no simple graphic approach to identify the nongravitational distribution of ventilation/perfusion ratios in the lung. That requires very complicated procedures done only in a few specialized pulmonary function laboratories. However, one can examine the effect of mismatching of ventilation to perfusion in a general way by determining the alveolar-arterial oxygen tension difference $(A - a)\Delta P_{O_2}$.

Notice that P_{O_2} in Figure 8-8B varies by more than 40 mmHg from the bottom to the top of the lung. Blood leaving units near the bottom has a lower P_{O_2} and consequently a lower S_{O_2} than blood leaving units near the top. Also, there is more flow to the bottom of the lung. You have already learned that increasing alveolar P_{O_2} above normal does not have much effect on blood oxygen saturation or concentration because the HbO_2 equilibrium curve is so flat above a P_{O_2} of 70 mmHg. Therefore, when there is any $\dot{V}_A/\dot{Q}$ mismatching, the mixed arterial P_{O_2} will always be less than the ideal value. To make a precise calculation, one must know the blood flow through each of the nine different regions.

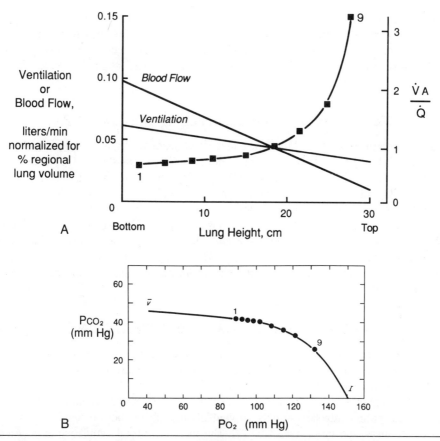

Fig. 8-8. Regional distribution of ventilation to perfusion in the normal lung. **(A)** Figures 8-7 and 8-5C are combined. The left-hand y-axis represents ventilation or perfusion in liters per minute. The right-hand y-axis is $\dot{V}A/\dot{Q}$. The x-axis is distance up the lung. The curved line is the distribution of $\dot{V}A/\dot{Q}$ obtained by dividing ventilation by perfusion at nine different points. Over the lower part of the lung, $\dot{V}A/\dot{Q}$ does not change much, whereas over the upper part of the lung, it changes dramatically. There is only one point, about halfway between the bottom and top of the lung, where the $\dot{V}A/\dot{Q}$ ratio equals the overall normal value of 0.84. **(B)** O_2-CO_2 diagram with the ventilation/perfusion points from Figure 8-8A added. Pa_{O_2} varies by more than 40 mmHg over the height of the lung, whereas Pa_{CO_2} varies by 14 mmHg.

In the normal human lung, although venous admixture due to venous blood bypassing the lung (anatomic shunt) is only 1 to 2% of cardiac output, the $\dot{V}A/\dot{Q}$ mismatch contribution to venous admixture may be 4 to 5%. Thus, the normal systemic arterial P_{O_2} in humans is about 90 mmHg, giving an $(A - a)\Delta P_{O_2}$ of about 10 mmHg. It is not necessary to learn exact numbers because they vary so much among individuals. $(A - a)\Delta P_{O_2}$ values of 20 mmHg or less are considered to be normal.

Remember: Most of the normal $(A - a)\Delta P_{O_2}$ is due to $\dot{V}A/\dot{Q}$ variations on a regional basis.

The consequence of the normal distribution of $\dot{V}_A/\dot{Q}$ is to decrease arterial oxygen saturation slightly to about 96.9% (Pa_{O_2} = 90 mmHg); that is, about 0.5% less than the ideal arterial oxygen saturation of 97.4%. At normal blood flow and oxygen consumption, mixed venous blood saturation must also be reduced by 0.5% to a value of 74.5%, instead of 75%. That reduces the $P\bar{v}_{O_2}$ by about 1 mmHg.

Ventilation/Perfusion Mismatching and Arterial P_{CO_2}

Although everything discussed thus far about $\dot{V}_A/\dot{Q}$ mismatching is stated in terms of arterial oxygen tension, there must be a comparable effect on Pa_{CO_2}, as the O_2-CO_2 diagram (Fig. 8-8B) shows. If the lung has a reduced efficiency for oxygen uptake, it must also have a reduced efficiency for CO_2 output. However, one can see immediately from looking at the O_2-CO_2 diagram in Figure 8-8B that the effects on Pa_{CO_2} are much less than the effects on Pa_{O_2}. Indeed, many people with fairly severe lung disease and considerable $\dot{V}_A/\dot{Q}$ mismatching may have nearly normal Pa_{CO_2}. As discussed in Chapters 9 and 11, this occurs because the CO_2 equilibrium curve of blood is almost linear and because of the overriding effect of arterial P_{CO_2} on ventilation. Contrary to what one might think, regulatory mechanisms of ventilation are far more sensitive to Pa_{CO_2} than to Pa_{O_2}.

COMPENSATION FOR $\dot{V}_A/\dot{Q}$ MISMATCHING

Obviously, the situations represented in Figure 8-1 are unstable. There is an enormous wasted ventilation in Figure 8-1, bottom, and wasted blood flow in Figure 8-1, top, so that Pa_{CO_2} and Pa_{CO_2} are adversely affected.

Fortunately, a number of compensatory mechanisms come into play. Initially, these are centrally mediated (brain controller) effects on ventilation, which in both examples shown rises as a result of the increased Pa_{CO_2} (see Ch. 11). But increasing total ventilation is only a stopgap because the wasted ventilation fraction is not affected.

Local factors, however, also come into play, and these are of great importance. When ventilation is wasted, the local Pa_{CO_2} falls. This lowers the hydrogen ion concentration [H^+] in and around the associated airway smooth muscle, which leads to airway constriction and a shift of ventilation away from the terminal respiratory units with high $\dot{V}_A/\dot{Q}$. The compensation can be very effective depending on how large the affected lung unit is and how much its time constant increases.

If blood flow is reduced to a terminal respiratory unit, then the local alveolar cell metabolism, notably surfactant production or its release, will be affected. A rising air-liquid interfacial tension reduces the lung unit's compliance, and its FRC volume decreases. This is an effective compensatory mechanism for severely underperfused units. It is a slow mechanism, however (hours to days), compared with the very fast changes in total ventilation (seconds) and local airway tone (seconds to minutes) caused by changes in P_{CO_2}.

When alveolar P_{O_2} decreases because of hypoventilation, low inspired P_{O_2}, or excessive local blood flow, the hypoxia leads to local pulmonary arterial vasoconstriction (hypoxic vasoconstriction), which reduces local blood flow, provided the mass of lung involved is not too large. Thus, compensation for altered $\dot{V}_A/\dot{Q}$ usually is remarkably effective, if the mass of lung involved is not too large or if the remaining lung is not too damaged. The human lung is so good at compensating for $\dot{V}_A/\dot{Q}$ mismatching that relying on arterial blood gas tensions alone may lead one to seriously underestimate the degree of abnormality.

READINGS

Books

1. Forster RE II, Dubois AB, Briscoe WA, Fisher AB: The Lung: Physiologic Basis of Pulmonary Function Tests. 3rd Ed. Year Book Medical Publishers, Chicago, 1986
   Chapter 7 contains a clear description of ventilation/perfusion including quantitative analyses of several examples. The alveolar-arterial P_{O_2} and P_{CO_2} differences are described. The multiple inert gas method is introduced. Be sure to read this before reading the paper by Wagner et al. (reference 6).
2. Nunn JF: Applied Respiratory Physiology. 3rd Ed. Butterworths, London, 1987
   Chapter 7 is useful, especially about time constants and local $\dot{V}A/\dot{Q}$ mismatching.
3. West JP: Ventilation/Blood Flow and Gas Exchange. 3rd Ed. Blackwell, Oxford, 1977
   The definitive and readable description of $\dot{V}A/\dot{Q}$ in the lung.

Reviews

4. Lenfant C: Measurement of ventilation/perfusion distribution with alveolar arterial differences. J Appl Physiol 18:1090–1094, 1963
   Describes how mismatching of $\dot{V}A/\dot{Q}$ affects the $(A - a)\Delta P_{O_2}$ and $(A - a)\Delta P_{CO_2}$.
5. Milic-Emili J, Henderson JAM, Dolovich MB, et al: Regional distribution of inspired gas in the lung. J Appl Physiol 21:749–759, 1966
   The classic description of uneven ventilation distribution in humans.
6. Wagner PD, Saltzman HA, West JF: Measurement of continuous distribution of ventilation perfusion ratios: theory. J Appl Physiol 36:588–599, 1974
   Description of the multiple inert gas method for determining the continuous description of $\dot{V}A/\dot{Q}$ ratios. You may find this very difficult.
7. West JF: Ventilation-perfusion relationships. Am Rev Respir Dis 116:919–943, 1977
   Readable up-to-date review with human examples.

QUESTIONS*

Drill

1. Use the $\dot{V}A/\dot{Q}$ equation for the whole lung (Eq. 8-1) to calculate the missing variable. State what you can deduce about the $\dot{V}A/\dot{Q}$, $\dot{V}A$, and $\dot{Q}$ in each condition and give specific reasons.

	$\dot{V}A$, liters/min	$\dot{Q}$, liters/min	R	$Ca - C\bar{v}_{O_2}$, ml O_2 /liter	Pa_{CO_2}, mmHg
a.	?	?	0.80	50	80
b.	?	?	0.84	40	36
c.	?	?	1.00	75	40
d.	?	?	0.80	46	40
e.	?	12.0	0.70	100	50
f.	10.0	?	0.80	50	20

Problems

2. In Figure 8-1 (bottom), one-half of the alveolar ventilation is wasted. Calculate the steady-state mean mixed PA_{CO_2} (combination of the alveolar ventilation of both units) if total alveolar ventilation, blood flow, $\dot{V}_{O_2}$, and R have their normal resting values.

3. In Figure 8-1 (top), one-half of the blood flow is shunted by the lung. Calculate mean mixed PA_{O_2} and then the Ppv_{O_2} of blood leaving the perfused lung if total ventilation, blood flow, $\dot{V}_{O_2}$, and R have their normal resting values.

4. a. Is static lung compliance affected by the rate of breathing? Explain your answer. b. If dynamic compliance is affected by frequency over the breathing rate of 10 to 40 breaths per min, does it increase or decrease as frequency rises? Explain.

5. The figure below shows data obtained in a normal adult human at rest and during moderate exercise. Assuming the distribution of ventilation is the same as shown in Figure 8-5C, describe the effect of exercise on $\dot{V}A/\dot{Q}$.

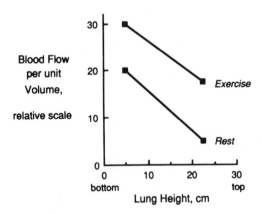

In the following two questions draw the time course of filling of both lung units in a manner analogous to Figure 8-5.

6. The resistance to one lung unit is doubled and the compliance is halved, as shown in the figure below.

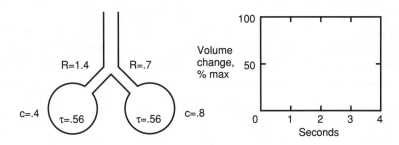

7. The compliance and resistance of one lung unit are each doubled, as shown in the accompanying figure.

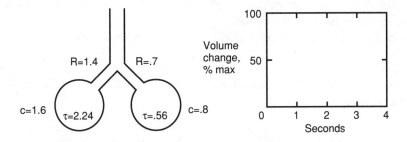

8. In which of the following $\dot{V}_A/\dot{Q}$ disturbances is Pa_{O_2} likely to be increased?
   a. Increased alveolar ventilation
   b. Decreased alveolar ventilation
   c. Increased cardiac output at constant oxygen consumption
   d. Decreased cardiac output at constant oxygen consumption
   e. Decreased alveolar ventilation and increased cardiac output at constant oxygen consumption

The next two problems require some calculations to determine the effect of $\dot{V}_A/\dot{Q}$ mismatching on the $(A - a)\Delta P_{O_2}$ and $(A - a)\Delta P_{CO_2}$. Determining mean alveolar composition by using the mixing equations is much easier than determining mean arterial gas tensions. It is also easier to calculate the CO_2 gradient because the $C_{CO_2} - P_{CO_2}$ equilibrium curve is essentially linear compared with the complex HbO_2 equilibrium curve.

9. The lungs of a normal, resting, upright human can be approximated by a three-compartment $\dot{V}_A/\dot{Q}$ model as shown below. One does not need the actual ventilation or flow to each compartment, only the fraction.

Compartment	$\dot{V}_A/\dot{Q}$	$\dot{V}_A$, %	$\dot{Q}$, %	$P_{A_{O_2}}$, mmHg	$P_{A_{CO_2}}$, mmHg
1	1.7	20	10	120	35
2	0.9	35	33	102	40
3	0.7	45	57	93	41

Assuming normal values for any unstated parameters you need, calculate:

a. Mean $P_{A_{CO_2}}$ and $P_{A_{O_2}}$

b. Mean $P_{a_{CO_2}}$ and $P_{a_{O_2}}$ (assume a linear $C_{CO_2} - P_{CO_2}$ equilibrium curve)

c. $(A - a)\Delta P_{CO_2}$ and $(A - a)\Delta P_{O_2}$ (either use Figure 1-2 and calculate bound and dissolved O_2 or look ahead to Figure 9-1, which has a table of blood oxygen concentration)

10. One way to analyze more complex ventilation/perfusion problems is to set up three "as if" compartments, as shown below, with $\dot{V}_A/\dot{Q} = \infty$ (wasted ventilation), 0 (right-to-left shunt), and 0.84 (normal). In this example, the mixed venous gas tensions and saturation and the absolute values for $\dot{V}_A$ and $\dot{Q}$ rather than the alveolar gas tensions are given.

Compartment	$\dot{V}_A$, liters/min	$\dot{Q}$, liters/min	$\dot{V}_A/\dot{Q}$	$P_{A_{CO_2}}$, mmHg	$P_{A_{O_2}}$, mmHg
1	1.0	0	0		
2	4.2	5.0	0.84		
3	0	1.0	∞		
Total	5.2	6.0	0.87		

Given that $P\bar{v}_{O_2}$ is about 38 mmHg and $S\bar{v}_{O_2}$ is about 71% and assuming normal values for other parameters as needed, calculate:

a. Mean $P_{A_{CO_2}}$, $P_{a_{CO_2}}$, and $(A - a)\Delta P_{CO_2}$ (assume a linear $C_{CO_2} - P_{CO_2}$ equilibrium curve)

b. Mean $P_{A_{O_2}}$, $P_{a_{O_2}}$, and $(A - a)\Delta P_{O_2}$ (for the latter, either use Figure 1-2 and calculate bound and dissolved O_2 or look ahead to Figure 9-1, which has a table of blood oxygen concentration)

Transport of Oxygen and Carbon Dioxide

THE BOTTOM LINE

Oxygen Transport

Hemoglobin quickly and reversibly binds with oxygen. The oxygen capacity of normal human blood (150 g Hb/liter) is 201 ml O_2/liter. The position of the hemoglobin-oxygen (HbO_2) equilibrium curve is well suited for the loading of oxygen in the lungs and its unloading in systemic tissue capillaries. Normal physiologic factors affecting the HbO_2 curve are hydrogen ion concentration, P_{CO_2}, temperature, and the concentration of 2,3-diphosphoglycerate in erythrocytes. An increase in any of these factors shifts the position of the HbO_2 curve to the right, reflecting decreased hemoglobin affinity for oxygen and increased partial pressure for half saturation (P_{50}). A decrease in any of the physiologic variables increases the affinity of hemoglobin for oxygen (shifts the curve to the left) and decreases the P_{50}. A small (2- to 3-mmHg) shift to the right (decreased affinity) occurs as blood passes through systemic capillaries because P_{CO_2} and hydrogen ion concentration increase. This shift increases O_2 unloading in the systemic capillaries; a reverse shift occurs in the lung, favoring O_2 uptake. The shape of the HbO_2 equilibrium curve is such that variations in $P_{A_{O_2}}$ (± 30 mmHg) have little effect on the amount of oxygen carried by arterial blood, whereas in systemic capillaries hemoglobin releases large quantities of oxygen as P_{O_2} falls below 70 mmHg. The shape of the curve can be affected by genetic variants of the hemoglobin molecule. The most common hemoglobin variant is fetal hemoglobin (HbF). Another clinically important variant is sickle cell hemoglobin (HbS). The marked leftward shifts of the HbO_2 curve caused by most other hemoglobin variants make them almost useless as oxygen transporters. Carbon monoxide (CO) has 250 times greater affinity for hemoglobin than does oxygen. Even in very low concentrations, it combines avidly with hemoglobin, interferes with oxygen binding, and markedly lowers the P_{O_2} (left shift) at which O_2 is unloaded in systemic capillaries.

Diffusion

Diffusion is the process by which respiratory gas molecules move by random kinetic energy from the regions of high to regions of low partial pressure. The transport of

(Continues).

(Continued).

oxygen between body compartments is governed by diffusion at a rate dependent on the P_{O2} gradient. Diffusion across the alveolus-blood barrier in the lung is seldom a serious problem because the barrier is so thin (1.5 μm). The principal diffusion limitation for oxygen is from the systemic capillaries through a several-micrometers-thick layer of interstitial liquid to the mitochondria of the respiring cells.

Carbon Dioxide Transport

Metabolic carbon dioxide is produced by aerobic metabolism in mitochondria, diffuses into systemic capillary blood, and is transported to the lungs, where it diffuses into alveolar gas and is exhaled. CO_2 is 20 times as soluble in water as is oxygen. It combines chemically with water to produce carbonic acid but at a slow rate. In erythrocytes the enzyme *carbonic anhydrase* catalyzes this reaction. Once formed, carbonic acid dissociates almost instantly into hydrogen ions (H^+) and bicarbonate ions. The hydrogen ions are removed by combining chemically with the enormous amount of hemoglobin within the red blood cells. The bicarbonate ions diffuse out of the red blood cells in exchange for chloride ions. Some of the CO_2 combines chemically with the hemoglobin molecule to form carbaminohemoglobin.

This chapter reviews the hemoglobin-oxygen (HbO_2) equilibrium curve, the metabolic and pathophysiologic factors that affect it, and their physiologic significance. Oxygen diffusion from the alveolar gas into the hemoglobin in the pulmonary capillaries and, more importantly, the oxygen pathway from the systemic capillaries into the tissue cell mitochondria are briefly described. Last, the transport of metabolic CO_2 to the lungs is discussed, mainly the forms by which CO_2 is carried in venous blood. In a break from tradition, a separate chapter (Ch. 10) discusses the role of CO_2 in the regulation of hydrogen ion concentration [H^+].

OXYGEN TRANSPORT

The Hemoglobin-Oxygen Equilibrium Curve

Earlier chapters discussed oxygen transport in blood, especially the reversible binding of O_2 to hemoglobin, and how to calculate hemoglobin-oxygen saturation (S_{O_2}) by using the HbO_2 equilibrium curve (Fig. 1-2). These initial paragraphs are by way of review, to tidy up some loose ends and to collect the information in one place for easy retrieval.

Figure 9-1 shows the HbO_2 equilibrium curve of normal human blood at 37°C and at a hydrogen ion concentration [H^+] of 40 nmol/liter (40×10^{-9} mol/liter; pH 7.40). A table of O_2 transport data for normal whole blood is shown below the curve. Row A shows the total O_2 concentration (milliliters per liter) as a function of P_{O_2} in steps of 10 mmHg. Row B shows the small quantity of O_2 dissolved in whole blood, since O_2 is not very soluble in plasma or in interstitial or intracellular liquid. Row C shows the concentration of O_2 chemically bound to hemoglobin, and row D shows the percentage saturation, which is the amount of O_2 bound relative to the hemoglobin capacity.

If we had to depend on dissolved O_2 to sustain the normal resting oxygen consumption of 250 ml/min, cardiac output would have to be more than 80 liters/min, even if all the oxygen could be extracted from the blood. At $P_{O_2} = 100$ mmHg, 1 liter of blood holds only 3 ml O_2 in physical solution. Fortunately, blood carries the iron-containing red protein hemoglobin packed into erythrocytes. Hemoglobin, at its normal concentration of 150 g/liter, permits whole blood to carry 65 times more oxygen at a P_{O_2} of 100 mmHg than does plasma.

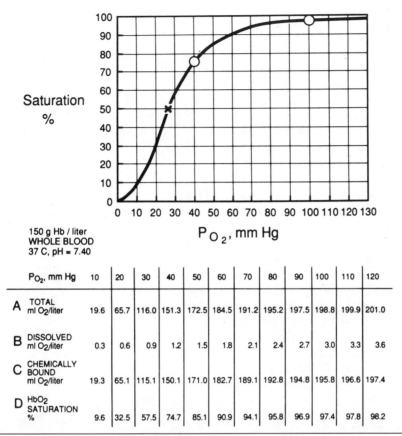

P_{O_2}, mm Hg	10	20	30	40	50	60	70	80	90	100	110	120
A TOTAL ml O$_2$/liter	19.6	65.7	116.0	151.3	172.5	184.5	191.2	195.2	197.5	198.8	199.9	201.0
B DISSOLVED ml O$_2$/liter	0.3	0.6	0.9	1.2	1.5	1.8	2.1	2.4	2.7	3.0	3.3	3.6
C CHEMICALLY BOUND ml O$_2$/liter	19.3	65.1	115.1	150.1	171.0	182.7	189.1	192.8	194.8	195.8	196.6	197.4
D HbO$_2$ SATURATION %	9.6	32.5	57.5	74.7	85.1	90.9	94.1	95.8	96.9	97.4	97.8	98.2

Fig. 9-1.   Standard hemoglobin-oxygen equilibrium curve for normal human blood (hemoglobin type A), [H$^+$] = 40 nmol/liter (pH 7.40), P_{CO_2} = 40 mmHg, temperature = 37°C and [2,3-DPG] = 15 μmol/g Hb. The two open circles are the ideal systemic arterial and mixed venous points at rest, ignoring the slight displacement of the mixed venous blood point caused by increased hydrogen ion concentration and P_{CO_2} in venous blood. The small cross ($\times$) indicates that the half-saturation point (P$_{50}$) is 26 mmHg. In the table below the graph are shown, as a function of P_{O_2} in steps of 10 mmHg: total oxygen concentration, dissolved oxygen, chemically bound oxygen, and percent saturation (S$_{O_2}$).

Hemoglobin consists of four O$_2$-binding heme molecules (iron-containing porphyrin rings) and globin (protein) chains, with one heme group per chain. The molecular weight of hemoglobin is 66,500. It appears to have evolved from myoglobin (the skeletal muscle heme protein) by the attachment of four myoglobin chains together. There are three important physiologic properties of the chemical binding of hemoglobin with O$_2$.

Hemoglobin Binding of Oxygen

Hemoglobin combines rapidly and reversibly with O$_2$. The O$_2$-containing form is called oxy-hemoglobin (HbO$_2$), and the unoxygenated form is called deoxyhemoglobin (Hb). The iron in the four heme pigments is in the ferrous (Fe^{2+} or reduced state).

Obviously, HbO$_2$ saturation (S$_{O_2}$) is not limited to multiples of 25, 50, 75, or 100%. Thus, when arterial blood is 90% saturated, it follows that some of the Hb molecules must have four oxygens bound and some must have three or two. There is even a small probability that a few of the molecules will have one or no oxygen molecules bound. In whole animal physiology, we do not consider individual hemoglobin molecules or even individual red blood cells because there are so many of them (4 to 5 billion erythrocytes per milliliter of whole blood normally). The statistical average of the amount of oxygen bound to hemoglobin molecules relative to the total amount that can be bound is its **oxygen saturation** (S_{O_2}).

The HbO_2 equilibrium curve (Fig. 9-1) does not contain any direct information about the **rate** at which oxygen associates with (joins) or dissociates from (leaves) its chemical attachment to hemoglobin. These reactions have been measured, however, and are rapid (milliseconds).

The sigmoid (S-shaped) HbO_2 equilibrium curve is well suited both for the *loading* of O_2 in the lungs ($P_{A_{O_2}} = 100$ mmHg) and the *unloading* in the tissue capillaries ($Pcap_{O_2} = 100 \rightarrow 40$ mmHg). The shape of the curve maximizes the quantity of O_2 transported from the lungs and the quantity released at a reasonably high P_{O_2} in the systemic capillaries. At $P_{A_{O_2}} = 100$ mmHg, HbO_2 is 97.4% saturated. Thus, increasing the $P_{A_{O_2}}$ above 100 mmHg does not add much additional oxygen (100% S_{O_2} corresponds to about 200 mmHg). Likewise, when alveolar oxygen tension falls below 100 mmHg, there is little change in the amount of O_2 chemically bound to hemoglobin until the P_{O_2} falls below 70 mmHg.

The functional importance of the flat upper portion of the curve is that the arterial oxygen concentration (Ca_{O_2}) does not change much when $P_{A_{O_2}}$ falls because of ventilation/perfusion mismatching, global hypoventilation, or low ambient P_{O_2} (high altitude). For example, at $P_{O_2} = 70$ mmHg, $S_{O_2} = 94.1\%$, a trivial decrease of 3%.

The sigmoid shape of the HbO_2 equilibrium curve results from *interaction* among the four globin chains. Oxygenation of any three of the iron atoms in the four heme rings (equivalent to 75% HbO_2 of a given molecule) greatly facilitates the combination of oxygen with the fourth iron atom (100% saturation) by means of a conformational (shape) change in the hemoglobin molecule that makes the fourth heme group more accessible to O_2.

Modifying Factors

The HbO_2 equilibrium curve (that is, the equilibrium of the chemical reaction, $Hb + O_2 \rightarrow HbO_2$) is modified by hydrogen ion concentration $[H^+]$, P_{CO_2}, temperature, and certain other chemicals (Fig. 9-2A). The HbO_2 equilibrium curve can be affected in two ways—by a change in its **position** (called a *right* or *left shift*) or by a change in its **shape** (e.g., carbon monoxide hemoglobin; genetic variants of the hemoglobin molecule).

The maximum amount of O_2 that can be bound to Hb ($S_{O_2} = 100\%$) per unit of blood is called its **oxygen capacity**. Since 1 g of functional Hb combines with 1.34 ml O_2, the O_2 capacity of normal blood is 150 g Hb/liter × 1.34 ml O_2/g Hb = 201 ml O_2/liter.*

Although the normal hemoglobin concentration in blood is 150 g/liter, it is lower in individuals with anemia (reduced concentration of erythrocytes or hemoglobin) and higher in persons with polycythemia (many blood cells). For example, normal premenopausal women have an average hemoglobin concentration of about 120 g/liter, since menstruation is a form of chronic blood loss leading to a mild iron deficiency anemia. Hematocrits below 30% (or <100 g Hb/liter) are usually associated with a disease process affecting erythrocyte turnover.

The erythrocyte concentration (hematocrit) affects the viscosity of blood as it flows through small vessels. The power requirement for the heart to transport the normal quantity of oxygen is at a minimum at a hematocrit of about 40% and is only slightly increased between hematocrits

---

* For those interested in exact stoiciometry, 150 g Hb/liter = (150 g/liter)/(66,500 g/mol) = 2.26×10^{-3} mol/liter = 2.26 mmol/liter; 1.34 ml O_2/g Hb × 150 g Hb/liter = 201 ml/liter × 1 mol/22,400 ml = 8.97 mmol/liter. The molar ratio of O_2/Hb = 8.97/2.26 = 3.97 (that is, 4 mol O_2/mol Hb).

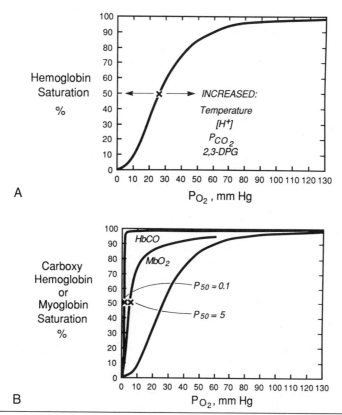

Fig. 9-2. (A) Effect of four normal metabolic factors on the affinity of hemoglobin for oxygen. The standard HbO_2 curve is shown. *Increased* P_{CO_2}, [H^+], temperature, or [2,3-DPG] increases the P_{50} (shift to the right), meaning decreased affinity of hemoglobin for oxygen. A *decrease* of any of the four factors decreases the P_{50} (shift to the left), signifying an increase in the affinity of hemoglobin for oxygen. The shifts affect only the position, not the shape, of the curve. (B) In addition to the standard HbO_2 equilibrium curve, the oxygen equilibrium curve of myoglobin (MbO_2) and of hemoglobin-carbon monoxide (HbCO) are shown. Both the MbO_2 and HbCO curves are hyperbolas, in contrast to the sigmoid shape of the normal HbO_2 equilibrium curve. The P_{50} for MbO_2 is 5 mmHg and that for HbCO is 0.1 mmHg. The affinities of myoglobin for O_2 and of hemoglobin for CO are, respectively, about 5 and 250 times the affinity of hemoglobin for O_2.

of 30 to 50%. Outside that range, the heart has to do much more work to pump adequate quantities of blood to meet the oxygen demands of the tissues. Even in persons who are polycythemic as a result of chronic hypoxemia (reduced Pa_{O_2} for whatever cause), the hematocrit does not usually rise above 55%. Only in serious disease (polycythemia vera or chronic high altitude sickness) will higher hematocrits (up to 80%) be found.

Myoglobin and Carboxyhemoglobin

Separately, each of the four heme rings combines with O_2 in a manner similar to that of the single-chain heme pigment myoglobin in skeletal muscle cells. The myoglobin oxygen equilibrium curve (MbO_2), a hyperbola, is compared with that of normal hemoglobin in Figure 9-2B. Myoglobin accepts O_2 readily enough but releases it only at low P_{O_2}. It is unsuited for O_2 transport in blood. It is useful, however, in skeletal muscle cells, where the P_{O_2} is normally in the range at which myoglobin is only partly saturated. In fact, one can use a value of 5 mmHg for the half-saturation partial pressure (P_{50}) of oxymyoglobin as a reasonable estimate of the P_{O_2} existing in the mitochondria of resting skeletal muscle cells.

Figure 9-2B also shows the equilibrium curve for carbon monoxide hemoglobin (HbCO). Compared with oxygen, carbon monoxide has more than 250 times the affinity for Hb and 50 times the affinity for Mb because carbon monoxide combines readily with Hb or Mb but does not dissociate from the complex unless the P_{CO} is very low. This can be a deadly relationship, about which more will be said later.

Factors Affecting the HbO$_2$ Equilibrium Curve

The standard HbO$_2$ equilibrium curve shown in Figure 9-1 is exactly correct only for human hemoglobin type A, a hydrogen ion concentration [H$^+$] of 40 nmol/liter (pH 7.40), a P_{CO_2} of 40 mmHg, a temperature of 37°C, and a 2,3-diphosphoglycerate concentration [2,3-DPG] of 15 µmol/g Hb.

When the concentration of any of the last four factors ([H$^+$], P_{CO_2}, temperature, [2,3-DPG]) *increases*, the affinity of hemoglobin for oxygen decreases. It is customary to describe the effect in terms of the P_{50} (P_{O_2} for 50% saturation), which in this instance increases, as shown by the arrow pointing to the right in Figure 9-2A.

The whole HbO$_2$ curve is shifted to the right of the standard curve. The change is in the position of the curve, not its shape; that is, every P_{O_2} value along the curve is multiplied by a constant, which is the ratio of $P_{50,change}/P_{50,normal}$ (the changed to the normal P_{50}). Conversely, when the value of any of these factors falls, the affinity of hemoglobin for oxygen increases and the P_{50} decreases. The entire HbO$_2$ curve is shifted to the left of the standard curve. Again, the change is in the position of the curve, not its shape.

Hydrogen Ions and P$_{CO_2}$

The effect of [H$^+$] is also called the Bohr effect (for Christian Bohr, a pioneer pulmonary physiologist). It is due to the fact that hydrogen ions have a greater affinity for Hb than for HbO$_2$.

Temperature

The temperature effect is the usual one for chemical equilibria, namely, increased temperature favors dissociation and decreased temperature favors association of O$_2$ with Hb.

2,3-Diphosphoglycerate

The compound 2,3-DPG is in erythrocytes in high concentration relative to other cells because mature red blood cells have no mitochondria. They respire by anaerobic metabolism (glycolysis), which produces 2,3-DPG as a side reaction. 2,3-DPG binds to Hb more strongly than to HbO$_2$. [2,3-DPG] increases in hypoxemia (decreased Pa_{O_2}) and when blood [H$^+$] decreases, whereas [2,3-DPG] decreases in blood stored for transfusions.

In everyday life, shifts in [H$^+$], P_{CO_2}, temperature, and [2,3-DPG] are small. For example, venous blood has a higher P_{CO_2} (46 mmHg) and [H$^+$] concentration (42 nmol/liter; pH 7.38) than does arterial blood, in which P_{CO_2} = 40 mmHg and [H$^+$] = 40 nmol/liter (pH 7.40) (Table 9-1). This means that the HbO$_2$ curve of mixed venous blood is shifted slightly to the right relative to that of arterial blood. The P_{50} increases from 26 to 28 or 29 mmHg, too small to warrant drawing a separate HbO$_2$ curve for venous blood.

In disease and some physiologic situations, large shifts in the position of the HbO$_2$ curve may occur. For example, the temperature of blood flowing to the hand from the brachial artery may

Table 9-1. Transport of CO_2 per Liter of Normal Whole Blood

	Arterial	Mixed Venous	a − v̄ Difference
Normal values			
[Hb], g/liter	150	150	
S_{O_2}, %	97.4	72.4	25
P_{CO_2}, mmHg	40	46	−6[a]
[H^+], nEq/liter	40	42	−2
pH, no units	7.40	7.38	0.02
α_{CO_2}, mmol/(liter × mmHg)	0.03	0.03	
CO_2 in blood			
Dissolved, mmol/liter	1.10	1.27	−0.17
Carbamino, mmol/liter	1.09	1.69	−0.60
HCO_3^-, mmol/liter	19.30	20.33	−1.03
Total CO_2, mmol/liter	21.50	23.30	−1.80
Total CO_2, ml/liter	482	522	−40

[a] The negative sign means *added* to blood during systemic capillary transit. (Data from Davenport AW: The ABC of Acid-Base Chemistry. 5th Ed. University of Chicago Press, 1969; and Nunn JF: Applied Respiratory Physiology. 3rd Ed. Butterworths, London, 1987.)

decrease by several degrees Celsius (centigrade) on a cold winter day. The falling temperature shifts the HbO_2 curve to the left (increased affinity), which lowers the P_{O_2} necessary to unload O_2. Thus, less oxygen is unloaded in the cold capillary blood at normal P_{O_2}. Fortunately, the temperature decrease also lowers the oxygen consumption of the hand, and the two effects tend to cancel.

Hemoglobin Variants

Another factor that may affect the HbO_2 equilibrium curve is genetic variants of the hemoglobin molecule. Normal adult human hemoglobin is called **type A**. The most common variant is **fetal hemoglobin** (HbF), which is the major hemoglobin present in the fetus. It is normally replaced soon after birth by hemoglobin A. HbF has slightly less affinity for O_2 (shift to the right), but it is less affected by [2,3-DPG], so that functionally (that is, in fetal blood) HbF has a greater affinity for O_2 (shift to the left), which is beneficial to the fetus, whose Pa_{O_2} is low (about 40 mmHg). Most genetic variants of hemoglobin shift the curve to the left. The effect may include a change in the shape of the curve as well as a change in its position. Some hemoglobin variants destroy the interaction among the globin chains, causing hemoglobin to revert toward its ancestral myoglobin behavior (Fig. 9-2B). One special form called **hemoglobin S** (HbS) crystallizes into long rods when P_{O_2} is low and [H^+] is increased. The rods distort the shape of the erythrocytes into what are called *sickle cells*. Although purified HbS binds O_2 as does HbA, erythrocytes containing it have more 2,3-DPG, so the HbO_2 curve is shifted to the right.

Remember: When Hb affinity for O_2 changes, P_{50} changes in the opposite direction.

How the Position of the HbO_2 Curve Affects O_2 Transport

What does a shift in the *position* of the HbO_2 equilibrium curve mean in terms of oxygen transport in blood? A shift to the right (decreased affinity) tends to reduce the quantity of oxygen that can be taken up at any specified PA_{O_2} as blood flows through the lung capillaries. But, the

the HbO_2 equilibrium curve is nearly flat above $P_{O_2} = 70$ mmHg. Except for extreme conditions, positional shifts in the curve have little effect on arterial oxygen concentration. A shift of the HbO_2 equilibrium curve to the right, however, reflects an increase in the quantity of oxygen that can be dissociated (given up) by blood as it flows through the systemic tissue capillaries. This has the beneficial effect of increasing the delivery of oxygen at a given partial pressure. There is a normal slight shift to the right (2 to 3 mmHg) caused by the rising P_{CO_2} and $[H^+]$ in systemic capillary blood (Bohr effect).

Conversely, a shift to the left (increased affinity) means an increase in the binding of oxygen by hemoglobin at any specified partial pressure. Such a slight shift (2 to 3 mmHg) occurs in the lung capillaries. In systemic capillaries, however, a leftward shift means a decrease in the amount of oxygen that can be unloaded at any given partial pressure. This could lead to tissue hypoxia (insufficient O_2 for aerobic metabolism) unless compensation (such as increased blood flow) occurs.

It may be helpful to compare normal exchange in the lung and in the capillaries of the heart. As mixed venous blood flows through the pulmonary capillaries, its P_{CO_2} and $[H^+]$ decrease as CO_2 diffuses out of the blood into the alveolar gas. This shifts the equilibrium curve slightly to the left, which means an increase in the affinity of hemoglobin for oxygen (reverse Bohr effect). When the blood flows through the coronary capillaries, tissue temperature, P_{CO_2}, and $[H^+]$ rise. These shift the HbO_2 equilibrium curve slightly to the right, thereby augmenting the delivery of oxygen at any given P_{O_2} (Bohr effect). This is especially useful in the myocardium because O_2 extraction is 50% or more even at rest, so that the 2- to 3-mmHg right shift is important.

How the Shape of the HbO_2 Curve Affects O_2 Transport

Changes in the shape of the HbO_2 curve almost always reflect deleterious effects on oxygen transport because the shape changes usually mean increased hemoglobin affinity for O_2, which means that the unloading of oxygen in systemic capillaries must occur at a lower P_{O_2}.

Carbon monoxide (CO) poisoning is the most important clinical example of this phenomenon. Acute and chronic carbon monoxide poisoning is by no means a rare event. Recent U.S. government statistics listed 3,800 confirmed diagnoses of CO poisoning in 1986. Figure 9-2B showed the HbCO curve shifted far to the left. The affinity of CO for Hb is so great relative to that of O_2 (>250-fold) that even at very low concentrations of CO in alveolar gas, there will be a substantial quantity of HbCO in blood in the steady state. Interestingly, the body produces small quantities of CO during hemoglobin metabolism so that carbon monoxide hemoglobin saturation may be 2 to 3% in normal blood. Cigarette smokers may have HbCO concentrations in excess of 10% of hemoglobin capacity.

The combustion of hydrocarbon fuels has increased the concentration of CO in the air of large cities. The advent of the catalytic converter for automobile emissions has reduced carbon monoxide air pollution in the United States and Canada, but one is likely to breathe substantial amounts of CO in large cities in most countries outside North America or in districts where heavy industries are concentrated.

The problem with CO is not only that it displaces oxygen from binding with hemoglobin but that it shifts the oxygen equilibrium curve far to the left and changes its shape. HbCO interferes with the interaction among the globin chains, which is responsible for the functionally beneficial shape of the HbO_2 equilibrium curve.

Anemia

Another less obvious factor that affects the HbO_2 equilibrium curve is the O_2 capacity of blood. As mentioned in Chapter 1, the breathing apparatus does not regulate the Hb concentration

(O_2 capacity) of arterial blood. Breathing only affects the Pa_{O_2}. Other factors (dietary iron, vitamin B_{12}, the hormone *erythropoietin*) regulate blood hemoglobin concentration. Blood loss, especially chronic loss as from a bleeding duodenal ulcer, also affects blood O_2 capacity.

Unfortunately, the usual HbO_2 equilibrium curve (Fig. 9-1) does not show changes in blood O_2 capacity, since the y-axis has a relative percentage scale. If one changes the y-axis to reveal the absolute concentration of oxygen (in milliliters per liter), then one can see the effect of changes in O_2 capacity. Figure 9-3 is such a graph. It shows the effect of moderately severe anemia ([Hb] decreased by one-half). The uppermost line in Figure 9-3 is the normal HbO_2 equilibrium curve (Hb = 150 g/liter, HbCO = 0%) in terms of O_2 concentration at the normal oxygen capacity of blood (201 ml O_2/liter) (100% S_{O_2}). The arterial point (Pa_{O_2} = 100 mmHg; Ca_{O_2} = 195 ml/liter), the mixed venous point ($P\bar{v}_{O_2}$ = 40 mmHg; $C\bar{v}_{O_2}$ = 150 ml/liter), and the P_{50} (26 mmHg) are shown.

If a person has a 50% reduction in hemoglobin concentration (75 g Hb/liter), the HbO_2 curve shown as the lowest line in Figure 9-3 is the result. The curve is changed neither in position nor in shape. It is only moved *down* to reflect the reduction in the O_2 capacity to 100 ml O_2/liter. The arterial point and P_{50} are not affected, but the mixed venous point has moved. How much it has moved depends on how much the cardiac output has increased to compensate for the loss of O_2-carrying capacity. In the example shown, cardiac output was constant. Thus, for a normal $\dot{V}_{O_2}$, the (a − v) ΔO_2 concentration difference must be doubled (see Fick equation for blood flow in Ch. 3). The mixed venous point is at 50 ml O_2/liter and P_{O_2} is 26 mmHg, which happens to be the 50% saturation point and overlies the P_{50} (purely fortuitous).

The middle line in Figure 9-3 represents the HbO_2 equilibrium curve for 50% HbCO in blood with a normal hemoglobin concentration. The arterial point is the same as for the anemic person, but the mixed venous point is moved far to the left at P_{O_2} = 13 mmHg, which is the same as the new P_{50} (again fortuitous). There are two reasons for the very low $P\bar{v}_{O_2}$. The HbCO decreased the O_2 capacity by 50% (moved the curve downward). More importantly, the curve

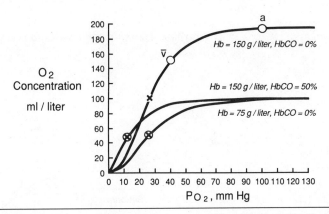

Fig. 9-3. Three HbO_2 concentration (not saturation) curves. Normal curve (top line), anemia (bottom line; hemoglobin concentration decreased by one-half), and 50% carbon monoxide hemoglobin (HbCO) (middle line). All are under standard metabolic conditions and at constant oxygen consumption and cardiac output. The arterial (a) and mixed venous (v̄) points and the P_{50} (×) are shown for normal blood. For *anemic* blood ([Hb] = 75 g/liter), the only difference is that the oxygen concentration at each point is reduced by one-half. The P_{50} (○) is normal; neither the position nor the shape of the curve is changed. The curve for *carbon monoxide* hemoglobin (HbCO = 50%), however, is shifted far to the left because HbCO changes both the shape and the position of the HbO_2 equilibrium curve. The P_{50} (○) is 13 mmHg for the same (a − v̄) oxygen concentration difference of 50 ml/liter.

is shifted to the left of the normal and anemia curves because of the effect of CO binding to two of the four iron atoms in each hemoglobin molecule. That markedly disturbs the chemical equilibrium between the association and dissociation of oxygen (increased affinity for O_2).

Another factor affecting the position, shape, and O_2 capacity is oxidation of the iron to its ferric state (Fe^{3+}) from the ferrous condition (Fe^{2+}). Oxidation is a continuing phenomenon in normal red blood cells. Fortunately, there are at least three reducing enzymes present in erythrocytes that convert oxidized hemoglobin back to ferrous (functional) hemoglobin. Certain chemicals can sharply increase oxidized hemoglobin and cause a condition known as **methemoglobinemia**. Oxidized hemoglobin does not bind or transport oxygen.

Oxygen Diffusion

Figure 9-4 shows the mean P_{O_2} at major points along the oxygen pathway from ambient air to the mitochondria of systemic tissue cells. I have already discussed the obligatory decrease in P_{O_2} as air goes from ambient atmosphere (dry room air) to the trachea (BTPS), the further decrease in alveolar gas due to the removal of oxygen by the pulmonary capillary blood flow and by the obligatory output of CO_2 (alveolar gas equation), and the decrease of P_{O_2} between alveolar gas and systemic arterial blood due to ventilation/perfusion mismatching and to the small right-to-left anatomic shunt.

Alveolocapillary Diffusion

One possibility for a disparity between $P_{A_{O_2}}$ and Pa_{O_2} is a limitation to the diffusion of oxygen across the alveolus-blood barrier. Chapter 2 described the structure of the alveolar wall and how the erythrocytes flowing through the capillaries are brought into intimate contact with alveolar gas, separated by a barrier only 0.5 to 1.5 μm wide.

For respiratory gases, the diffusion equation is

$$\dot{V} = \frac{\text{diffusion coefficient} \times \text{area} \times (P_{A_{O_2}} - Pcap_{O_2})}{\text{distance}} \tag{9-1}$$

where $\dot{V}$ is the volume flow of gas by diffusion. The *diffusion coefficient* is a quantity dependent

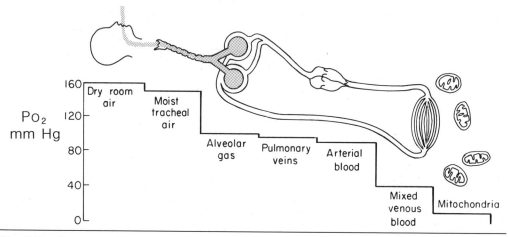

Fig. 9-4. Oxygen partial pressure cascade from room air to systemic tissue mitochondria at normal sea level barometric pressure (760 mmHg). Of the total decrease, 38% occurs between room air and systemic arterial blood. The remainder occurs between the systemic capillary blood and the tissue mitochondria.

on the molecular size and solubility of the gas, among other parameters; *area* is the effective alveolar surface across which the diffusion occurs; and *distance* is the path length along which diffusion occurs. The mean O_2 pressure in the pulmonary capillary blood ($Pcap_{O_2}$) is a complex function, not only of the passive diffusion across the air-blood barrier but also of the process of diffusion and chemical reaction that occurs when oxygen penetrates the erythrocytes and chemically reacts with hemoglobin.

Under normal resting conditions—and indeed even with considerable deviations from normality, such as heavy exercise or in patients with a variety of cardiac and pulmonary diseases—there is adequate time during red blood cell transit through the capillaries for the hemoglobin in the red blood cells to come into complete equilibrium with the alveolar gas, so that there is no detectable diffusion limitation.

> **Remember:** The capillary blood volume in the lungs is usually about the same as the stroke volume of the right ventricle, so that at rest the erythrocytes have one cardiac cycle for gas exchange.

Inert gases (nitrogen, anesthetic gases, etc.) equilibrate between alveolar gas and pulmonary capillary blood extremely rapidly (milliseconds). The transfer rate of oxygen is slower because of the enormous unfilled O_2 capacity of mixed venous blood (50 ml/liter). In other words, the "effective" solubility of oxygen in blood is markedly increased by hemoglobin, even though mixed venous blood is 75% saturated with O_2.

When physiologists or physicians refer to a pulmonary diffusion limitation, they are not referring only to the passive diffusion of oxygen molecules across the alveolocapillary barrier, because that proceeds as rapidly as for any inert gas. They are referring to the time necessary for the combined process of diffusion and the chemical reaction of oxygen with hemoglobin. Although the chemical reaction $Hb + O_2 \rightarrow HbO_2$ is rapid (milliseconds), it adds a significant delay to the equilibration time because of the low solubility of O_2 in water within the alveolar wall tissue and plasma and the fact that the O_2 uptake by hemoglobin must proceed sequentially.* Thus, much of the limitation to O_2 diffusion between alveolar gas and capillary blood is within the red blood cells, not in the barrier.

An example of a real diffusion limitation for oxygen is when someone exercises heavily (increased oxygen demand) while breathing a very low inspired oxygen pressure (alveolar hypoxia). Under those conditions, the driving pressure for oxygen diffusion across the alveolus-capillary barrier is reduced at the same time the demand for oxygen is increased (because of lower $C\bar{v}_{O_2}$) and cardiac output is increased (resulting in less time for O_2 exchange in the lung capillaries). Although there are a number of compensatory factors, the result is that the blood may leave the capillaries without coming into complete equilibrium with alveolar gas.

Some clinical physiologists believe that an O_2 diffusion limitation can be demonstrated in certain lung diseases in which there is thickening or scarring of the alveolar walls. Unfortunately, it is not easy to separate the diffusion component from the ventilation/perfusion mismatching or capillary obliteration that the disease has caused. Measuring Pa_{O_2} during oxygen breathing is of no help in trying to make the distinction because the high Pa_{O_2} eliminates both the diffusion

---

* An analogy is as follows. A group of 100 people walking side by side (parallel transport) can cross a field in 1 minute. But if at some point there is a wall with narrow gates, it will take longer for them to cross because only a few people at a time can pass through the gates (sequential transport).

limitation and the ventilation/perfusion mismatching. One should not invoke the diffusion process as a cause of decreased Pa_{O_2} until all other causes have been ruled out.

Oxygen Diffusion to the Mitochondria

Diffusion is, however, the rate-limiting process in the peripheral tissues, where the diffusion equation is

$$\dot{V} = \frac{\text{diffusion coefficient} \times \text{area} \times (\text{Pcap}_{O_2} - \text{Pt}_{O_2})}{\text{distance}} \tag{9.2}$$

Here *area* is the capillary surface area and *distance* is the path length from the capillaries through the tissues to the mitochondria in the cells. Pcap_{O_2} and Pt_{O_2} are the mean P_{O_2} values in the systemic capillary and the tissue, respectively.

Arterial blood enters the systemic capillaries at a P_{O_2} of 100 mmHg. But according to Figure 9-1, Pcap_{O_2} must fall substantially before any significant quantity of O_2 dissociates from hemoglobin. Thus, the mean capillary P_{O_2} (about 55 mmHg) is closer to 40 mmHg than to 100 mmHg. Oxygen diffusion to the tissue cells depends on a modest (<50 mmHg) partial pressure difference between the capillary blood and the most distant mitochondria. Fortunately, mitochondria are able to carry out oxidative metabolism at P_{O_2} values as low as 1 to 2 mmHg.

Attempts to determine tissue oxygen tension (Pt_{O_2}) are fraught with technical difficulties. However, using devices known as micro-oxygen electrodes, reasonable P_{O_2} measurements have been made in several tissues (skeletal muscle, myocardium, and brain). Under normal resting conditions, it is unusual to find Pt_{O_2} <5 mmHg, which means that all mitochondria are receiving adequate oxygen. A reasonable estimate of mean resting Pt_{O_2} is about 10 mmHg; however, the mean value is probably not as useful as the lowest value. Pt_{O_2} falls not only along the capillary but in the radial direction away from the capillary.

Perhaps the most important factor affecting tissue O_2 diffusion is the *distance* over which oxygen must diffuse to reach the cells. In the myocardium, a critical tissue and one that requires a large oxygen supply, the capillaries are about 25 μm apart—the width of one left ventricular muscle fiber. Thus, from each capillary oxygen has to diffuse outward within a tissue cylinder of about 13 μm radius. That seems little enough, but it is 10 times further than across the alveolus-capillary barrier in the lung. Since the diffusion rate is affected by the square of the path length, oxygen molecules require about 100 times longer to diffuse the 13 μm from the capillary to the furthest heart muscle mitochondria than from the alveolar gas to the red blood cells in the pulmonary capillaries. In addition, along the way mitochondria are extracting oxygen so that tissue P_{O_2} falls in a complex manner. In brain cortex the capillaries are some 40 μm apart, and in resting skeletal muscle they are about 80 μm apart.

The most effective way to improve oxygen delivery to tissue cells is to decrease the diffusion path length by recruitment of more capillaries, which also increases the surface area of the capillaries across which oxygen diffusion occurs. This occurs in skeletal muscle, where functional capillary density increases threefold in heavy exercise.

Although the rate of dissociation of oxygen from hemoglobin is slower than the association reaction, under most conditions the P_{O_2} of venous blood leaving an organ is very close to the P_{O_2} of the end-capillary blood.

The normal arteriovenous oxygen concentration difference is 50 ml O_2/liter (Fig. 9-5). In Figure 9-5, note that net O_2 transport occurs only from the alveolar capillaries to the systemic capillaries. The remaining 150 ml O_2/liter circulates around and around without any apparent function. But it does have value: (1) it maintains the P_{O_2} of systemic capillary blood at a high level (>40 mmHg), which is necessary for adequate tissue O_2 diffusion, and (2) it provides a

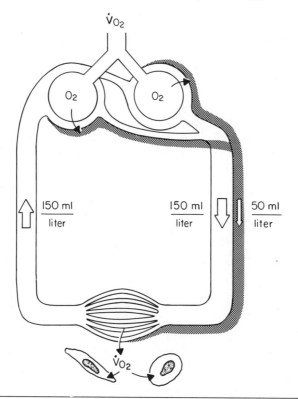

Fig. 9-5.   Blood transport of O_2 represented as independent streams. The metabolic oxygen (cross-hatched path) enters the pulmonary capillaries and is transported in *arterial* blood to the systemic capillaries, where it dissociates from hemoglobin and diffuses to the tissue cell mitochondria. The transport of metabolic O_2 is 50 ml/liter at rest ($\dot{V}_{O_2}$ = 250 ml/min; blood flow = 5 liters/min). The transport of metabolic O_2 is only a function of arterial blood. Most of the oxygen in blood (ordinarily 150 ml/liter) recirculates endlessly (large open path). It functions as an emergency reserve and to maintain a reasonable P_{O_2} in the systemic capillaries.

reserve of O_2 (bound to hemoglobin) for use in emergencies (transient inadequate blood flow). The emergency supply of O_2 is part of what is called **aerobic O_2 debt**; that is, no glycolysis (lactate production) occurs.

Under maximum steady-state exercise conditions, the $(a - \bar{v})\Delta C_{O_2}$ difference increases to about 100 ml O_2/liter blood. When this is multiplied by the threefold rise in cardiac output, it accounts for a sixfold increase in oxygen consumption. It is uncommon for steady-state mixed venous oxygen saturation to fall below 50% ($P\bar{v}_{O_2}$ = 26 mmHg).

The normal myocardium extracts the maximum quantity of oxygen per volume of blood even at rest; that is, the coronary sinus (venous) oxygen saturation is about 50%. Increases in oxygen demand by the heart are met by a one-for-one increase in blood flow.

CARBON DIOXIDE TRANSPORT

CO$_2$ Concentration in Blood

One of the chief products of cellular metabolism is carbon dioxide (CO_2). It is carried by venous blood to the lung, where it is eliminated in the expired gas. The total amount of CO_2

thus transported, $\dot{V}_{CO_2}$, averages 200 ml/min in a resting adult but may increase sixfold in steady-state exercise. Normally, the quantity transported per liter of cardiac output is 40 ml (5 liters/min × 40 ml/liter = 200 ml/min).

But there is far more CO_2 in blood than that. In fact, at a normal Pa_{CO_2} of 40 mmHg, the total CO_2 concentration in arterial blood is about 480 ml/liter and that in mixed venous blood is about 520 ml/liter (Fig. 9-6). What is all that excess CO_2 there for? Carbon dioxide in blood and other body liquids is inexorably bound up with the maintenance of the hydrogen ion concentration $[H^+]$ of the internal environment, which must be carefully regulated because protein enzyme activity is very sensitive to it (see Ch. 10). Although the two processes (transport of metabolic CO_2 and hydrogen ion regulation) occur simultaneously and interact in venous blood, it is useful for the beginning student to think of them as two separate physiologic processes.

Mechanisms of CO_2 Transport by Blood

In the metabolic sense, CO_2 elimination begins with its formation during the aerobic metabolism of cells. As CO_2 is formed, it increases tissue P_{CO_2} above that of arterial blood entering

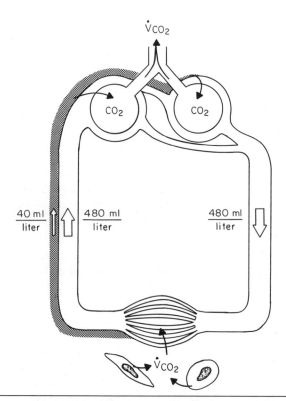

Fig. 9-6.   Blood transport of CO_2 represented as independent streams. The metabolic CO_2 produced by tissue cells ($\dot{V}_{CO_2}$) enters the capillaries and is transported by *venous* blood to the lungs (crosshatched path), where it diffuses into the alveolar gas and exits from the lung. The transport of metabolic CO_2 is 40 ml/liter at rest ($\dot{V}_{CO_2}$ = 200 ml/min; blood flow = 5 liters/min). The transport of metabolic CO_2 is only a function of venous blood. Most of the CO_2 in blood (ordinarily 480 ml/liter) recirculates endlessly. Its function is to help stabilize blood hydrogen ion concentration by providing the anion HCO_3^- to balance the excess cations in plasma (discussed fully in Ch. 10).

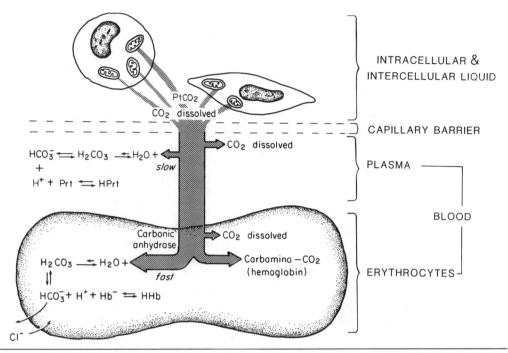

Fig. 9-7.   Schematic representation of the forms of CO_2 transport by blood. The CO_2 produced by aerobic metabolism of cells is dissolved in intracellular and intercellular liquids at an average tissue partial pressure (Pt_{CO_2}) of 50 mmHg, that is, higher than the P_{O_2} of either arterial or venous blood. Since dissolved CO_2 is soluble not only in water but also in lipids, it diffuses readily through cell membranes and easily crosses the capillary barrier to enter plasma. In plasma, a small amount of CO_2 reacts slowly (no carbonic anhydrase is present) with water to produce carbonic acid, which rapidly but reversibly dissociates into hydrogen ions (H^+) and bicarbonate (HCO_3^-). Nearly all the hydrogen ions are removed from solution by reaction with plasma proteins. Most of the CO_2 entering capillary plasma diffuses into the erythrocytes, where the CO_2 forms a vast amount of carbonic acid rapidly because of the high concentration of carbonic anhydrase. As fast as the carbonic acid is formed, it dissociates into hydrogen ions and bicarbonate. Hemoglobin present in high concentration (150 g Hb/liter) is a weak acid and combines with the hydrogen ions. In addition, some of the CO_2 combines with the amino side chains on hemoglobin to form carbamino-CO_2. As the bicarbonate accumulates in the interior of the red blood cell, it diffuses into plasma along its concentration gradient. To maintain electrical neutrality, some of the chloride (Cl^-) in plasma diffuses into the red blood cells along its concentration gradient. The net effect is that two-thirds of the metabolically produced CO_2 is transported in plasma, mainly in the form of bicarbonate.

the capillaries. If we assume an average normal mean resting Pt_{CO_2} of 50 mmHg, dissolved CO_2 molecules diffuse from the tissue into the plasma and into the red blood cell along the P_{CO_2} partial pressure gradient from $50 - 40 = 10$ mmHg at the arterial end of the tissue capillary to $50 - 46 = 4$ mmHg at the venous end.

How is the CO_2 in blood transported? As Figure 9-7 shows, it is carried in three forms: **dissolved CO_2** (a tiny fraction of which is converted to carbonic acid [H_2CO_3]), **bicarbonate ion** (HCO_3^-), and bound to hemoglobin and plasma proteins (**carbamino-CO_2**).

The hydration of CO_2 to form carbonic acid takes place according to the reaction

$$CO_{2,\ dissolved} + H_2O \rightleftharpoons H_2CO_3 \qquad (9\text{-}3)$$

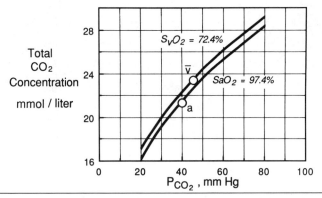

Fig. 9-8. Carbon dioxide equilibrium curve of whole blood. The y-axis is in absolute concentration units (millimoles per liter of blood). The CO_2 equilibrium curve is approximately linear over the range shown. Two curves are shown: one for arterial blood (Sa_{O_2} = 97.4%) and one for mixed venous blood ($S\bar{v}_{O_2}$ = 72.4%). The normal arterial (a) and mixed venous ($\bar{v}$) points are shown as 21.5 and 23.3 mmol CO_2/liter, respectively.

This reaction has a slow half-time (>5 seconds) in plasma but is markedly accelerated (half-time in milliseconds) inside the red blood cell because of the enzyme **carbonic anhydrase**, which is present in red blood cells but is virtually absent in plasma and interstitial liquid.*

What is not so obvious from Eq. 9-3 is that the equilibrium is far to the left in the direction of dissolved CO_2. Thus, there is very little carbonic acid; only about 0.2% of the dissolved CO_2 is in the form of H_2CO_3. Carbon dioxide is moderately soluble in blood; α_{CO_2}, 37°C = 0.03 mmol/liter × mmHg) or 0.7 ml/(liter × mmHg), that is, about 20 times greater than for oxygen (α_{O_2} = 0.03 ml/[liter × mmHg]) (don't confuse the 0.03 *mmol* CO_2 with 0.03 *ml* O_2).

As carbonic acid is formed, it rapidly dissociates into ions

$$H_2CO_3 \rightleftharpoons H^+ + HCO_3^- \tag{9-4}$$

This reaction is spontaneous (not catalyzed by carbonic anhydrase or any enzyme) and very fast (microseconds). It would not proceed far, however, unless the ions produced were removed from the reaction site. The hydrogen ions are removed from solution by combining chemically with the enormous amount of hemoglobin within the red blood cells (150 g/liter whole blood) and to a lesser extent with the plasma proteins (70 g/liter). This is part of [H^+] regulation (discussed in Ch. 10). The bicarbonate ion (HCO_3^-) diffuses out of the red blood cells into plasma in exchange for Cl^- because the erythrocyte cell membrane is permeable to both molecules. Thus, the total CO_2 reaction may be written as

$$CO_{2,dissolved} + H_2O \rightleftharpoons H_2CO_3 \rightleftharpoons H^+ + HCO_3^- \tag{9-5}$$
$$+$$
$$Hb \rightleftharpoons HHb$$

It proceeds rapidly and far to the right, even though at any instant there is very little H_2CO_3 because the ionization reaction (right) is so fast relative to the hydration reaction (left) and because there is so much hemoglobin.

---

* There is some carbonic anhydrase associated with cell surfaces and in plasma, probably owing to the continual slow breakdown of red blood cells. But for practical purposes, the plasma carbonic anhydrase is zero.

Figure 9-8 shows the CO_2 equilibrium curve of blood. Over the range of P_{CO_2} usually encountered in humans, it is nearly linear. Two lines are shown because the CO_2 equilibrium curve is significantly affected by the oxygen saturation of hemoglobin (this is the Haldane effect, named after another pioneer pulmonary physiologist). The Haldane effect has to do with the fact that deoxygenated hemoglobin (Hb) is a weaker acid (less dissociated into H^+ and Hb^- ions) than oxygenated hemoglobin (HbO_2), at the normal $[H^+]$ of human blood. As blood becomes deoxygenated in the systemic capillaries, its ability to bind with CO_2 (to form carbamino-CO_2) is increased. This is the reciprocal of the effect that CO_2 has on the HbO_2 equilibrium curve (Bohr effect). The Bohr and Haldane effects work simultaneously and are beneficial in both systemic and lung capillaries. In the systemic capillaries, the P_{O_2} remains higher (better diffusion gradient) and the P_{CO_2} lower (lower $[H^+]$) than otherwise would be the situation. In the lung the reverse interaction occurs.

The fact that the CO_2 equilibrium curve is nearly linear whereas the HbO_2 equilibrium is markedly curvilinear over the useful ranges of P_{CO_2} and P_{O_2}, respectively, partially explains why, when there is mismatching of ventilation/perfusion, the $(A - a)\Delta P_{O_2}$ is much greater than the $(A - a)\Delta P_{CO_2}$. Over the range of 20 to 80 mmHg, if part of the lung is underventilated (low $\dot{V}A/\dot{Q}$), the high P_{CO_2} in the blood leaving that unit may be compensated for by another part of the lung that is overventilated (high $\dot{V}A/\dot{Q}$) and therefore has low P_{CO_2} in the blood leaving it.*

Table 9-1 shows average normal data for the transport of carbon dioxide per liter of blood. The total quantity is large. Standard values are listed for arterial and mixed venous blood and their $(a - \bar{v})$ differences. Of the metabolic CO_2 transported in mixed venous blood to the lungs (1.81 mmol/liter; 40 ml/liter), about 65% is carried as bicarbonate, 30% as carbamino-CO_2, and 5% as dissolved CO_2.

READINGS

Books

1. Comroe JH Jr: Physiology of Respiration. 2nd Ed. Year Book Medical Publishers, Chicago, 1974
   Chapter 14 on oxygen transport, Chapter 15 on tissue oxygen exchange, and Chapter 16 on carbon dioxide transport cover the subject in detail.
2. Murray JF: The Normal Lung. 2nd Ed. WB Saunders, Philadelphia, 1986
   Chapter 6 is useful, but there is no need to read the section on lung diffusion. Good summary of O_2 and CO_2 transport by blood from the viewpoint of a chest physician.
3. Nunn JF: Applied Respiratory Physiology. 3rd Ed. Butterworths, London, 1987
   Although Chapter 8 on oxygen diffusion is excessive considering its limited import, the review of oxygen transport and metabolism (Chapter 10) is good. Chapter 9 on CO_2 transport is thorough, as one would expect from an anesthetist.
4. Schmidt RF, Thews G: Human Physiology. (English Ed.) Springer-Verlag, Berlin, 1983
   Chapter 21 on tissue respiration and P_{O_2} gradients is good.
5. Stryer L: Biochemistry. 2nd Ed. WH Freeman, New York, 1981
   A standard modern text of biochemistry. Oxidative metabolism is discussed in Chapters 13 and 14 and glycolytic metabolism is covered in Chapter 12.

---

* Differences in blood flow to the different regions of the lung, however, prevent complete compensation.

Reviews

6. Wasserman K, Whipp BJ: Exercise physiology in health and disease. Am Rev Respir Dis 112:219–249, 1975
The classic review of this important physiologic function. O_2 and CO_2 transport and energy utilization are clearly yet succinctly covered.

Articles

7. Crowell JW, Smith EE: Determinants of the optimal hematocrit. J Appl Physiol 22:501–504, 1967
Describes how blood rheology (viscosity) affects O_2 transport, vascular resistance, and blood flow distribution.
8. Staub NC: Alveolar arterial oxygen tension due to diffusion. J Appl Physiol 18:673–680, 1963
Summarizes the process of O_2 uptake in the pulmonary capillaries and why diffusion is rarely a rate-limiting problem in the lungs.

QUESTIONS*

Drill

1. All variables are normal, except as noted.
   a. What is S_{O_2} at P_{O_2} = 18.6 mmHg when P_{50} is decreased by 10 mmHg?
   b. What is Pa_{O_2} if the HbO_2 equilibrium curve is shifted 10 mmHg to the left?
   c. What is C_{O_2} at P_{O_2} = 55 mmHg when P_{50} is increased by 10 mmHg?
   d. What is $P\bar{v}_{O_2}$ if the position of the HbO_2 curve is shifted 5 mmHg to the right?
   e. What is S_{O_2} at P_{O_2} = 63.5 mmHg when O_2 affinity for Hb decreases by 7 mmHg?
   f. What is S_{CO}, if P_{ACO} = 0.4 mmHg and P_{AO_2} = 100 mmHg?
2. If there are 5×10^6 erythrocytes per microliter of whole blood, what is the [Hb] of one erythrocyte? How many milliliters of O_2 can be carried by one erythrocyte?
3. The circulating blood volume of humans is about 7% of body weight. What is the total *emergency* oxygen content of blood in a normal 70-kg adult?
   a. 97.5%
   b. 750 ml
   c. 200 ml/liter
   d. 75%
   e. 1,000 ml

Problems

4. The $(a - \bar{v})\Delta O_2$ concentration difference across the heart (myocardium) is 100 ml/liter (assume Ca_{O_2} = 200 ml O_2/liter). If the HbO_2 equilibrium curve is shifted 3 mmHg to the right in the myocardial capillaries: a. What is the P_{O_2} of coronary venous blood? b. If the mean P_{O_2} of myocardial muscle fibers is 5 mmHg, what effect does the Bohr shift have on the mean P_{O_2} gradient between coronary capillary blood and myocardial mitochondria. [*Hint*: The mean P_{O_2} of capillary blood is the P_{O_2} at half O_2 unloading, not $(Pa_{O_2} + P\bar{v}_{O_2})/2$.]
5. Some physiologists believe that the reactions of CO_2 within red blood cells may be too slow to permit complete equilibration between PA_{CO_2} and whole blood in the pulmonary capillaries under some conditions. If that did occur, the likely consequence is:
   a. $Pa_{CO_2} < PA_{CO_2}$
   b. $Pa_{CO_2} > PA_{CO_2}$
   c. $Pa_{CO_2} = PA_{CO_2}$
   d. Slight inhibition of ventilation
   e. Slight decrease in systemic arterial $[H^+]$
6. An anemic ([Hb] = 100 g/liter), resting, elderly woman has a normal HbO_2 equilibrium curve. Relative to normal values, it is most likely that her:
   a. Cardiac output is decreased
   b. $(a - \bar{v})\Delta O_2$ is increased
   c. O_2 consumption is decreased
   d. Hemoglobin affinity for O_2 is decreased
   e. Mixed venous P_{O_2} is increased

---

* Answers begin on p. 211.

7. In a man suffering from carbon monoxide poisoning such that 25% of his hemoglobin is in the form HbCO, the most effective treatment is to
   a. Have him breathe 100% oxygen
   b. Advise him not to smoke
   c. Make him hyperventilate on room air
   d. Advise him not to take any trips to high altitude
   e. Make him breathe air with 5% CO_2 added

Answer the following three questions based on the figure below, which shows the normal HbO_2 equilibrium curve and nine points. Select the point that best fits the description in each question and write out your explanation.

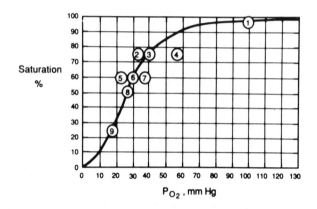

8. Mixed venous blood of a normal person breathing air during moderate steady-state exercise.
9. Arterial blood in a resting person with polycythemia ([Hb] = 180 g/liter) breathing air, who is otherwise normal.
10. Pulmonary arterial blood in a normal person breathing air at sea level, while hyperventilating to $P_{A_{CO_2}} = 20$ mmHg.

10

Acid-Base Balance

THE BOTTOM LINE

Central Role of CO_2 in Hydrogen Ion Regulation

P_{CO_2} is controlled by breathing (alveolar ventilation equation). Ventilation can change $P_{A_{CO_2}}$ rapidly (seconds or minutes) when blood or cerebrospinal fluid acid-base status is altered.

Definitions

A solution is *acid* if its $[H^+] > [OH^-]$. *Strong electrolytes* such as Na^+Cl^- are completely ionized. *Weak electrolytes*, chiefly the weak acid proteins, especially hemoglobin, are only partially ionized. The total weak acid concentration ($[A_{tot}]$) differs widely among body liquid compartments. In acid-base balance, the concentration of electrolytes is expressed in hydrogen ion *equivalents* for each ion species. CO_2 in solution is considered to be a weak acid, but it is regulated separately from the other weak acids. *Buffers* are solutions that limit changes in $[H^+]$. pH is the symbol for $-\log[H^+]$.

Strong Ion Difference

The strong ion difference ($[SID]$) is the deficit in strong electrolyte anions compared with cations. At $P_{CO_2} = 40$ mmHg, $[A_{tot}] = 20$ mEq/liter, $[SID] = 24.5$ mEq/liter, and the normal systemic arterial blood $[H^+] = 40$ nEq/liter. The strong ion difference is chiefly determined by the kidney's ability to regulate plasma sodium concentration. $[SID]$ changes slowly (hours or days) in response to acid-base changes.

Three Independent Variables Determine Hydrogen Ion Concentration

The P_{CO_2}, total weak electrolytes $[A_{tot}]$, and $[SID]$ completely determine the $[H^+]$ of blood and other body liquids. The difference between $[SID]$ and the ionized portion of A_{tot} gives the bicarbonate concentration: $[HCO_3^-] = [SID] - [A^-]$. The ratio $[HCO_3^-]/[CO_2]$ is determined by the $[H^+]$.

Hydrogen Ion Concentration

$[H^+]$ is expressed as nanoequivalents (10^{-9}), not milliequivalents. The Henderson-Hasselbalch equation uses logarithmic pH notation to relate $[H^+]$ to the HCO_3^-/CO_2 ratio.

$$pH = 6.10 + \log \frac{[HCO_3^-]}{0.03 \times P_{CO_2}}$$

(Continues).

(Continued).

Cerebrospinal Fluid

The cerebrospinal fluid (CSF) contains no protein (weak acid); therefore, $[HCO_3^-]$ = [SID]. The CSF is poorly buffered, so its $[H^+]$ is changed more than that of blood for a given change in P_{CO_2}.

Acid-Base Disorders

"Pure" acid-base disorders are divided into two groups: *respiratory* (P_{CO_2} changes) and *metabolic* ([SID] changes). Each group can be further divided into *acidosis* ($[H^+]$ increased) or *alkalosis* ($[H^+]$ decreased). Acid-base balance in blood is usually obtained by measuring $[H^+]$ and P_{CO_2} with suitable electrodes and then using a graph, such as the *Siggaard-Anderson nomogram*, to obtain $[HCO_3^-]$ and to determine the deviation of [SID] from normal. The respiratory *compensation* for acid-base disturbances ordinarily begins almost immediately. Metabolic compensation is much slower. In either case, the net effect is to return the $[H^+]$ toward normal (buffering). Full understanding of acid-base balance requires knowledge of renal as well as respiratory physiology.

In previous chapters, I referred to the normal arterial hydrogen ion concentration, $[H^+]a$, as 40 nmol/liter and the normal mixed venous blood, $[H^+]\bar{v}$, as 42 nmol/liter.* This chapter describes how the respiratory system helps to maintain these hydrogen ion concentrations. The area of physiology called **acid-base balance** is not complicated, but it often appears so to beginning students. Fortunately, in the last decade a much clearer approach to understanding acid-base balance has emerged, largely through the work of Stewart (see books by Stewart and Jones in the reading list). I use Stewart's approach in this chapter. Of course, to fully understand acid-base balance requires knowledge of renal physiology. Thus, this chapter is a beginning only.

Following a brief review of the central role of CO_2 in hydrogen ion regulation, some definitions necessary for the understanding of acid-base balance in modern respiratory physiology will be given. I will describe those variables that are independently regulated and that act to determine hydrogen ion concentration in the various body compartments, although mostly I will confine my examples to whole blood. Finally, I will describe the conversion of $[H^+]$ to pH notation by use of the widely known Henderson-Hasselbalch equation, briefly mention hydrogen ion regulation in one special compartment (cerebrospinal fluid), and conclude with a description of the fundamentals of acid-base disorders and their graphic display on the Siggaard-Anderson nomogram.

THE CENTRAL ROLE OF CO_2 IN HYDROGEN ION REGULATION

If carbon dioxide was only transported from the systemic capillaries to the lungs (Fig. 9-6), its physiology would be simple. But what are we to make of the enormous quantity of CO_2 carried around the circulation for no obvious *metabolic* function? The amount of metabolic CO_2 being transported per liter of mixed venous blood is less than 8% of its total CO_2 concentration.

---

* Nanomoles (10^{-9}), not millimoles, are used in defining the concentration of H^+ in body liquids, which is one-millionth the concentration of other ions.

Why do we need a huge reservoir of CO_2 in the blood and other body liquids? The obvious reason is that carbon dioxide is one of the important independent variables controlling blood, interstitial, intracellular, and transcellular hydrogen ion concentrations ($[H^+]$).

Normally, alveolar ventilation is regulated so that despite wide fluctuations in metabolic CO_2 production, $P_{A_{CO_2}}$ (Pa_{CO_2}) is held constant, as defined by the alveolar ventilation equation (Eq. 4-3). However, in terms of metabolic CO_2 and O_2 transport, one could function adequately with a Pa_{CO_2} of 30 or 50 mmHg. The small changes in Pa_{O_2} that would follow because of altered alveolar ventilation have trivial effects on oxygen transport (see Ch. 9). Therefore, $P_{A_{CO_2}}$ is held at 40 mmHg for a more important function, which is the regulation of $[H^+]$ in body liquids. In fact, the normal $P_{A_{CO_2}}$ is necessary to offset the huge quantity of CO_2 in body liquids, mainly in the form of bicarbonate ion (HCO_3^-), which in turn is essential to maintain the high concentration of sodium in plasma and extracellular liquid.

There are some conditions (for example, severe chronic obstructive pulmonary disease) in which one cannot readily change $P_{A_{CO_2}}$ by altering ventilation. Therefore, one must rely on other mechanisms to control the $[H^+]$ in body liquids. The kidneys and to a lesser extent the gastrointestinal tract do this by slowly (hours to days) adjusting the amount of sodium ion ($[Na^+]$) in extracellular liquids (plasma and interstitial liquid).

Remember: Regulation of $[H^+]$ by ventilatory regulation of $P_{A_{CO_2}}$ is normally fast (seconds to minutes). Regulation of $[H^+]$ by renal adjustment of plasma sodium concentration is slow (hours to days).

DEFINITIONS

Acids and Bases

A substance is an acid if, when it is added to a solution, it increases the $[H^+]$ or decreases the $[OH^-]$ of the solution. A substance is a base if, when it is added to a solution, it decreases the $[H^+]$ or increases the $[OH^-]$ of the solution. These definitions are compatible with the Brønsted definition of an acid as a proton (H^+) donor and a base as a proton acceptor. The way acids and bases are defined here is the way most physicians and physiologists actually think of them.

According to the above definitions, metallic sodium is a base because when added to water it causes a decrease in the hydrogen ion concentration, even though the sodium does not accept an H^+ in the strict sense. Each sodium atom donates an electron, which reacts with an H^+ in the water to form a hydrogen atom, which combines with another hydrogen atom to form hydrogen gas (H_2). The H^+ ion came from the small amount of ionized water, and therefore the hydroxyl ion concentration ($[OH^-]$) increased.

Chlorine (Cl_2) is considered to be an acid because when it reacts with water, it extracts two electrons to form two chloride ions ($2Cl^-$) and thereby generates hydrogen ions.

Acid-Base Status of a Solution

A solution is neutral if its $[H^+] = [OH^-]$; acidic if its $[H^+] > [OH^-]$; and basic (alkaline) if its $[H^+] < [OH^-]$. By these definitions, all body liquids are alkaline except gastric acid and urine.

Electrolytes

When dissolved in water, some molecules break apart (dissociate) into charged particles (ions), which are relatively independent in their behavior, although they do maintain electrical neutrality in the bulk solution as required. Not all substances dissociate. For example, neither CO_2 nor glucose molecules dissociate.

Substances that form ions are capable of carrying electrical current in water. They are called *electrolytes*. It is convenient to divide them into two groups—*strong electrolytes*, which are completely dissociated and therefore have no finite equilibrium constant, and *weak electrolytes*, which are only partially dissociated and therefore have a finite equilibrium constant.

Equivalents

The concentrations of substances in body liquids are generally expressed as millimoles per liter. For electrolytes, concentration can also be expressed in terms of equivalent ionic charge. Monovalent ions (Na^+, Cl^-, HCO_3^-, H^+) have the same value in molar and equivalent units. But for the divalent ions (Mg^{2+}, Ca^{2+}, SO_4^{2-}, CO_3^{2-}), the ionic equivalency (normality) is twice the molarity. Thus, 1 mmol/liter of magnesium ion equals 2 mEq/liter.

Weak Electrolytes

Weak electrolytes are important because when they dissociate they produce a hydrogen ion (H^+) and an anion (A^-). In terms of body acid-base status, the interesting weak acid anions are proteins ($[Prt^-]$); in blood mainly $[Hb^-]$. At all hydrogen ion concentrations compatible with human life, proteins behave as weak acids. The total concentration of weak acids ($[A_{tot}]$) equals the concentration in the un-ionized form ($[HA]$) plus the concentration in the ionized form ($[A^-]$).

$$[A_{tot}] = [HA] + [A^-] \qquad (10\text{-}1)$$

The concentration of weak acids can be fixed independently of any other parameter. Thus, in this introduction to acid-base analysis, we will assume they remain constant at whatever value is given (see Table 10-1 footnote).

Carbon Dioxide

CO_2 is regulated by ventilation independently of any other parameter. When dissolved in water, CO_2 also behaves as a weak acid. Actually, carbonic acid (H_2CO_3) is a fairly strong acid. But H_2CO_3 is present in very low concentration, although in equilibrium with dissolved CO_2 (Eq. 8-1). Thus, it is useful to think of CO_2 (the molecule) as a weak acid. It is treated separately from all other weak electrolytes.

Buffers

Buffers are solutions that are able to limit changes in $[H^+]$ when either acid or base is added to them. The weak acids (A_{tot}) (proteins) and CO_2 act as buffers. The buffering activity of a weak electrolyte is described by the ratio of the ionized to the un-ionized form. Thus, for the anionic proteins (Hb, plasma protein, intracellular protein), for intracellular and extracellular phosphate and sulfate, and for CO_2 at any hydrogen ion concentration compatible with life, the $[H^+]$ is proportional to the following ratios:

$$[H^+] \propto \frac{[HCO_3^-]}{[CO_2]} \sim \frac{[A^-]}{[HA]} \sim \frac{[HPO_4^{2-}]}{[H_2PO_4^-]} \sim \frac{[Hb^-]}{[HHb]} \sim \frac{[Prt^-]}{[HPrt]} \qquad (10\text{-}2)$$

The relations shown in Eq. 10-2 are not equations. There are no equal signs. The ratios do not determine $[H^+]$; that is, the ratios are not independent variables. The $[H^+]$ determines the ratios. The ratio $[HCO_3^-]/[CO_2]$ is used experimentally and clinically because it is easy to measure P_{CO_2} with electrodes and because there is such a large quantity of CO_2 in body liquids. CO_2 is less important inside cells, where the proteins (A_{tot}) are the principal weak acid buffers.

pH

The symbol pH is used widely to represent $[H^+]$. It is defined as follows:

$$pH = -\log[H^+] \qquad (10\text{-}3)$$

pH came into popular use because it is a positive number and a linear function in the Henderson-Hasselbalch equation. Two serious difficulties in using it instead of $[H^+]$ are that (1) when hydrogen ion concentration rises, pH falls, and (2) $[H^+]$ is not a linear function of pH. For example, at the normal $[H^+]$a of 40 nEq/liter, the pH is 7.40. If the $[H^+]$ increases to 100 nEq/liter, the pH falls to 7.00, but if $[H^+]$ falls to 16 nEq/liter, the pH rises to 7.80. The pH changes from normal are the same (0.40 unit), but the $[H^+]$ changes are markedly different (60 and 24 nEq/liter, respectively).

The widespread use of pH is unfortunate because it is a rather *insensitive* and *misleading* representation of $[H^+]$. In this chapter, I use hydrogen ion concentration, $[H^+]$, but I sometimes include pH in parentheses: $[H^+] = 40$ nEq/liter (pH 7.40). One should be able to switch between the two systems.

STRONG ION DIFFERENCE

The strong ion difference* is the *difference* between the sum of all the strong positive ions (cations) and the sum of all the strong negative ions (anions). At hydrogen ion concentrations compatible with life, the strong ion difference ([SID]) is nearly always a positive number; that is, the sum of strong cations > sum of strong anions. Obviously, the [SID] must be balanced by something to achieve electrical neutrality. This balance is provided by weak acids, namely, proteins ($[A^-]$) and bicarbonate ($[HCO_3^-]$). The strong ion difference can be set independently of any other acid-base parameter, usually by renal regulation of Na^+ plasma concentration.

In plasma, the $[HCO_3^-]$ is about 24 mEq/liter and accounts for most of the huge excess quantity of CO_2 in blood, as represented by the wide stream in Figure 9-6.†

Remember: The reason for the huge excess of CO_2, as HCO_3^-, in blood is to partially compensate for the strong ion difference ([SID]).

Another way of describing the importance of the strong ion difference ([SID]) is as follows. If one takes a bottle of club soda (which is CO_2 dissolved in water under pressure), places it in a chamber, and reduces the pressure, all the CO_2 will escape into the gas phase. On the other hand, if one takes a sample of plasma, places it in a chamber, and reduces the pressure,

---

* The strong ion difference is essentially the same as what is called "buffer base" in previous textbooks. Strong ion difference is preferred because it makes a positive identification of this important independent variable.

† Do not confuse plasma with whole blood because the status of their acid-base balance is not identical.

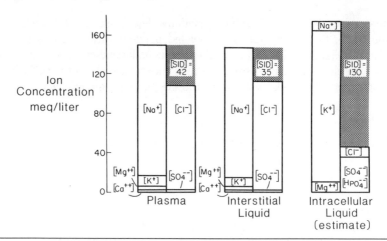

Fig. 10-1. Bar graphs representing the concentrations of positive ions (cations) and negative ions (anions) of plasma, interstitial liquid, and estimated average intracellular liquid. The difference between strong electrolyte cations and anions is the strong ion difference ([SID]). The [SID] in intracellular liquid is enormous. To read the bar graph, place a straight-edge on the top and bottom lines of any desired ion and read the difference between the two values on the y-axis. For plasma, the total of positive ions is about 150 mEq/liter, of which [Na$^+$] is 150 − 10 = 140 mEq/liter. Similarly, the interstitial [Cl$^-$] is 114 − 2 = 112 mEq/liter.

one cannot extract much CO_2. This is because the law of electrical neutrality keeps the bicarbonate in solution to balance the sodium ions.

The only way to reduce the CO_2 content of the plasma is to reduce the [SID] by adding a strong acid that will provide more strong electrolyte anions to balance the cations. The bicarbonate will react with the added H$^+$ to form carbonic acid, which will break down into CO_2 and H_2O.

Figure 10-1 shows the [SID] in bar graph form for plasma, interstitial, and estimated intracellular liquids. Figure 10-2 shows a completely balanced ion diagram produced by adding ad-

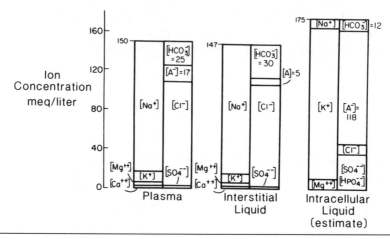

Fig. 10-2. The two components of the strong ion difference, namely, weak acids (proteins, [A$^-$]) and bicarbonate, [HCO$_3$$^-$]. Interstitial liquid has a low protein concentration but an increased P$_{CO_2}$. The increased [HCO$_3$$^-$] necessary to balance the strong ion difference is set by the interstitial liquid [H$^+$]. The intracellular strong ion difference is balanced mainly by weak acids (proteins) rather than by bicarbonate.

ditional negatively charged ions to achieve electrical neutrality. There are two weak electrolytes that contribute anions to provide electrical neutrality, namely, bicarbonate (HCO_3^-) and protein (A^-). The bar graphs in Figures 10-1 and 10-2 are in standard clinical use. They are called gamblegrams (after J. Gamble, who popularized their use).

The strong ion difference ([SID]) can be set by adding (diet, metabolism, or injection) or removing (vomiting, diarrhea, or kidney) strong electrolyte ions, either cations (Na^+, K^+, Ca^{2+}) or anions (Cl^-, SO_4^{2-}, acetoacetate$^-$).

THREE INDEPENDENT VARIABLES DETERMINE HYDROGEN ION CONCENTRATION

I have defined three independent variables (CO_2, strong ion difference, total weak acid). They are independent because each can be set separately without regard to the others. When these three parameters are set, all other acid-base variables are determined, namely, hydrogen ion concentration ($[H^+]$), bicarbonate concentration ($[HCO_3^-]$), and all the weak acid buffer ratios that were described by the proportions in Eq. 10-2.

The remainder of this chapter describes the regulation of $[H^+]$ in whole blood. Although we are vitally interested in the regulation of *whole body* hydrogen ion concentration, it is more complex, even though it follows the same pattern. It is customary to reserve extended discussion of whole body acid-base balance until the fundamentals of renal physiology have been learned.

In Figure 10-1, the [SID] of plasma is 42 mEq/liter. Figure 10-2 shows that the ionized side chains of plasma proteins (A^-) contribute 17 mEq/liter, leaving the required $[HCO_3^-]$ of 25 mEq/liter. The total weak acid concentration ($[A_{tot}] = 20$ mEq/liter) is thus 85% dissociated (17/20) at normal arterial blood $[H^+]$. Since the normal adult plasma protein concentration is about 70 g/liter (0.70 mmol/liter), the number of anionic side chains per protein molecule averages 23 (17 mEq/0.70 mmol).

HYDROGEN ION CONCENTRATION

Units

Although I have frequently mentioned $[H^+]$ and expressed it as nanoequivalents per liter, these units need to be stressed. The hydrogen ion concentration in body liquids is one-millionth that of any other ion. It is so small that it cannot be shown in Figure 10-2. Although the $[H^+]$ is very low, it has important effects on protein function because hydrogen ions (protons) are very tiny, have a high charge density, and generate large electrical field gradients. They are important in hydrogen bonding, which helps to determine tertiary (three-dimensional) protein conformation. In addition, $[H^+]$ affects enzyme activity.*

The Importance of Water in H^+ Reactions

Water is such a ubiquitous substance (60% body weight) that we tend to forget that it is an important component of the chemical reaction upon which acid-base regulation is based. In Chapter 9, I included water in the mass action Eqs. 9-3 to 9-5. In a neutral solution of pure water ($[H^+] = [OH^-]$ at 37°C), $[H^+] = 210$ nEq/liter. The neutrality of plasma occurs at $[H^+] = 158$ nEq/liter.†

---

* Comparative physiologists believe that body acid-base balance is regulated to maintain a constant net protein ionization (charge), not to keep $[H^+]$ constant. This is consistent with the decrease in $[H^+]$ observed as body temperature decreases. This need not concern us because body temperature in humans remains nearly constant (37°C; range 33 to 41°C).

† The commonly stated neutral $[H^+]$ of plasma is 100 nEq/liter (pH = 7.00). That is the neutral $[H^+]$ of water at 25°C.

[H$^+$], the Henderson-Hasselbalch Equation, and pH

Acid-base status is measured by taking a sample of arterial blood and measuring its [H$^+$] and P_{CO_2}. Thus, we must examine the relationship between [H$^+$], P_{CO_2}, and carbonic acid. We begin by setting up the mass action equation for the weak electrolyte carbonic acid (H_2CO_3) as follows:

$$K_A \times [H_2CO_3] = [H^+] \times [HCO_3^-] \tag{10-4}$$

where K_A is the equilibrium constant for this reaction and equals 0.000338 mEq/liter. However, the carbonic acid concentration ($[H_2CO_3]$) cannot be easily measured. H_2CO_3 is in equilibrium with the dissolved CO_2, although the carbonic acid represents only 0.235% of the total dissolved CO_2. The exact relationship is

$$[H_2CO_3] = \frac{[CO_2,\text{dissolved}]}{426} \tag{10-5}$$

The $426 = 100\%/0.235\%$. Now substitute Eq. 10-5 into Eq. 10-4 to obtain

$$\frac{K_A}{426} \times [CO_2,\text{dissolved}] = [H^+] \times [HCO_3^-] \tag{10-6}$$

The ratio $(3.38 \times 10^{-4}/426)$ is defined as a new *effective* equilibrium constant for *dissolved* CO_2. Most textbooks refer to it as an "apparent" equilibrium constant, K'_A. The prime indicates that it is the equilibrium constant of dissolved CO_2, not H_2CO_3. K'_A equals 794 nEq/liter. Next, rearrange Eq. 10-6 to isolate [H$^+$]

$$[H^+] = K'_A \times \frac{[CO_2]}{[HCO_3^-]} \tag{10-7}$$

Taking logarithms of each term to the base 10 and multiplying the whole equation by -1, one obtains the following equation:

$$-\log[H^+] = -\log K'_A - \log \frac{[CO_2]}{[HCO_3^-]} \tag{10-8}$$

The logarithm of the equilibrium constant, $K'_A = 794$ nEq/liter, is negative: $\log K'_A = -6.10$. Thus, the negative logarithm of K'_A is a positive number, which is called $pK'_A = 6.10$. Similarly, the negative logarithm of the [H$^+$] is called pH (Eq. 10-2). Making these substitutions, we arrive at the equation

$$pH = pK'_A + \log \frac{[HCO_3^-]}{[CO_2]} \tag{10-9}$$

I have inverted the $[CO_2]/[HCO_3^-]$ ratio to restore a positive sign to the log ratio. There is only one more step, which is to recall that the dissolved CO_2 is defined in terms of P_{CO_2} and its solubility coefficient in blood is

$$[CO_2] = \alpha_{CO_2} \times P_{CO_2} \tag{10-10}$$

Making the final substitution, one obtains the Henderson-Hasselbalch equation.

HENDERSON-HASSELBALCH EQUATION

The Henderson-Hasselbalch equation is as follows:

$$pH = 6.10 + \log \frac{[HCO_3^-]}{[0.03 \times P_{CO_2}]} \qquad (10\text{-}11)$$

Without thinking about its source (Eq. 10-7), the vast majority of physicians and physiologists use pH synonymously with $[H^+]$, even though they are not linearly related and move in opposite directions. Such is human contrariness.

The Henderson-Hasselbalch equation is exactly correct only at 37°C, since CO_2 solubility and the equilibrium constant K'_A vary with temperature. However, since human life exists within a fairly narrow range (33°C to 41°C), the equation is quite accurate.

In modern pulmonary function laboratories, blood pH is measured by using an H^+-sensitive glass electrode and P_{CO_2} is measured by using a CO_2-sensitive electrode. The Henderson-Hasselbalch equation is used to compute the blood bicarbonate concentration.

The hydrogen ion concentration ($[H^+]$) determines the ratio $[HCO_3^-]/[0.03 \times P_{CO_2}]$. The absolute value of $[HCO_3^-]$ is determined by the two principal independent variables, [SID] and $[A_{tot}]$ (Fig. 10-2), as shown in the following relationship:

$$[HCO_3^-] = [SID] - [A^-] \qquad (10\text{-}12)$$

The relationship includes only the ionized weak acids (A^-; proteins), not the total weak acids. ($[A^-]$ is also called the "anion gap" in the old clinical literature.) If we knew the equilibrium constant for the weak acids, we could write a Henderson-Hasselbalch equation using the ratio $[A^-]/[HA]$.

CEREBROSPINAL FLUID

Cerebrospinal fluid (CSF) (or brain interstitial liquid) is a special problem because the only weak acid present is carbonic acid. There is no significant concentration of protein in brain extracellular liquid because the blood-brain barrier prevents any protein escape from plasma at the capillary walls within the brain or at the choroid plexus. Thus, $[A_{tot}] = 0$ and [SID] = $[HCO_3^-]$ by Eq. 10-12.

CSF behaves in a manner somewhat similar to interstitial liquid (Fig. 10-1), which has a reduced protein concentration. However, the $[H^+]$ of normal CSF is greater than that of interstitial fluid: $[H^+]_{CSF} = 48$ nEq/liter (pH 7.32). Assuming that the CSF P_{CO_2} is 50 mmHg, the bicarbonate concentration ($[HCO_3^-]$), calculated by using the Henderson-Hasselbalch equation, is 25 mEq/liter. This is slightly higher than in blood plasma but lower than that of average interstitial liquid (Fig. 10-2). In part, this is because CSF is a *transcellular* liquid, meaning that active metabolic processes affect $[SID]_{CSF}$ and, consequently, $[HCO_3^-]_{CSF}$.

Suppose the $P_{CO_2,CSF}$ fell rapidly to 30 mmHg, which can happen if a person hyperventilates for several minutes. Since there is no weak acid other than CO_2 and since there can be no change in the bicarbonate concentration as long as the strong ion difference (SID) is constant, $[H^+]_{CSF}$ must fall. The new $[H^+]$ is 29 nEq/liter (pH 7.54).

Of course, the [SID] will eventually change through metabolically dependent processes (active transport), but that takes time (hours or days).

Chapter 11 shows that $[H^+]$ and P_{CO_2} of CSF and brain interstitial liquid have important influences on breathing through their action on chemosensitive respiratory control areas near the ventral surface of the brain stem.

Table 10-1. Independent and Dependent Variables in the Four Pure Acid-Base Disturbances

Variable	Respiration Acidosis	Respiration Alkalosis	Metabolic Acidosis	Metabolic Alkalosis
Independent[a]				
P_{CO_2}	↑	↓	NC[b]	NC
[SID]	NC	NC	↓	↑
Dependent				
[H$^+$]	↑	↓	↑	↓
pH	↓	↑	↓	↑
[HCO$_3^-$]	↑	↓	↓	↑

^{a} The other independent variable, the total weak acid ([A_{tot}], mainly hemoglobin and plasma proteins in blood) is considered constant in any given circumstance.
^{b} NC, no change.

ACID-BASE DISORDERS

As we saw in Eq. 10-2, [H$^+$] is proportional to the ratio of the ionized to the un-ionized form of each weak acid. The Henderson-Hasselbalch equation makes use only of [HCO$_3^-$]/[CO$_2$]. Many textbooks refer to that ratio as kidney/lung, signifying that ventilation alters P_{CO_2} (which it does) and that the kidney alters [HCO$_3^-$]. Actually, the kidney has little to do with blood bicarbonate concentration. What the kidney regulates is the strong ion difference ([SID]) through its retention or elimination of sodium. But, since most of the sodium is reabsorbed as NaHCO$_3$ (for electrical neutrality), it is reasonable to say that the kidney regulates [HCO$_3^-$].

There are other ways to alter the strong ion difference, for example, uncontrollable vomiting (loss of Cl$^-$) or severe diarrhea (loss of Na$^+$). It is useful to consider two main forms of acid-base disturbance, *respiratory* and *metabolic*.

In view of the wide availability of pocket calculators, we should be able to calculate [H$^+$] directly using Eq. 10-7. But the Henderson-Hasselbalch equation is too deeply ingrained to be rooted out easily. In fact, most physicians do not even use the Henderson-Hasselbalch equation, preferring its graphic representation. Figure 10-2 shows a modified version of a graph called the Siggaard-Anderson nomogram in which log P_{CO_2} is plotted as a function of [H$^+$] (pH).*

There are several graphic systems representing the Henderson-Hasselbalch equation. It really does not matter which one is used, since all contain essentially the same information. The main limitation of the Siggaard-Anderson nomogram is that it was designed to describe the acid-base status of whole blood.

Before applying the Siggaard-Anderson nomogram, I must mention the common forms of acid-base disturbance. Since there are two main variables, P_{CO_2} and [SID], there must be two main forms of disturbance, and since each variable can be either increased or decreased, there must be two components to each type of disturbance. Thus, there are four "pure" acid-base disturbances: *respiratory* acidosis and alkalosis and *metabolic* acidosis and alkalosis.

Table 10-1 shows the relative variations in the independent variables (P_{CO_2} and [SID]) and the dependent variables ([H$^+$] and [HCO$_3^-$]) in each of the pure acid-base disturbances. The

---

* Until about 20 years ago, most analyses of acid-base disorders were made in terms of a graphic representation of the Henderson-Hasselbalch equation in which the bicarbonate concentration ([HCO$_3^-$]) was plotted as a function of [H$^+$] in graphs called Davenport diagrams (named after the famous physiologist who promoted them). It was a clear and easy way to express variations in acid-base balance. One may still see such diagrams in some textbooks. Why this switch? Because the P_{CO_2} electrode came into common use and greatly simplified acid-base evaluation.

changes are shown by directional arrows. Everything is fairly self-evident, as long as one keeps in mind that $[H^+]$ and pH vary in opposite directions.

Remember: In respiratory disturbances, $[HCO_3^-]$ varies in the same direction as P_{CO_2}; in metabolic disturbances, it varies in the same direction as $[SID]$.

Siggaard-Anderson Nomogram

To become familiar with the Siggaard-Anderson nomogram (Fig. 10-3A), find the point that represents normal arterial blood ($[H^+]$ = 40 nEq/liter [pH 7.40] and P_{CO_2} = 40 mmHg). The line representing P_{CO_2} = 40 mmHg is also marked by slanting tick marks, which are labeled "plasma bicarbonate, mEq/liter." At the normal blood point, the plasma bicarbonate concentration is 24.5 mEq/liter. The box surrounding the ideal arterial blood point represents the range of normal $[H^+]$ (35 to 45 nEq/liter; pH 7.45 to 7.35) and P_{CO_2} (35 to 45 mmHg).

In the upper left quadrant is a short, curving line labeled "Hb, g/liter." This line is necessary because of the variability of $[A_{tot}]$ with [Hb] among humans.*

For normal blood, a straight line drawn between the mean blood point ($[H^+]$ = 40 nEq/liter; P_{CO_2} = 40 mmHg) to Hb = 150 g/liter represents the blood acid-base balance or blood buffer line. If you change P_{CO_2}, the $[H^+]$ concentration moves along this line before any compensation occurs.

If [Hb] = 0 (for example, in plasma), a line drawn between [Hb] = 0 and the arterial point represents the acid-base line of plasma (Fig. 10-3B [solid line]). The slope of the plasma line is not quite as steep as the slope of the whole blood line (dashed line), which means that plasma does not buffer against changes in $[H^+]$ as well as whole blood does.

If there is no plasma protein (that is, $[A_{tot}]$ = 0, as in CSF, the $[HCO_3^-]$ must be constant and equal to the strong ion difference ($[SID]$). The line representing this condition is called an **isobicarbonate** line because every point on it represents a single bicarbonate concentration. It is indicated by a line at a 135-degree angle to the P_{CO_2} = 40 mmHg line, as shown by the dotted line in Figure 10-3B. The slope of the isobicarbonate (HCO_3^-/CO_2 titration) line is less steep than the slope of the plasma line, indicating a further decrease in the buffering power of bicarbonate solutions compared with plasma or whole blood. In other words, transcellular solutions (such as CSF with no protein) are not as well buffered against changes in P_{CO_2} as is blood, plasma, or interstitial liquid. Thus, during acute respiratory acidosis or alkalosis, cerebrospinal fluid $[H^+]$ changes more than does arterial blood $[H^+]$ before any compensation occurs.

The four *primary* acid-base disturbances are easily represented on the Siggaard-Anderson nomogram (Fig. 10-4).† *Respiratory* disturbances occur along the blood buffer line. As P_{CO_2} rises, the arterial point moves up and to the left. For example, if P_{ACO_2} increased by 20 mmHg to 60 mmHg, the $[H^+]$ would increase to 52 nEq/liter (pH 7.28), representing pure respiratory

---

* Plasma proteins in normal whole blood (hematocrit [Ht] = 0.45) amount to 38.5 g/liter [70 g/liter plasma × (1 − Ht)]. Thus, [Hb] of 150 g/liter represents 80% of $[A_{tot}]$.

† If you dislike reading graphs, please remember it is not necessary to use them. They are a tool, not an end in themselves, intended to make determinations of acid-base status quick and easy. But with a pocket calculator, you can easily solve Eq. 10-7 (the H^+ mass balance equation) or its offspring, the Henderson-Hasselbalch equation, to calculate $[HCO_3^-]$ or pH.

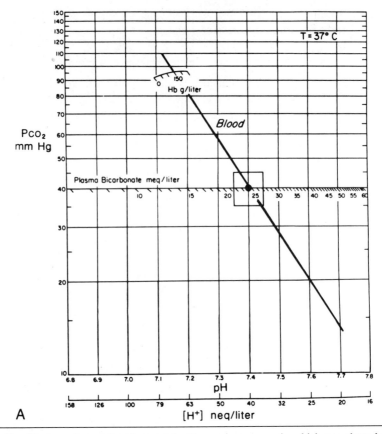

Fig. 10-3. Simplified version of the Siggaard-Anderson nomogram, in which are plotted two variables from the Henderson-Hasselbalch equation: log P_{CO_2} on the y-axis and $[H^+]$ (pH) on the x-axis. The normal mean arterial point is at $[H^+]$ = 40 nEq/liter (pH 7.40) and P_{CO_2} = 40 mmHg. The box represents the normal range of P_{CO_2} and $[H^+]$ in humans. **(A)** The line represents the normal whole blood buffer line (between the normal arterial point and Hb = 150 g/liter). (*Figure continues.*)

acidosis. To obtain the $[HCO_3^-]$ at the new $[H^+]$ and P_{CO_2}, use Eq. 10-7 or the Henderson-Hasselbalch equation (Eq. 10-11) or draw a 135-degree line from the new blood point to intersect the P_{CO_2} = 40 mmHg (isobicarbonate) line. Any method should give the same answer, namely, 27.2 mEq/liter. Thus, the blood buffers (A_{tot}) have acted to release strong cations, which caused the 3 mEq/liter rise in $[HCO_3^-]$; that is, $[A^-]$ decreased. Likewise, if one hyperventilated so as to decrease P_{ACO_2} quickly to 20 mmHg, the $[H^+]$a would fall to 25 nEq/liter (pHa 7.60), representing pure respiratory *alkalosis*. The $[HCO_3^-]$ would decrease to 19.0 mEq/liter. Again, the superior buffering power of whole blood is evident; $[HCO_3^-]$ is reduced because of the increased $[A^-]$. If the P_{CO_2} had been reduced in CSF ($[HCO_3^-]/[CO_2]$ solution), the $[H^+]$ would have decreased to 20 nEq/liter (pH 7.70). Pure respiratory acid-base disturbances can exist if the only variable that changed is P_{CO_2} and [SID] and [A_{tot}] remain constant (that is, no compensation).

Primary metabolic disturbances consist of all points along the horizontal line at P_{CO_2} = 40 mmHg in Figure 10-4B. Points to the left of the normal $[H^+]$ represent pure metabolic acidosis,

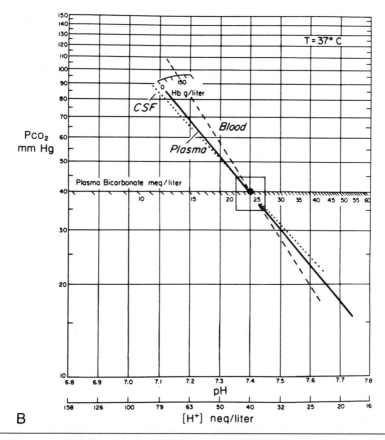

Fig. 10-3 (*Continued*). **(B)** The plasma buffer line (between the arterial point and Hb = 0) (solid) and the line for CSF (dotted), which represents a constant [HCO$_3^-$] buffer line, have been added to the blood buffer line (dashed). The steeper the slope of the line, the greater the buffering power of the liquid, that is, the greater is [A$_{tot}$]. Thus, whole blood is a better buffer than plasma, which is a better buffer than cerebrospinal fluid.

and points to the right represent pure metabolic alkalosis. In moving along the iso-P$_{CO_2}$ line, the plasma bicarbonate changes, representing changes in [SID]. For example, take metabolic acidosis with [H$^+$] = 56 nEq/liter (pH 7.25). The plasma bicarbonate concentration is 17 mEq/liter, a reduction of 7 mEq/liter in [HCO$_3^-$]. This occurred because of an increase in strong acid anions (SO$_4^{2-}$, HPO$_4^{2-}$, or keto acids).

Metabolic alkalosis is shown by moving to the right along the P$_{CO_2}$ = 40 mmHg line. As indicated in Table 10-1, as the [H$^+$] falls due to an increase in [SID], the plasma bicarbonate concentration also rises.

Compensatory Changes

Pure disturbances of acid-base balance last only briefly before compensation begins. There are very few acid-base disturbances in which the data fall on either the pure respiratory or the pure metabolic line. But it is inappropriate to discuss extensively the compensations that occur

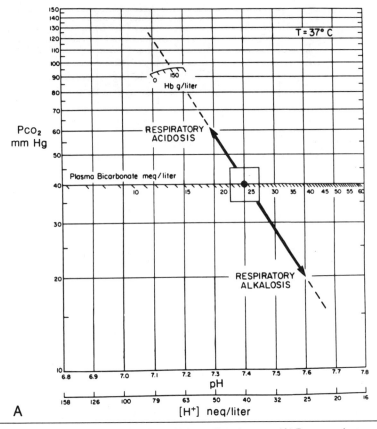

Fig. 10-4. Representation of the four primary acid-base disturbances. **(A)** Pure respiratory disturbances, caused by changes in P_{CO_2}. Plasma bicarbonate changes moderately due to the weak acid buffers (Hb and plasma protein). (*Figure continues.*)

following primary acid-base disturbances, since neither renal function nor control of breathing have been discussed. However, there are a few intuitive points that can be made.

The two lines of primary respiratory and metabolic disturbances correspond to a limited set of points on the Siggaard-Anderson nomogram. There are infinitely more points off the lines than on them. All these other points represent *combinations* of metabolic and respiratory disturbances. Two examples are plotted in Figure 10-5.

When a primary respiratory disturbance occurs, it is not long before other mechanisms begin to restore $[H^+]$ toward normal. The compensation is never complete, however, since that would remove the restoring stimulus, but in some long-term acid-base disturbances, the degree of restoration of $[H^+]$ is remarkable.

The main compensatory mechanism for respiratory disturbances is renal retention or excretion of sodium. In other words, the kidney adjusts the ratio $[HCO_3^-]/[CO_2]$ toward normal by changing the strong ion difference ([SID]).

Let us examine the compensation for respiratory acidosis in which P_{ACO_2} increased by 20 mmHg. If the P_{ACO_2} remains at 60 mmHg, the blood $[H^+]$ would soon start to fall; that is, the arterial blood point would move to the right along the line $P_{CO_2} = 60$ mmHg. How much the

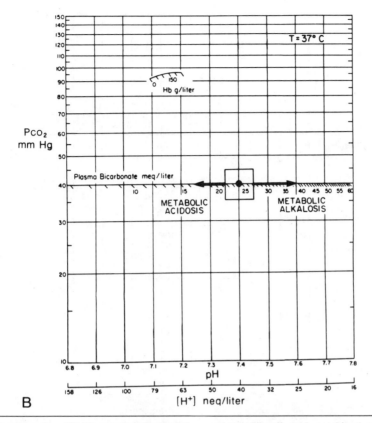

B

Fig. 10-4 (*Continued*).   **(B)** Pure metabolic disturbances markedly affect plasma bicarbonate, since they directly change the strong ion difference ([SID]).

$[H^+]$ will decrease depends on how efficient the kidneys are in retaining sodium or excreting chloride, either of which increases the strong ion difference and therefore increases $[HCO_3^-]$. Suppose the $[H^+]$ decreased to 42 nEq/liter (pH 7.38). A 135-degree (isobicarbonate) line drawn through the new compensated blood point should intersect the plasma bicarbonate line $P_{CO_2} = 40$ mmHg at 34.3 mEq/liter, indicating a further increase in [SID] by 7.1 mEq/liter. The total increase in $[HCO_3^-]$ from normal (24 mEq/liter) is 9.9 mEq/liter.

A second example is provided by a patient who has developed severe metabolic acidosis (as in uncontrolled diabetes). If fixed ventilation were provided so that P_{CO_2} could not change, the $[H^+]$ would shift along the pure metabolic acidosis line. Fortunately, acidosis (increased P_{CO_2} or increased $[H^+]$) usually alters breathing (see Ch. 11), so that ventilation increases and P_{ACO_2} decreases. Suppose the subject had a $[H^+]$ of 56 nEq/liter (pH 7.25). In the uncompensated condition, $[HCO_3^-] = 17.0$ mEq/liter at $P_{CO_2} = 40$ mmHg, which stimulated ventilation sufficiently to lower P_{ACO_2} to 30 mmHg. By now, you should be able to calculate the increase in the alveolar ventilation that would cause such a change in P_{ACO_2}, using the alveolar ventilation equation (Eq. 4-3). As a result, $[H^+]$ would fall along a line parallel to the normal blood buffer line (constant $[A_{tot}]$) until it intersected the line $P_{CO_2} = 30$ mmHg. The compensated

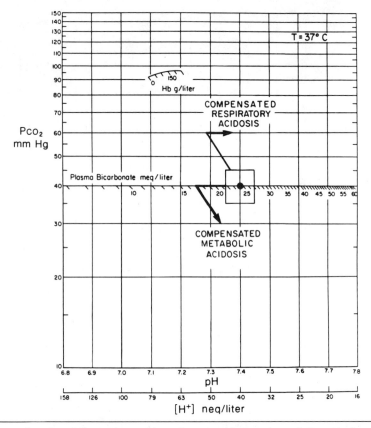

Fig. 10-5.   Examples of partially compensated respiratory acidosis and metabolic acidosis, as represented on the Siggaard-Anderson nomogram. The compensation for the primary respiratory acidosis is renal retention of sodium or excretion of chloride creating a metabolic alkalosis, as indicated by the increase in the plasma bicarbonate concentration. The metabolic acidosis is compensated by increased ventilation, which reduces P_{CO_2} to partially match the decrease in plasma bicarbonate.

$[H^+]$ would be 47 nEq/liter (pH 7.33); that is, the $[H^+]$ would be reduced by 9 nEq/liter. The $[HCO_3^-]$ would decrease further to 15.3 mEq/liter for a total decrease from normal (24.5 mEq/liter) of 9.2 mEq/liter.

READINGS

Books

1. Davenport HW: The ABC of Acid-Base Chemistry. 5th Ed., revised. University of Chicago Press, 1969
   A masterful, thorough, yet simple description of acid-base balance. It was the acid-base bible until Stewart's book (reference 3) was published. The introduction of the P_{CO_2} electrode in 1960 made the famous Davenport diagram (graph of pH versus HCO_3^-) obsolete.
2. Jones NL: Blood Gases and Acid-Base Physiology. 2nd Ed. Thieme, New York, 1987
   In the second edition of this programed text, Jones switched completely to the Stewart

approach to acid-base physiology, thoroughly described in 17 very brief, easy-to-read chapters (Chapters 18 to 34).
3. Stewart PA: How to Understand Acid-Base. Elsevier, New York, 1981
The modern approach to acid-base balance. Naturally, the old guard acid-base physiologists don't like it.

Reviews

4. Stewart PA: Independent and dependent variables of acid-base control. Respir Physiol 33:9–26, 1978
A brief introduction to modern acid-base balance.

Articles

5. Siggaard-Anderson O: The pH-log pCO_2 blood acid-base nomogram revised. Scand J Clin Lab Invest 14:598–604, 1962
Slight modification to bring the nomogram to its current form. The complete diagram is more complex than the version used in this chapter. The buffer base line $= [SID] + [A_{tot}]$ and the base excess line $= [SID]_{normal} - [SID]_{altered}$. The lines are empirical, that is, based on measurements, not theory.
6. Siggaard-Anderson O, Engel K: A New Acid-Base Nomogram. Scand J Clin Lab Invest 12:177–186, 1960
The source of the nomogram.

QUESTIONS*

Drill

1. Use Eq. 10-7 to calculate the missing quantity. Name the acid-base disturbance.

	$[H^+]$, nEq/liter	P_{CO_2}, mmHg	$[HCO_3^-]$, mEq/liter
a.	?	40	24
b.	?	60	27.2
c.	25	15	?
d.	45	35	?
e.	30	?	35.9

2. Use the Henderson-Hasselbalch equation to calculate the missing variables. Name the acid-base condition.

	$[H^+]$, nEq/liter	pH	P_{CO_2}, mmHg	$[HCO_3^-]$, mEq/liter
a.	?	7.45	35	?
b.	?	7.35	?	23.5
c.	72	?	?	33
d.	25	?	40	?
e.	?	7.31	40	?

Problems

3. a. How much does the hydrogen ion concentration ($[H^+]$) change between pH 7.40 and pH 6.95? b. How much does pH change between $[H^+]$ = 55 nEq/liter and $[H^+]$ = 30 nEq/liter?

4. In the normal stomach containing pure gastric acid (HCl), the $[H^+]$ = 100 mEq/liter. a. what is the pH? b. what is P_{CO_2}? c. what is [SID]? (Careful, this one is tricky.) d. what is $[HCO_3^-]$?

5. When the strong ion difference ([SID]) decreases,
   a. Metabolic acidosis must be present
   b. Respiratory acidosis must be present
   c. Pa_{CO_2} always rises
   d. Total weak acid ($[A_{tot}]$) decreases
   e. pH rises

6. If one increases the blood bicarbonate concentration of a normal person by infusing sodium bicarbonate, which of the following is most likely to occur?
   a. $[H^+]$a will increase
   b. $[H^+]$a will decrease
   c. Metabolic acidosis with a compensatory rise in Pa_{CO_2} will occur
   d. Respiratory alkalosis with a compensatory metabolic acidosis will occur
   e. Pa_{CO_2} will fall as respiratory compensation for the increased $[H^+]$a

7. On the Siggaard-Anderson nomogram shown here, plot the arterial blood acid-base status of the following conditions. (The status may be a point, a line, or an area on the nomogram.)

---

* Answers begin on p. 211.

a. A normal woman who has voluntarily hyperventilated for a few minutes.
b. A normal man who has lived for a year at high altitude (above 10,000 feet).
c. A baby with pyloric stenosis who has been vomiting repeatedly over 3 days.
d. A person with emphysema (chronic obstructive pulmonary disease) whose effective $\dot{V}_A$ is decreased by 25% suddenly develops diabetic ketosis (acidosis).

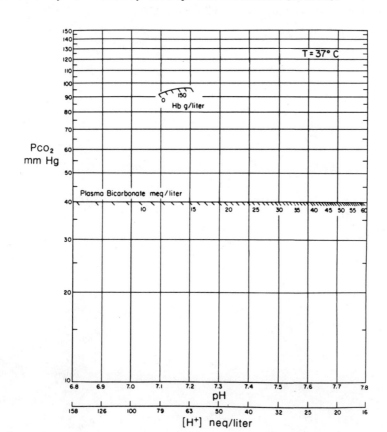

8. The shift in the position of the HbO_2 curve that occurs in metabolic acidosis would
   a. Increase the ability of hemoglobin to take up O_2 in the lung
   b. Be in the same direction as that produced by decreased temperature
   c. Have no effect on tissue P_{O_2}
   d. Increase $P\bar{v}_{O_2}$
   e. Decrease the partial pressure at which O_2 is delivered to tissue cells
9. Which of the following statements is most nearly correct for CSF?
   a. [SID] is the same as in systemic arterial blood.
   b. [SID] is much greater than in systemic arterial blood.
   c. $pH_{CSF} > pHa$, normally.
   d. For equal changes in P_{CO_2}, $[H^+]_{CSF}$ changes less than does $[H^+]a$.
   e. An acute change in $P_{CO_2,CSF}$ is accompanied by a change in $[HCO_3{}^-]_{CSF}$ that is less than would occur in systemic arterial blood for the same $[H^+]$ change.

10. Raising a normal person's Pa_{CO_2} acutely to 60 mmHg by adjusting inspired P_{CO_2} and keeping it there for 15 min would increase systemic arterial blood
    a. $[H^+]$ by more than a factor of 3/2 from control
    b. $[H^+]$ by less than a factor of 3/2 from control
    c. $[HCO_3^-]$ by a factor of 3/2 from control
    d. $[HCO_3^-]$ by more than a factor of 3/2 from control
    e. pH

11

Control of Breathing

THE BOTTOM LINE

General Plan

There are two main schemes for the regulation of breathing. *Metabolic* (automatic) control is concerned with oxygen delivery and with acid-base balance ($P_{A_{CO_2}}$). *Behavioral* (voluntary) control is related to coordinated activities in which breathing may be temporarily suspended or altered. The control system consists of a *central controller* (driver) located in the brain stem (medulla and pons), an *effector* (mainly the muscles of the chest wall but also the smooth muscle of the airways), and various *sensors* that report back to the central controller the results of the intended action.

Timing Diagram of Breathing

Breathing is a kinetic event. The duration of each breath (T_{tot}) depends on the frequency of breathing. The force of inspiratory muscle contraction and the duration of inspiration (T_I) control the tidal volume. Expiration is normally passive during the time available (T_E).

Brain Stem Controller

The central controller includes not only the brain stem neuron pools and spinal cord motor neurons but also the reticular activating system (which regulates the alertness of the brain). The modern view of the brain stem controller is that it contains a tonically active inspiratory neuron pool that receives input from a wide variety of sensors. The summed sensory input generally inhibits inspiratory activity. These inhibitory impulses are subsumed under the term *inspiratory cutoff switch*. Higher centers regulate behavioral breathing by temporarily overriding the brain stem pattern generator.

Sensors

The sensory component includes **central chemoreceptors** (brain stem surface), **peripheral chemoreceptors** (carotid bodies), and **proprioceptors** (lung stretch, irritant, and C-fiber receptors, as well as diaphragm, intercostal, and abdominal muscle spindles and tendon organs). The brain stem surface receptors are most sensitive to $P_{A_{CO_2}}$, which affects arterial, cerebrospinal fluid, and brain interstitial and intercellular liquid P_{CO_2} and $[H^+]$. The initial ventilatory response to CO_2 is large and occurs rapidly. Cerebral blood flow also affects the central chemoreceptors because brain metabolism (aerobic, anaerobic) generates CO_2 or lactic acid, which need to be removed. The

(Continues).

189

(Continued).

peripheral chemoreceptors in the carotid bodies are mainly sensitive to reduced arterial oxygen tension, although they are also affected by local blood flow, $[H^+]$, and Pa_{CO_2}. The response to hypoxia comes into play only at low Pa_{O_2} (<60 mmHg). There are interactions between P_{O_2} and P_{CO_2} that affect the threshold and sensitivity of the chemical regulators. Mechanical receptors send information about lung and chest wall position and so limit inspiratory expansion. Irritant receptors in the large airways protect the delicate alveolar surfaces from particles, chemical vapors, and physical factors. C-fiber receptors in the terminal respiratory units are stimulated by distortion of the alveolar walls (lung vascular congestion or edema).

Exercise

Many factors influence ventilation in exercise in a manner incompletely understood, but there is no doubt that the controlled variable is Pa_{CO_2}.

Sleep

Sleep is a complex phenomenon consisting of several phases during which breathing control varies. Sensitivity to both CO_2 and O_2 is diminished, possibly because the reticular activating system is depressed.

Hypoxia

Acute and chronic hypoxia affect breathing somewhat differently because of slow adjustments in cerebrospinal fluid $[H^+]$, which alters CO_2 sensitivity.

Under a variety of conditions, both the rate and depth of breathing change (as in exercise, during sleep, or in chronic hypoxia) in such a manner that $P_{A_{CO_2}}$ (or its equivalent, Pa_{CO_2}) is maintained close to 40 mmHg.

Why should this be? One might think that the arterial oxygen tension, Pa_{O_2}, ought to be the control signal for the regulation of alveolar ventilation (see Ch. 1), but recall from the shape of the hemoglobin-oxygen equilibrium curve (see Ch. 9) that the oxyhemoglobin saturation in arterial blood is rather insensitive to Pa_{O_2}. In addition, when $P_{A_{CO_2}}$ is regulated, the $P_{A_{O_2}}$ is automatically set (alveolar gas equation).

On the other hand, if arterial oxygen tension were to decrease below 60 mmHg ($Sa_{O_2} =$ 91%), the supply of oxygen to the systemic tissue mitochondria might be impaired due to a reduced oxygen diffusion gradient. Therefore, there ought to be a controller that senses very low Pa_{O_2} and stimulates breathing.

Indeed, both $P_{A_{CO_2}}$- and low Pa_{O_2}-regulating mechanisms do exist and interact to control alveolar ventilation. The $P_{A_{CO_2}}$-sensitive mechanism is the main controller, operating on a breath-by-breath basis as we go about our daily business, scarcely ever giving a thought to our breathing patterns. But the $P_{A_{CO_2}}$ controller can be overridden in systemic arterial hypoxemia (for example, acclimatization to living at high altitude) by the Pa_{O_2}-sensitive controller. In addition, we must allow for all the ancillary actions related to breathing (talking, swallowing, straining, coughing, etc.). These require a controller that will break through the normal regulating pattern and temporarily, at least, match breathing to the expected voluntary or behavioral activity. Thus, there must be two kinds of controls—a **metabolic controller**, which serves basic body needs and a **behavioral controller**, which can temporarily override the metabolic control system.

This chapter describes the basic organization of ventilatory control, including a description of various types of sensory information and ancillary controllers. To assist understanding of control, three common conditions are considered. Unfortunately, we cannot delve too deeply into the subject before it becomes complicated and controversial, as do most aspects of homeostasis that involve multiple levels of integration within the central nervous system. Even with an expert knowledge of neuroscience and long experience, physiologists and physicians are sometimes faced with apparent contradictions concerning how breathing is controlled in specific conditions, such as exercise.

THE GENERAL PLAN

The modern view of the control of breathing begins with the commonsense notion that two separate but overlapping patterns are involved in breathing. These are the **metabolic** (automatic, regular) control pattern and the **behavioral** (voluntary, irregular) control pattern. Metabolic breathing is concerned with oxygen delivery to the mitochondria and with acid-base balance ($P_{A_{CO_2}}$). Behavioral breathing is related to volitional activities such as talking, singing, suckling, swallowing, coughing, sneezing, defecation, and parturition and emotional states such as anxiety or fear. Our daily experience teaches us that we can override metabolic breathing at any time we desire but only briefly. Within several seconds—a minute or two at most—the metabolic control system usually reasserts its authority. Normal persons cannot hold their breath until they die.

We know less about the behavioral control system than about the metabolic system. Indeed, this is one area in which "natural experiments" (clinical studies of patients with neurologic disorders) often give important insights.

At the most fundamental level, all control systems are the same. They consist of a controller (driver), an effector (output), and a sensor to report back to the controller the results of the effector (Fig. 11-1). Figure 11-2 is a considerably more complex reworking of the basic control system, but it is about the minimum organization necessary for this introductory description.* Refer to Figure 11-2 when reading the next few pages.

The metabolic controller is primitive (evolved early) and resides within phylogenetically ancient structures, the brain stem and spinal cord. It was once thought that control of inspiration and control of expiration were precisely located in specific brain stem centers, but as now conceived, the organization is much looser. In addition, surrounding and interdigitating throughout the brain stem is a loose network of interneurons known as the **reticular activating system**. It influences the brain stem and spinal cord controllers by affecting the state of alertness (wakefulness) of the brain. The reticular activating system becomes quiescent during sleep.

The **higher-center controllers** (thalamic and cerebral cortex) are concerned with behavioral regulation of breathing in relation to the many complex motor activities that make use of the lungs and chest walls. Their influence feeds down to the brain stem controller. There is also a direct path to the spinal cord motor neurons of the muscles of breathing (effectors). The spinal cord is the interface between the central controllers and the peripheral effectors. Most of the output from the controllers feeds into the motor neurons that affect the muscles of breathing at spinal cord levels C5–T8.

The **effectors** are the diaphragm, abdominal, intercostal, and accessory muscles of breathing (see Ch. 5). Although the lung does not breathe on its own, there are regulatory influences impinging on the lung (airways) from the central controllers, especially through the parasympathetic branch of the autonomic nervous system (vagus nerve).

At the **sensory** level, there are inputs from the muscles of breathing (proprioceptors), which feed information about the results of any intended action back to the central controllers. The

---

* Some parts of this chapter, especially the organization and levels of control in the brain, may be confusing to students who are not familiar with neuroscience.

main function of these proprioceptors (muscle spindles and tendon organs) is to gauge the appropriateness of a particular breathing activity relative to the central controllers' output. One example is during Müller's maneuver (the attempt to inspire against a closed glottis), in which a great effort is associated with no useful ventilation of the lung; that is, the thorax does not enlarge appropriately, and a very unpleasant sensation develops. Try it.

Sensory receptors abound in the lung. Indeed, the vagus nerve is predominantly a sensory nerve (90%). The sensory nerve fibers carry information about the condition of the airways and of the terminal respiratory units. The main classes of airway and lung receptors are:

Stretch receptors: These are associated with the smooth muscle of the bronchi and possibly of the bronchioles. They are activated mainly by lung expansion, which dilates and stretches the airways and alveoli.

Irritant receptors: These are located in or adjacent to the airway epithelium, especially in the larynx, trachea, and main bronchi. They activate the cough reflex. Their primary stimuli are chemical or physical interactions of materials (vapors, particles, etc.) with the mucociliary (epithelial) cells.

C-fiber receptors: Most of the *afferent* neurons in the vagus nerve are tiny, unmyelinated fibers. Many originate in the lung, especially in the terminal respiratory units, where they lie within the alveolar walls. They are activated by certain chemicals arriving via the pulmonary circulation and also by distortion of alveolar tissue (vascular congestion, as in heart failure).

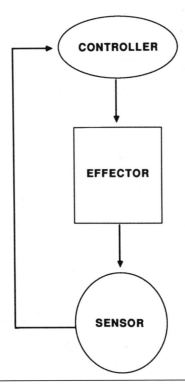

Fig. 11-1. Basic block diagram for a feedback control system (same as in Fig. 1-3). The controller drives the effector to give a response. The sensor detects the response and reports back to the controller. The controller determines whether the response was adequate for the stimulus and makes necessary adjustments in its output.

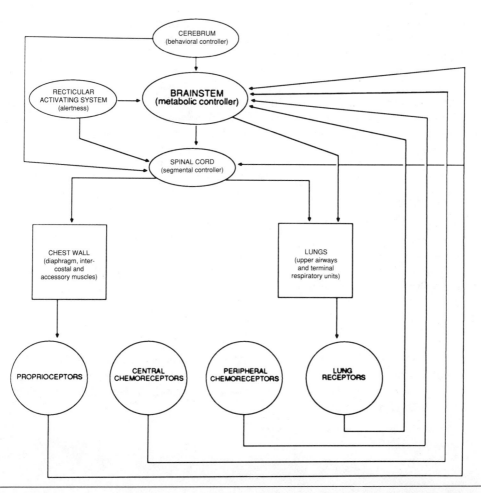

Fig. 11-2.   Control system for breathing organized as in Figure 11-1. This is about the simplest diagram that permits an integrated discussion of the control of breathing. There are four controllers. The **brain stem controller** is the main one, but the other three controllers have important modulating actions. The main effectors are the **chest wall muscles,** but there are some effects in the lung, notably on airway smooth muscle tone through the vagus nerve. There are four kinds of sensory receptors. These feed back to the brain stem controller or spinal cord. Two receptors, the **central** and **peripheral chemoreceptors,** do not directly sense effector action. They sample systemic arterial blood.

Two groups of important **chemoreceptors** located in special areas remote from the lungs and chest wall evaluate the results of breathing on the arterial blood gases. The **peripheral** chemoreceptors are the oxygen-sensitive cells of the carotid bodies. To a lesser degree, they are also sensitive to P_{CO_2}. These cells lie adjacent to, but distinct from, the carotid sinus on either side of the neck at the bifurcation of the common carotid arteries. The **central** chemoreceptors lie on or near the ventral surface of the brain stem (medulla). They are sensitive to Pa_{CO_2} and, on a delayed basis, systemic arterial $[H^+]$.

THE TIMING DIAGRAM OF BREATHING

The first phase of the breathing cycle consists of increasing contraction of the diaphragm or intercostal muscles, which enlarges the thoracic cavity, lowers the pleural and alveolar pressures, and causes air to flow down the airways to the alveoli. After some time, these neural stimuli greatly diminish or cease, at which point expiration begins. Expiration is normally passive in that the chest and lungs, because they have been distorted from their equilibrium position, will return to FRC without any external energy being applied.

Figure 11-3 shows the timing diagram of the normal breathing process (solid line) in which the inspiratory time (T_I) does not occupy more than 40% of the total time, T_{tot}, of each breath (see also Fig. 6-3). The duration of expiration (T_E) is longer because resistance to airflow is increased during expiration. The last 0.5 second or so of expiration is a period of no airflow (expiratory pause). The frequency of breathing is the reciprocal of the duration of each breath ($1/T_{tot}$). At a breathing frequency of 12 breaths per minute, $T_{tot} = 5$ seconds, of which $T_I < 2$ seconds.

Go back to Eq. 4-4, the alveolar ventilation equation

$$\dot{V}_A = \frac{\dot{V}_{CO_2} \times 0.863}{P_{ACO_2}} \tag{11-1}$$

Since minute alveolar ventilation is equal to the breathing rate times the alveolar ventilation per breath (Eq. 4-3), the alveolar ventilation equation can be rewritten as

$$f \times (V_T - V_D) = \frac{\dot{V}_{CO_2} \times 0.863}{P_{ACO_2}} \tag{11-2}$$

where f is frequency, V_T is tidal volume, and V_D is the anatomic dead space, which can be considered constant for practical purposes. This modified form of the alveolar ventilation equation reveals that the only ways by which alveolar ventilation can be regulated are by changing the frequency or the tidal volume.

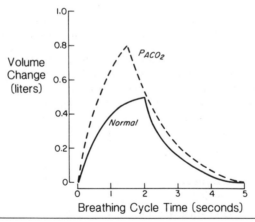

Fig. 11-3. Timing diagram of breathing. Because breathing is a kinetic event, the time is important. In a normal breath, inspiratory time (T_I) takes no more than 40% of the total breathing cycle. The effect of increasing alveolar carbon dioxide (P_{ACO_2}) is shown by the dashed line. In this example, the CO_2 has increased the stimulus output from the central brain stem controller to the inspiratory muscles, which increased the rate of lung volume expansion. The increased lung expansion is sensed by lung and chest wall mechanical receptors. These feed impulses back to the brain stem controllers, which stop inspiration. When P_{ACO_2} is increased, inspiration may cut off sooner than normally, but tidal volume is greater than normal because the rate of volume change is faster.

One way to change ventilation is by alterating the timing of each breath. As T_{tot} decreases, frequency increases. Changes in frequency usually affect both T_I and T_E.

Another way to change ventilation is to alter the rate at which lung volume increases during inspiration. If the muscles of breathing contract more vigorously, inspiration will proceed more rapidly. This may or may not be modified by a shortening of T_I.

An increase in $F_{I_{CO_2}}$ mainly affects the rate of volume change during inspiration, whereas the stimulus from decreased Pa_{O_2} (hypoxemia) affects mainly the frequency of breathing. Figure 11-3 shows the CO_2 effect as a dashed line. Note that inspiratory time is slightly shortened, but tidal volume is increased anyway. The slowly adapting lung stretch receptors, whose afferents travel to the brain in the vagus nerve, and the proprioceptor afferents in the intercostal and diaphragmatic sensory nerves impinge on the brain stem control system to stop inspiration before the lung becomes overexpanded. The overall activities of these receptors make up what is called the **inspiratory cutoff switch**.

THE BRAIN STEM CONTROLLER

As Figure 11-4 shows, the **pons** and **medulla** are the portions of the brain that are continuous with the spinal cord. Phylogenetically, they are the most primitive parts of the brain. This is where the metabolic breathing controller is located, as well as where the cardiovascular centers lie, and where the 9th through 12th cranial nerves, which contain most of the sensory (afferent) information about breathing (lung, central, and peripheral chemoreceptors), enter the brain. In other words, the primitive brain (without the thalamus, hypothalamus, cerebellum, or cerebral cortex) contains sufficient organization to maintain a basic breathing pattern.

In a modification of the formal concepts of classical physiology (inspiratory center, expiratory center, pneumotaxic center, apneustic center),* it is now generally accepted that the medullary and pontine controllers are spatially dispersed. There is no "ultimate neuron," that is, no pacemaker neuron, to start a breathing cycle. Compare Figure 11-4A (classical view) with Figure 11-4B (modern view).

Figure 11-5 is a more functional representation of the putative interactions among the main groups (pools) of brain stem breathing controller neurons. Consult it when reading the following description.

A group of neurons (pool A; dorsal respiratory group), located bilaterally in the *nucleus tractus solitarius*, contains upper motor neurons. Their axons partially cross and project down the spinal cord to the lower motor neuron pools (C3–C5) of the phrenic nerve (diaphragm) and of the intercostal muscles (T1–T8). The pool A neurons receive excitatory stimuli from the central and peripheral chemoreceptors. Pool A is reasonably analogous to the classical "inspiratory center" since, when excited, these neurons cause inspiration to occur.

Some of the output of the pool A neurons connects directly to a second group of neurons (pool B; ventral respiratory group) associated with the caudal portion of the *nucleus retroambiguus*. Pool B also sends axons down the spinal cord to the accessory muscles of breathing. In that sense pool B is also an inspiratory center. But pool B also receives input from the lung stretch receptors and probably the chest wall proprioceptors. Some of the output of pool B activates another group of neurons in the rostral portion of the *nucleus retroambiguus* (pool C).

---

* The concept of *pneumotaxis* ("arrangement of breath," meaning to modulate breathing), which dates from the nineteenth century, is based on the view that a special center coordinates inspiratory and expiratory activities. *Apneusis* ("without breath") is a type of breathing in which long periods of inspiration are broken at irregular intervals by brief expiratory gasps.

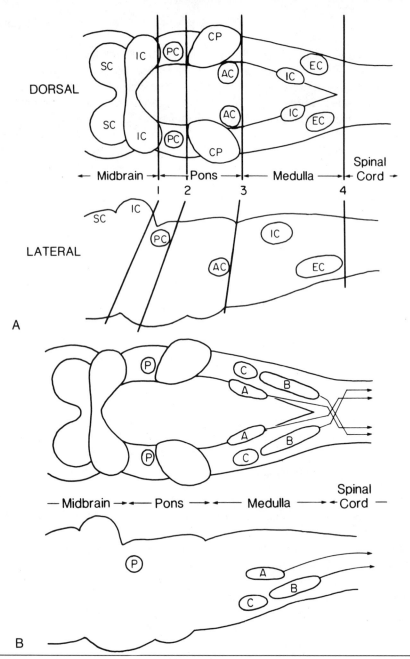

Fig. 11-4. Comparison between the classical and modern views of the brain stem controller mechanisms. **(A)** The classical description included an **inspiratory** center (IC) and an **expiratory** center (EC) in the medulla and an **apneustic** center (AC) and a **pneumotaxic** center (PC) in the pons. The pontine centers were believed to modulate breathing. The existence of the various centers was deduced by brain stem sectioning (lines 1, 2, 3, and 4). (Adapted from Comroe JH: Regulation of respiration—the respiratory centers. p. 25. In Physiology of Respiration. Year Book Medical Publishers, Chicago, 1974, with permission.) **(B)** According to the modern view, there are no well-defined inspiratory, expiratory, or apneustic centers. These are replaced by **neuron pools** (A, B, and C) in the medulla. Both pools A and B provide tonic inspiratory activity, whereas pool C is stimulated by multiple sensory impulses to inhibit pool A tonic activity. Pool C is identified as the **inspiratory cutoff switch**. A pneumotaxic center (P) exists in the anterior pons, which also feeds into the pool C group. It probably receives input from the higher centers such as the cerebral cortex.

When this neuron group is stimulated, it has a strong inhibitory effect on pool A (the inspiratory motor neuron group). Still more anteriorly in the *nucleus parabrachialis medialis* of the pons is the pneumotaxic center or pool P (pontine respiratory group). Its output stimulates pool C to inhibit pool A (inspiratory motor neurons). The source of stimuli to the pneumotaxic center (pool P) is not well known but probably includes output from higher centers (behavioral effects).

> **Remember:** There are three interconnected medullary neuron pools that receive external sensory information. They activate or inhibit the next pool in the loop in such a way that a basic respiratory rhythm (oscillation) is generated.

The external inputs—pneumotaxic center and sensory—appear to give timed "kicks" to the medullary neuron pools, thereby influencing the speed of the cycle (frequency) and the strength of the output to the effectors (depth of breathing). This fits fairly well with the timing diagram of breathing shown in Figure 11-3. The O_2 and CO_2 or $[H^+]$ chemoreceptors stimulate deeper breathing and increased inspiratory time, whereas the chest wall proprioceptor sensors and the lung stretch receptors stimulate neurons that lead to inhibition of inspiratory output.

This view of how the respiratory rhythm is maintained and modulated has led to the concept that the ratio of tidal volume to inspiratory time (V_T/T_I) is a physical analogue of the central inspiratory controller's activity.

Apneusis or apneustic breathing (see last footnote) was classically thought to require a special brain stem center (Fig. 11-4A). But the prevailing view is that apneusis is essentially a failure of the pool C neurons to inhibit pool A motor neuron activity (Fig. 11-5). In that sense, pool C is an antiapneustic center. When pool C is excited by the pneumotaxic center or pool B (lung

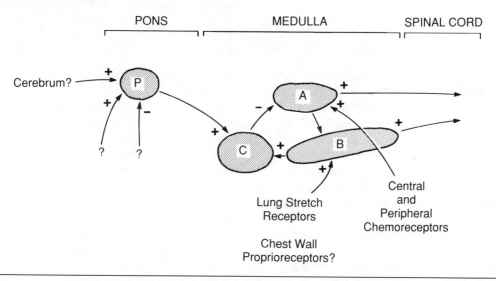

Fig. 11-5.   Basic wiring diagram of the brain stem ventilatory controller. The signs on the main outputs (arrows) of the neuron pools indicate whether the outputs are excitatory ($+$) or inhibitory ($-$). Pool A is tonically active, providing inspiratory stimuli to the muscles of breathing (apneusis). Other centers feed into pool C (inspiratory cutoff switch; antiapneusis), which sends inhibitory impulses to pool A. Pool B is stimulated by pool A and provides additional stimulation to the muscles of breathing, but pool B also stimulates pool C. Feedback from various sensors acts at different locations.

stretch receptor and chest wall proprioceptors), it *normally* inhibits inspiration (the inspiratory cutoff switch). When the pneumotaxic center is ablated (destroyed) and the vagus nerve is cut (lung stretch receptors), pool C is *depressed*. It does not inhibit pool A and does not stop inspiration. Thus, apneusis occurs.

The axons of neurons in the *nucleus tractus solitarius* (to the motor neurons of the phrenic nerve) and also the *nucleus retroambiguus* (to the motor neurons of the accessory breathing muscles) form the descending pathways that control automatic (metabolic) breathing. They partially cross within the brain stem and descend ipsilaterally and contralaterally in the ventro-lateral columns of the spinal cord to reach the lower motor neurons (C4–T8). The projections of the behavioral (voluntary) pathways from the cerebrum take a separate path (Fig. 11-2) down the spinal cord in the corticobulbar tracts.

It is important to know that diseases or injuries to the brain stem or the spinal cord may interfere with metabolic (automatic) breathing while leaving voluntary breathing intact (Ondine's curse).*

Remember: The brain stem breathing controller is mainly a tonically active inspiratory center. Expiration occurs when sufficient inhibitory stimuli reach the brain stem motor neurons to stop their activity or by direct thalamic or cortical input (behavioral control).

The control of breathing within the spinal cord is limited to integration of descending motor and segmental (proprioceptor) sensory inputs. These are not sufficient to generate a breathing rhythm. Integration at the cord level consists of inhibitory feedback from the chest wall pro-prioceptors to the lower motor neurons in the various cord segments. This allows for fast monitoring and regulation of the appropriateness of the breathing response to the breathing stimulus. In other words, spinal cord interactions prevent excessive contraction of the muscles of breathing.

SENSORS

Alveolar ventilation is controlled so that $P_{A_{CO_2}}$ (or Pa_{CO_2}) is maintained constant. In fact, control is so tight that, on the average, $P_{A_{CO_2}}$ does not deviate from its normal value (40 mmHg) by more than about $+2$ mmHg for more than a few minutes, under a wide variety of conditions. Since a deviation of $+2$ mmHg is only 5% of 40 mmHg, the feedback regulation is very good. Naturally, there is a price to pay for such high "gain control" (to borrow a term from control systems analysts). There is the danger of too much sensitivity, which might cause sequential breaths to vary excessively. Since that does not happen normally, we know that the P_{CO_2} sensor system is *damped*, because the signal is delayed and diluted so that the ventilatory response does not change too quickly or by too much.

Chemoreceptors are sensory elements (specific cells or nerve terminals) that are capable of responding to changes in the chemical composition of the liquid surrounding or within them. Some chemoreceptors are nonspecific, that is, they respond to many different stimuli. Some are specific. Both the central (brain) and the peripheral (carotid bodies) chemoreceptors are fairly specific for changes in the respiratory gases and hydrogen ion concentration.

---

* In Germanic mythology, Ondine was a sea nymph who was abandoned by her human husband. As punishment she cursed him by requiring that he had to remember to breathe. He died when he fell asleep.

Central Chemoreceptors

The main CO_2 sensors are located in the central nervous system on or close to the ventro-lateral surface of the medulla. They are near the brain stem controller but distinct from it.

When P_{ACO_2} varies owing to some change in alveolar ventilation, the control signal has to pass from the pulmonary capillaries (as a change of Pa_{CO_2}) through the left heart and arterial system to the brain before it is sensed. In addition to the transit delay of several seconds, the blood gas changes are also diluted in the left ventricle, where pulmonary venous outflow from two or three heartbeats (one-half of a breathing cycle) mix.

Early on (see Ch. 4) it was mentioned that although we say that alveolar $P_{CO_2} = 40$ mmHg, it actually varies slightly with breathing, rising during expiration because the delivery of CO_2 to the lungs in the mixed venous blood continues (even though expiration is occurring and alveolar volume is decreasing) and falling during inspiration as alveolar volume rises more rapidly than does the delivery of mixed venous blood. This waxing and waning of P_{ACO_2} (and also of P_{AO_2}) contributes to the modulation of breathing via the peripheral and central chemoreceptors because, in general, receptors are more sensitive to changes than to steady levels of stimulation.

The hydrogen ion concentration ($[H^+]$) of body liquids is partially controlled through changes in Pa_{CO_2}. Hydrogen ions, however, do not readily pass across cell membranes or the blood-brain barrier, whereas CO_2 (being water and lipid soluble and neutral) diffuses readily into and through cells. For example, the P_{CO_2} of cerebrospinal fluid (CSF) and of brain interstitial and intracellular liquids reflects changes in arterial blood CO_2 tension within several seconds. But changes in the hydrogen ion concentration of arterial blood are only slowly (hours) reflected by changes in the $[H^+]$ of CSF and brain liquids.

For many years, there has been a debate whether CO_2 sensors are located in the lungs or, at least, associated with the pulmonary circulation. No specific CO_2 receptors have been found, which is just as well because signals from receptors in the lung would reach the brain stem controller very quickly.* Ventilation might become unstable, with large and small tidal volumes alternating as the central controller tried to rapidly correct alveolar ventilation to hold Pa_{CO_2} constant. Since Pa_{CO_2} changes are not detected until arterial blood reaches the carotid bodies or the medullary surface receptors, breath-by-breath swings in P_{ACO_2} are smoothed into slower, continuous changes.

The steady-state ventilatory response (Eq. 11-1) to P_{ACO_2} (or Pa_{CO_2}) is hyperbolic, whereas the acute response to changes of inspired P_{CO_2} is a fairly linear function of the partial pressure of carbon dioxide above 40 mmHg, provided Pa_{O_2} is >100 mmHg (Fig. 11-6). Below $P_{ACO_2} = 40$ mmHg, however, the response curve bottoms out, meaning that breathing continues and is not much influenced by P_{ACO_2}. The line shown in Figure 11-6 is an average one. The variation among individuals is large, so the exact numbers are less important than the general shape and position of the curve.

There are two parameters used to describe a CO_2 response curve. These are the **set point**, which is the intercept on the P_{ACO_2} axis (x-axis) where minute ventilation would theoretically decrease to zero, and the **slope** of the main straight part of the line, which gives the change in ventilation per unit change in P_{ACO_2} (or P_{ACO_2}). The normal operating point ($P_{ACO_2} = 40$ mmHg and minute ventilation of 6 liters/min) is indicated by the open circle.

---

* Pa_{CO_2} may, however, affect the basal tone of airway smooth muscle and, consequently, affect various sensory modalities in the vagus nerve. In that sense, there are P_{CO_2} receptors in the lung, but their importance in ventilatory control is controversial.

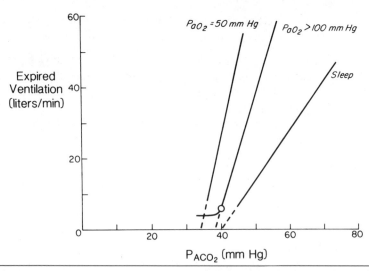

Fig. 11-6. CO_2-ventilation dose-response curve. Ventilation is sensitive to P_{ACO_2} (or P_{aCO_2}) as shown by the middle line (labeled $P_{aO_2} > 100$ mmHg). The normal operating point is shown by the open circle $P_{ACO_2} = 40$ mmHg and $\dot{V}_E = 6$ liters/min). The curve is defined by the slope of the straight portion and the extrapolated x-axis intercept. Increasing inspired CO_2 causes a steep rise in ventilation to about 60 liters/min at $P_{CO_2} = 55$ mmHg, giving a sensitivity of 3.6 liters/(min $\times$ mmHg P_{ACO_2}). P_{ACO_2} below normal decreases ventilation, but it does not stop. For low P_{aO_2}, the set point (x-intercept) is shifted to the left and there is an increase in the slope (sensitivity). Sleep is an example of a depressed dose-response curve in which the set point is shifted to the right and the slope is reduced, indicating decreased sensitivity.

There is an interaction between P_{aO_2} and the CO_2 response curve, as represented by the line to the left of the normal CO_2 response in Figure 11-6. As the ventilatory response curve during hypoxia is shifted to the left and is steeper, both the set point and the slope have changed. Thus, hypoxia decreases the threshold for CO_2 activity and increases the sensitivity (slope) of the response. Hyperoxia (increased P_{aO_2}) has a slight depressing effect on the CO_2 set point, that is, the normal line is shifted slightly to the right.

When the reticular activating system has decreased the background neural activity that keeps the brain stem controller neurons partially excited, the CO_2 response curve shifts to the right (higher set point) and has a less steep slope (decreased sensitivity), as shown by the right-hand line labeled *sleep* in Figure 11-6.

An increase in P_{CO_2} or [H^+] of CSF or medullary interstitial liquids excites the central chemoreceptors. Their output feeds into neuron pool A (Fig. 11-5) and increases the inspiratory motor neuron drive. The force of inspiration increases and tidal volume is increased. Inspiratory time (T_I) may be shortened, as shown in Figure 11-3.

The short-term ventilatory response to P_{aCO_2} occurs in two phases. The initial response (<2 minutes) is associated with rapid changes in alveolar, arterial, and CSF P_{CO_2}. But ventilation continues to change for some 10 to 20 minutes before a new quasi-steady state is achieved. The slower phase is believed to represent a delay in the adjustment of [H^+] within the brain interstitial liquid, CSF, and chemoreceptor intracellular liquids. Therefore, the steepness of the CO_2 response curve, as drawn in Figure 11-6, depends on how long one waits before making the ventilation determination. Nevertheless, most ventilatory control investigators believe that the action of P_{CO_2} on breathing is due to its role in changing [H^+] both intracellularly and extracellularly.

In Chapter 10, it was stated that CSF and brain interstitial liquid have only the $[HCO_3^-]/$ $[CO_2]$ weak acid buffer system. Therefore, changes of P_{CO_2} in the central nervous system cause a larger immediate change in $[H^+]$ than do the same changes of P_{CO_2} in blood or even in interstitial liquid elsewhere. CSF is not as good a buffer as is blood or interstitial liquid in other organs (see Fig. 10-3B).

Slow adjustment in ventilation continues for a long time after the initial P_{CO_2} response. These later adjustments tend to restore brain interstitial hydrogen ion concentration toward its normal value. Over a period of hours to 1 or 2 days following a rise in Pa_{CO_2}, there is a slow increase in the strong ion difference ([SID]) of brain CSF and brain interstitial liquid. This, of course, increases the $[HCO_3^-]$. Since the total concentration of strong cations (mainly sodium) is not increased (the body jealously controls total osmotic activity of intracellular, interstitial, and transcellular liquids), the change must be mediated by the removal of strong anions (Cl^-). How the chloride pump operates is not precisely defined, although it is unlikely to be markedly different from chloride pumps in other organs (airway epithelium, gastric epithelium, renal tubules). The result is that the $[H^+]$ slowly decreases and the central nervous system stimulus to breathing decreases until in the final steady state the hyperbolic relation between $\dot{V}A$ and Pa_{CO_2} is re-established (alveolar ventilation equation).

People who have been hypercapnic for a long time have a higher set point for their CO_2 response curve. Thus, patients with chronic obstructive pulmonary disease (emphysema) may not have a markedly increased minute ventilation, even though their Pa_{CO_2} is 50 to 60 mmHg or higher. This is partly due to the increased work of breathing caused by the disease but it is also partly due to a higher P_{CO_2} threshold.

At the peripheral chemoreceptor, stimulation also occurs when Pa_{CO_2} and $[H^+]a$ are increased. The effect on breathing (alveolar ventilation) is much less than the response to the central nervous system changes. The CO_2 drive to ventilation is apportioned as 67 to 80% to the central chemoreceptor and 20 to 33% to the peripheral chemoreceptors.

The response to altered $[H^+]a$ is different. This response has two phases and overall is much slower than the response to a change in P_{CO_2}. The hydrogen ion concentration of the peripheral chemoreceptors changes almost instantly because they are situated adjacent to the arterial bloodstream and blood flow through the carotid body is high relative to its size. The capillary barrier in the carotid body does not impose a significant limitation on hydrogen ion diffusion, whereas the capillaries of the brain have very tight intercellular junctions (blood-brain barrier) so that entry of hydrogen ions into brain interstitial liquid and CSF is very slow. Thus, the immediate response to a change in $[H^+]a$ comes entirely from the carotid bodies, followed later by a larger response from the central chemoreceptors.

Effect of Cerebral Blood Flow

The brain normally metabolizes aerobically and at a respiratory quotient of 1.0 (glucose). The CO_2 generated must be removed in brain venous blood. If cerebral blood flow is decreased (for example, by low cardiac output), the P_{CO_2} of brain interstitial and intracellular liquids and of CSF will rise and ventilation will increase. Fortunately, the arteriolar smooth muscle is sensitive to brain tissue P_{CO_2}. Thus, vasodilation will occur as Pt_{CO_2} rises, blood flow will be restored toward normal (autoregulation), and ventilation will decrease.

During hypoxia the brain produces lactic acid (by anaerobic metabolism), which increases the $[H^+]$ of brain interstitial liquid and CSF. This stimulates breathing, the more so because the lactic acid cannot easily cross the blood-brain barrier to be transported by blood to the liver for metabolism.

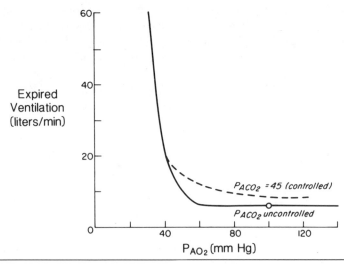

Fig. 11-7. The P_{AO_2}-ventilation dose-response curve. The solid line indicates the response to hypoxia when P_{ACO_2} is uncontrolled. The normal operating point is shown by the open circle at $P_{AO_2} = 100$ mmHg and $\dot{V}_E = 6$ liters/min. As P_{AO_2} is decreased, there is little ventilatory response until about 60 mmHg. The response is mediated through the carotid body chemoreceptors. If P_{ACO_2} is controlled (dashed line at 45 mmHg), ventilation is predictably increased at normal P_{AO_2} and the threshold for hypoxic stimulation is shifted to higher P_{O_2}.

Peripheral Chemoreceptors

The carotid bodies are well situated to sample systemic arterial blood. Although they respond mainly to changes in Pa_{O_2}, they are also stimulated by changes in Pa_{CO_2} and $[H^+]a$. Lack of oxygen is a stimulus to breathing. Since the direct effect of hypoxia on the brain is depression of neuronal activity, the drive to breathe caused by lack of oxygen comes entirely from the peripheral chemoreceptors.

The normal P_{AO_2}-ventilation dose-response curve is shown by the solid line in Figure 11-7. The key points that describe the relationship are as follows:

1. The ventilatory response threshold is at a low P_{AO_2} of <60 mmHg, although some impulse traffic can be recorded from the carotid body nerves even at higher P_{AO_2}.
2. The ventilatory response curve is hyperbolic, which means ventilation increases more and more rapidly as P_{AO_2} falls.
3. Pa_{O_2} is the stimulus, not arterial oxygen concentration (Ca_{O_2}), as long as blood flow to the carotid and aortic bodies is normal.
4. The P_{AO_2}-ventilation dose-response curve is sensitive to P_{ACO_2} (or Pa_{CO_2}), just as the CO_2-ventilation dose-response curve is sensitive to oxygen, as shown in the dashed line in Figure 11-7 for which P_{ACO_2} was controlled by varying F_{ICO_2}.
5. The stimulus to breathing by low Pa_{O_2} is persistent; that is, nerve impulses to the brain stem controllers continue even after irreversible damage has occurred to the brain and other organs. Some say that the carotid body is the last organ to die.

There are many interesting details that afford additional insight into the function of the peripheral chemoreceptors. For example, Pa_{O_2} is the specific stimulus, as is shown by the fact that anemia, carbon monoxide poisoning, and methemoglobinemia (oxidized Hb) do not stimulate breathing, even though they may markedly reduce the arterial oxygen concentration (Ca_{O_2}) (see Fig. 9-2B). But when carotid body blood flow decreases, as may occur in hemorrhagic shock or other low-cardiac-output states, the chemoreceptors may be stimulated even though Pa_{O_2} is nearly normal. In fact, the ventilatory response curve to Pa_{O_2} is essentially a mirror image of the hemoglobin-oxygen equilibrium curve; that is, the specific carotid body stimulus appears to be one of adequate oxygen delivery, even though it is detected as the P_{O_2} of the interstitial or intracellular liquids of the carotid body cells and nerve terminals.

The ventilatory response to low oxygen is damped over the short term by the decreased Pa_{CO_2} caused by any increased ventilation. For example, suppose the hypoxic drive to breathing doubled alveolar ventilation. This would cause a 50% decrease in Pa_{CO_2}, which would tend to decrease breathing. However, as Figure 11-6 shows, the drive to breathe is not completely eliminated when Pa_{CO_2} falls below the normal level. If Pa_{CO_2} is maintained constant as ventilation rises during acute alveolar hypoxia, the ventilatory response is greater and the hypoxic threshold is higher.

During longer exposure (days) to decreased inspired oxygen (for example, remaining at high altitude), the ventilatory response tends to increase as the body readjusts its $[H^+]_{CSF}$ to the decreased Pa_{CO_2}. This is how early acclimatization to high altitude occurs.

One would expect that the hypoxic drive to breathe would be very strong in a patient who is both severely hypoxic and hypercapnic, as in severe chronic obstructive pulmonary disease (emphysema). It is! But the breathing apparatus may not be able to respond appropriately, which some physicians and physiologists believe causes the unpleasant symptom of **dyspnea** (difficult or painful breathing).

The hypoxic drive to breathe appears to be lost in long-term high altitude residents who develop the syndrome called *chronic mountain sickness*. These people have severe arterial hypoxemia and are markedly polycythemic (hematocrit > 55%).

Mechanical Receptors

The various mechanical receptors in the lungs and chest wall feed into the brain stem controller, mainly at the level of the pool B neuron group (Fig. 11-5) but possibly also at the pneumotaxic center (pool P). The increased pool B impulses add to the excitation that feeds into the pool C neurons, the inspiratory cutoff switch.

One set of mechanical receptors in the lung consists of the **stretch receptors** located in the smooth muscle of the bronchi. These receptors are excited when the muscles are stretched, such as occurs with the increased transpulmonary pressure associated with inspiration. When these receptors reach their thresholds, they fire continuously and adapt very slowly, that is, their firing is persistent. The stretch receptors' afferent fibers travel in the vagus nerve and impinge upon the brain stem controller (pool B) where they act to inhibit inspiratory drive (via excitation of pool C). The pulmonary stretch receptor impulses do not directly inhibit the inspiratory neurons (pool A). Although they are important, the stretch receptors constitute only one of the sensory modalities feeding into the central control loop.

The stretch receptors act to help prevent overinflation of the lung. Also, in the presence of airway narrowing or slow inspiration, their delayed activation allows inspiration to last longer, so that an adequate tidal volume is achieved.

The inhibition of the inspiratory effort caused by activation of the pulmonary stretch receptors is called the **Hering-Breuer reflex**. Although this reflex is active in some anesthetized animals, it is relatively weak in the human adult except at tidal volumes above normal and apparently does not function at all in the human newborn.

The **irritant receptors**, located in the epithelium and subepithelium of the upper airways, are stimulated by particulate matter (dust particles, foreign bacteria), certain irritating chemical vapors (sulfur dioxide, nitrogen dioxide, and ammonia), and by a variety of physical factors (increased lung volume, airflow velocity, air temperature, and bronchial smooth muscle constriction). The irritant receptors may be related to periodic sighing, which produces a larger than normal breath and which helps to maintain normal lung volume (FRC) by reducing the air-liquid surface tension (see Ch. 5).

The **C fibers** are stimulated by several chemicals delivered via the pulmonary circulation. These chemicals are nonspecific irritants and, of course, are not the normal stimulus to C-fiber activation. Such chemical tests show that many C fibers are located close to the pulmonary (rather than the bronchial) microcirculation; that is, they are located in the terminal respiratory units (alveolar walls). There is some evidence that C fibers are activated by distortion of the alveolar walls, such as that caused by pulmonary vascular congestion or by interstitial liquid accumulation (pulmonary edema).

The effect of C-fiber stimulation is not entirely clear, although laryngeal and airway constriction and periods of apnea (no breathing) have been demonstrated experimentally. In the normal, resting adult, however, neither the irritant receptors nor the C fibers appear to be very active.

The **chest wall receptors** are located in the costochondral joints, in the tendons of the intercostal muscles, and in the intramuscular spindles. These receptors supply information via the intercostal nerves and ascending spinal tracks to the brain stem controllers, pool B neurons, and possibly the pneumotaxic center about the state of contraction of the muscles of breathing. For example, the receptors in the central tendon of the diaphragm monitor the force of its contraction. Their activation tends to inhibit inspiration.

The muscle spindles are not very active during quiet breathing, mainly because there are only a few of them in the diaphragm, which contribute most of the chest wall motion at rest. There are, however, abundant muscle spindles in the intercostal muscles, although these seem to be more related to postural changes and to the fine regulation of phonation (speaking, singing, etc.) than to automatic (metabolic) breathing.

Because the muscle spindle receptors are in parallel with the main intercostal muscle fibers, they are inhibited during active contraction of the intercostal muscles. However, if the muscle spindle fibers are stimulated via their γ motor neurons, they may continue to be active during muscle contraction and thereby enhance contraction. The neurons from the muscle spindle afferent receptors travel all the way to the cerebral cortex, apparently providing information about movements of the chest during behavioral control of breathing. Some physiologists believe these afferents are mainly responsible for the sensation of dyspnea when their signals are inappropriate to the breathing stimulus.

CONTROL OF BREATHING IN EXERCISE

The increase in alveolar ventilation in steady-state exercise is so closely matched to body metabolism ($\dot{V}_{CO_2}$) that Pa_{CO_2} scarcely changes. Upon that fact, however, hangs a dilemma. Since CO_2 is the main drive to ventilation, how is it that alveolar ventilation changes if Pa_{CO_2} does not? Nor does Pa_{O_2} decrease—on the contrary, Pa_{O_2} increases slightly owing to the improved matching of ventilation to perfusion throughout the lung as cardiac output and ventilation rise.

A number of accessory factors have been suggested as contributing to the increased ventilation seen in exercise. These include stimulation of muscle and joint receptors by motion, increased body temperature, increased spread of cerebrocortical electrical activity and cortical (volitional) stimuli, such as occurs in anticipation of exercise. None of these effects adequately explains the control of ventilation in exercise. Physiologists fall back on the rather vague statement that control of breathing is multifactorial.

But exercise ventilation is too closely matched to the CO_2 load (cardiac output $\times$ $\dot{V}_{CO_2}$) to be mere chance. It is known that the cyclic swings of alveolar and arterial P_{CO_2} and P_{O_2} with breathing are enhanced during exercise and that changes in arterial blood gas tensions drive ventilation.* Another possibility, of course, is that the set point (threshold) of the P_{CO_2}-ventilation dose-response curve is reduced so that what appears to be a normal Pa_{CO_2} is actually an increased Pa_{CO_2} relative to the new set point. Resistance to this explanation is that the set point does not change quickly (1 to 2 minutes) in CO_2 response tests. Finally, it is possible that standard CO_2 response curves underestimate the sensitivity of the central controller. This could mean that the changes in Pa_{CO_2} (<1 mmHg), which are not reliably detected by CO_2 electrodes, could greatly augment ventilation.

Remember: In steady-state exercise Pa_{CO_2} is tightly controlled, but a complete explanation of how that occurs is lacking.

Although work physiology cannot be described in any detail, it has been implied several times by the use of the term *steady-state* exercise that there must also be *non–steady-state* exercise. Non–steady-state exercise occurs in two common circumstances: during the first minute or two of the transition from rest to exercise, and when the metabolic demands of the working muscles exceed the ability of the lungs and cardiovascular system to supply substrate (oxygen, glucose). In non–steady-state exercise, the accumulation of lactic acid (anaerobic glycolysis) in blood disrupts the normal regulatory patterns. In terms of breathing, the main effect is a marked augmentation in ventilation, so that Pa_{CO_2} decreases, mainly as a result of the acute metabolic acidosis.

CONTROL OF BREATHING IN SLEEP

The study of breathing and its control during sleep is a relatively recent field of pulmonary physiology. However, a number of clinical syndromes (obstructive and central sleep apneas, sudden infant death, and certain types of insomnia) may be related to disordered regulation of breathing during sleep.

Sleep is a more complex phenomenon than generally supposed. Table 11-1 illustrates the main types and stages of sleep, including the awake condition. Sleep is organized temporally into stages that reoccur in a cyclic pattern throughout the night. These stages can be correlated with both neuromuscular and behavioral activities.

There are four stages (two light and two heavy) of quiet sleep. Every so often (1 to 2 hours) sleepers enter into a more active type of sleep, which is called REM (for *r*apid *e*ye *m*ovement) sleep, so named from the observation that led to its discovery. REM sleep also consists of two

---

*Cyclic changes in alveolar gas tensions may also influence the thresholds of intralung sensory receptors.

Table 11-1.   Control of Breathing in Sleep

Stage of Sleep	Main Control Factors[a]	Breathing Pattern
Awake		
Rest	Alertness, metabolic	Regular
Activity	Behavioral	Irregular
Sleep		
Non-REM		
Light	Alertness, metabolic	Periodic
Heavy	Metabolic	Regular
REM		
Tonic	Alertness, metabolic	Regular
Phasic	Behavioral	Irregular

[a] Alertness, state of reticular activating system; metabolic, brain stem controllers; behavioral, higher centers override metabolic control.
(Adapted from Phillipson EA: Control of breathing during sleep. Am Rev Respir Dis 118:909–939, 1978, with permission.)

types, tonic and phasic. All stages of sleep are described as *metabolic* with the exception of phasic REM sleep, which is thought to be behavioral (dreaming and body movements).

The breathing patterns that occur in sleep vary with the stage or phase. In early sleep, breathing may be periodic (with episodes of apnea), but then breathing becomes regular until phasic REM sleep occurs, during which the pattern is irregular.

A number of events occur during sleep that would be considered startling if they occurred in an awake person. For example, in the early stage of sleep all motor nerve activity in the hypoglossal and pharyngoglossal nerves ceases. Thus, the muscles of the mouth and throat relax, allowing the tongue and associated structures to narrow the pharyngeal airway. This not only contributes to snoring but may lead to complete upper airway obstruction (obstructive sleep apnea), from which the sleeper may be aroused, suddenly sitting up in bed wide awake without knowing what happened.

The problem of sleep apnea is that, although the ventilatory response to hypoxia is not diminished during normal metabolic sleep, spontaneous breathing during REM sleep is remarkably insensitive to peripheral chemoreceptor stimulation (hypoxemia). Investigations of arterial oxygen saturation during sleep show that it may fall to 70% ($Pa_{O_2} < 40$ mmHg).

The response to CO_2 during sleep shifts quickly, thus disproving the contention that such shifts take several hours. A representative CO_2 response curve during sleep is shown in Figure 11-6. The sensitivity of the central controller (that is, the slope of the P_{CO_2}-ventilation curve) is diminished, and the set point is shifted to the right. The sensitivity of the brain stem controller to mechanoreceptor or irritant receptor stimulation is normal during metabolic sleep but decreased during phasic REM sleep.

A possible explanation for most of these control changes is that the reticular activating system (controlling the state of the brain) is depressed during sleep. This has the general effect of decreasing the alertness (wakefulness) of the controller.

CONTROL OF BREATHING IN ACUTE AND CHRONIC HYPOXIA

The vast majority of the world's population has always lived within 100 miles of the sea, that is, near sea level. Nevertheless, some have moved to higher ground, even to altitudes in excess of 14,000 feet (4,500 m). Barometric pressure at 14,000 feet is approximately 435 mmHg with a P_{IO_2} of 91 mmHg. According to the alveolar gas equation (Eq. 4-5), $P_{AO_2} = 67$ mmHg if alveolar ventilation has doubled and Pa_{CO_2} fallen to 20 mmHg. The arterial S_{O_2} is reduced, even allowing for the leftward shift of the HbO_2 equilibrium curve due to the hypocapnia.

The hypoxia stimulates the peripheral chemoreceptors to increase ventilation, whereas the hypocapnia (decreased Pa_{CO_2}) and decreased $[H^+]a$ do not stimulate the peripheral chemoreceptors and the low P_{CO_2} of the CSF does not stimulate the central chemoreceptors. On the other hand, the low CO_2 causes cerebral vasoconstriction, which tends to raise the P_{CO_2} of brain tissue liquid and CSF.

After a few hours, the strong ion difference, which is equal to $[HCO_3^-]$ in brain interstitial liquid and CSF, is reduced by the rise in $[Cl^-]$CSF caused by an active metabolic mechanism across the blood-brain microvascular barrier. This change in the central chemosensory environment is manifested by a shift in the position and slope of the CO_2-ventilation dose-response curve (Fig. 11-6).

As the [SID] decreases, the $[H^+]$CSF returns toward normal and the hypoxic stimulus to breathing is enhanced; that is to say, the inhibition by the reduced P_{CO_2} is less. Each time, of course, that breathing increases, there is a further fall in P_{CO_2}. The change $[H^+]$CSF continues until the final steady-state level of 20 mmHg is reached (in the example being cited) at an alveolar ventilation of twice the normal level. The final $[H^+]$ in systemic arterial blood is less than normal, since compensation is never complete.

With long-term residence at high altitude, there is a stimulation of erythrocyte production (polycythemia), which increases the total weak acid buffers ($[A_{tot}]$) in blood. This allows for an additional decrease in the $[HCO_3^-]$ concentration of blood.

READINGS

Books

1. Comroe JH Jr: Physiology of Respiration. 2nd Ed. Chapters 3–9. Year Book Medical Publishers, Chicago, 1974
   Lucid and detailed discussion of every aspect of regulation. Comroe believed that the control of breathing was so important that he placed it at the beginning of his book.
2. Nunn FJ: Applied Respiratory Physiology. 3rd Ed. Butterworths, London, 1987
   A thorough but brief description including some historical aspects.

Reviews

3. Cherniack NS, Altose MD, Kelsen SG: Control of respiration. In Berne RB, Levy MN (eds): Physiology. CV Mosby, St. Louis, 1983
   Chapter 40 is a well-organized, terse statement of the modern view.
4. Coleridge JCG, Coleridge HM: Afferent vagal fibre innervation of the lung and airways and its functional significance. Rev Physiol Biochem Pharmacol 99:2–110, 1984
   A detailed account of the important but misunderstood C fibers.
5. Dempsey JA, Vidruk EH, Mitchell GS: Pulmonary control systems in exercise: update. Fed Proc 44:2260–2270, 1985
   Reviews some of the continuing controversial aspects of ventilatory control.
6. Lydic R: State-dependent aspects of regulatory physiology. FASEB J 1:6–15, 1987
   Brief review of the effect of wakefulness on the control of breathing and other body functions.

7. Mitchell RA, Burger AJ: Neural regulation of respiration. Am Rev Respir Dis 111:206–224, 1975

An authoritative account emphasizing the modern neurophysiology of the brain stem metabolic controller.

8. Phillipson EA: Control of breathing during sleep. Am Rev Respir Dis 118:909–939, 1978

A thorough up-to-date review which has been an important source for the present chapter.

9. Wasserman K, Whipp BJ: Exercise physiology in health and disease. Am Rev Respir Dis 112:219–249, 1975

A clear, concise review of this important physiologic condition.

QUESTIONS*

Use the following information to answer the next two questions.

Arterial Blood Acid-Base Data

[H^+], nEq/liter	Pa_{CO_2}, mmHg	[HCO_3^-], mEq/liter	Pa_{O_2}, mmHg
a. 40	40	24	100
b. 25	20	19	40
c. 40	40	24	40
d. 62	80	32	100
e. 63	40	15	100

1. Which of the arterial blood samples above would be likely to stimulate medullary chemo-receptors most?
   a. b. c. d. e.
2. Which of the arterial blood samples above would be likely to stimulate carotid body chemoreceptors most?
   a. b. c. d. e.
3. A 55-year-old molecular biologist with chronic obstructive pulmonary disease (emphysema) has a Pa_{CO_2} of 55 mmHg and a resting total ventilation of 6.3 liters/min. The subject's wasted ventilation is closest to:
   a. 1.8 liters/min
   b. 3.2 liters/min
   c. 3.9 liters/min
   d. 6.3 liters/min
   e. 9.4 liters/min
4. A normal subject breathing 15% O_2 ($F_{I_{O_2}}$ = 0.15) for 10 minutes is suddenly switched to a gas mixture containing $F_{I_{O_2}}$ = 0.15 and $F_{I_{CO_2}}$ = 0.03. The effect on the subject's minute ventilation is most likely to be
   a. An increase within 2 minutes
   b. An increase within 1 or 2 hours
   c. A decrease within 2 minutes
   d. A decrease within 1 or 2 hours
   e. No change
5. Not many years ago there was a treatment fad for severe asthma in which the carotid bodies were removed. A likely physiologic consequence of this procedure would be
   a. Loss of response to inhaled CO_2
   b. Greater than normal hypoxemia on ascent to high altitude
   c. Greater than normal decrease in [H^+]$_{CSF}$ on ascent to high altitude
   d. Fall in Pa_{CO_2} in steady-state exercise due to excessively increased ventilation
   e. Increased basal airway smooth muscle tone
6. Hysteria is a pyschoneurotic disorder characterized by marked emotional swings. Hyperventilation may be a prominent sign. a. Why are hysterical individuals prone to feeling dizzy or to fainting? b. Why is minute ventilation increased?
7. What are the expected differences in arterial blood gases, minute ventilation, and phrenic

---

* Answers begin on p. 211.

nerve motor neuron activity in a person who is suffocating following aspiration of vomitus compared with a person who is dying of severe hypoxemia at extremely highly altitude?
8. If the diaphragm contracts more vigorously but T_I and T_{tot} are not different from normal, what happens to $\dot{V}_A$, P_{ACO_2}, and slowly adapting lung stretch receptor activity?

The figure below shows a normal CO_2-ventilation dose-response curve with several added points. Which point best describes each of the following conditions?

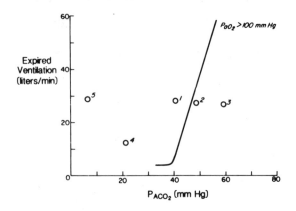

9. A normal person during sleep.
   1   2   3   4   5
10. A normal person breathing 10% oxygen for several minutes.
    1   2   3   4   5

Answers

The chapter questions, which include drill questions and problems, both quantitative and qualitative, are designed to help you review and remember what you have read and use the information to synthesize new relationships.

To obtain a clear understanding of what is being asked, please take time to read each question carefully. In answering, you are not limited to the material in the current or any previous chapter, but may use any source of information available.

CHAPTER 1. RESPIRATION AND BREATHING

1. This question, which covers nearly everything in this chapter, is open-ended, permitting you to be as terse or verbose as you wish. The essential words are in boldface.

Transport Step or Site	Possible Rate-Limiting Process or Factor
Atmosphere	O_2 supply depends on atmospheric **pressure** and **composition**. Rate limitation begins here, although the body has no direction control, as mountain climbers know.
Alveoli	**Ventilation** is a **convective** (mass transport) process, made possible by breathing. In chest wall weakness or with airway obstruction, inadequate ventilation may occur.
Pulmonary capillaries	Blood circulates around the body due to the energy imparted by cardiac pumping. Blood circulation is a **convective** process.
Ventilation/ perfusion	Imbalance is often the main rate-limiting process in lung disease.
Alveolocapillary diffusion	This process, driven by the O_2 partial pressure difference between alveolar gas and pulmonary capillary blood, may be rate limiting whenever the demand for oxygen is increased, as in exercise.
Blood	The respiratory system is not responsible for the composition of blood. In carbon monoxide poisoning or abnormal hemoglobinemias, this may be the rate-limiting step.
Systemic capillary blood	Passing through the tissue capillaries, blood must give up its oxygen. **Abnormal hemoglobin** may limit this process. **Perfusion imbalance** due to low cardiac output (shock) or arteriovenous shunts may fail to deliver adequate quantities of blood.

Tissue diffusion   If cells are **distant** (>100 μm) from a perfused capillary, they may receive inadequate oxygen.

Cell respiration   In cyanide poisoning blockade of the **respiratory enzymes** in the **mitochondria** occurs.

2. The brain and then the heart have the most critical oxygen needs of all organs. Irreversible changes may occur in a few minutes. In cardiopulmonary resuscitation (CPR), one establishes an airway, ventilates the lungs, and assists circulation. Least important are bone, skin, and muscle. In first aid courses one learns that even an arterial tourniquet placed on a bleeding arm or leg can be left for up to 1 hour without significant anoxic tissue damage. The kidneys, liver, and gastrointestinal tract are of intermediate sensitivity, whereas the lungs have plenty of oxygen available in the air spaces.

3. This arrangement represents the worst possible ventilation/perfusion imbalance. The ratio is infinite (ventilation/zero) for the right lung and zero (zero/perfusion) for the left lung. Obviously, no gas exchange occurs.

4 and 5. At $P_{O_2} = 40$ mmHg, read up to the hemoglobin-oxygen equilibrium curve and then horizontally to the y-axis. For **mixed venous blood** (pulmonary artery), 75% saturation is normal. For 50% oxyhemoglobin saturation, read horizontally to the hemoglobin-oxygen equilibrium curve and then down to $P_{O_2} = 27$ mmHg, the **half-saturation** pressure for normal human hemoglobin.

6. The y-axis is **relative,** not absolute. To determine the **quantity** of oxygen stored as oxyhemoglobin, you must know the **concentration** of normal hemoglobin. Look ahead to Figure 9-1.

7. The most logical and organized approach is to discuss oxygen transport control in relation to **oxygen** and **carbon dioxide.** Either molecule may be detected at any point along the O_2 or CO_2 transport path (see Question 1-1). Since the brain is the organ most sensitive to oxygen deprivation (Question 1-2) and is the controller, the most reasonable answer to the first three subquestions is to *detect the oxygen concentration of arterial blood going to the brain,* which is not far from actual practice (see Ch. 11). The carotid bodies, located adjacent to the carotid sinuses, detect arterial blood P_{O_2}, but these controllers are rather insensitive. The principal controlled molecule is CO_2, which not only is a respiratory gas but also is involved in another major regulatory process, acid-base balance (see Ch. 10). Moreover, CO_2 production is intimately connected to O_2 consumption (see Ch. 3, Eq. 3-4). The main controller is exquisitely sensitive to CO_2 and is located near the surface of the brain stem.

   To maintain oxygen transport, ideally the controller should detect a decrease in oxygen going to the brain and adjust breathing, cardiac output, blood hemoglobin concentration, tissue perfusion, etc. in response. In fact, not all this is accomplished by one controller. The central brain controller primarily adjusts ventilation to maintain arterial blood (brain surface) P_{CO_2} as near normal as possible, and many systems contribute (chronically) to the control of oxygen transport.

8. Holding the breath provokes a number of increasingly unpleasant sensations, the first being the absence of breathing. Since one usually inspires maximally before holding the breath, sensations related to the expansion of the chest are detected. The subject becomes increasingly uncomfortable, warm, and flushed and begins to wiggle. The nervous impulses from the lungs, diaphragm, abdomen, and rib cage, together with the rising P_{CO_2} and falling P_{O_2} in arterial blood, demand that one breathe.

   However, the question was to name the fail-safe mechanism. Since breath holding is a

voluntary function, it requires willpower and consciousness (wakefulness). Normal people break their breath hold when the reward no longer equals the discomfort. But the fail-safe mechanism is due to the fact that breathing is an **automatic** function. If one lost consciousness, breathing would commence again.

CHAPTER 2. STRUCTURAL BASIS FOR LUNG FUNCTION

1. From the text description and Figures 1-1 and 2-8, you can see that there is only one set of airways, through which air flows in both directions, which gives rise to the anatomic dead space. The pulmonary circulation, however, is continuous from right ventricle to left atrium. Flow is only in one direction, so there is no dead space.

2. Calculate the volume (in cubic centimeters) of a sheet 8×10^{-6} m (8 µm) thick (total alveolar wall thickness) and with a 50-m^2 surface. Remember that one-half of the surface is on each side of the alveolar wall (review Fig. 2-3). Thus, you want the volume of a sheet 25 m^2 by 8×10^{-6} m thick. The alveolar wall volume is 200×10^{-6} m^3 or 200 cm^3. If necessary, review conversion factors between units, specifically µm to m and m^3 to cm^3.

3. The differences are listed below roughly in order of importance.

Bronchi	**Bronchioles**
Diameter >1 mm	Diameter <1 mm
Cartilage in walls	No cartilage
Surrounded by lung but not attached to it	An integral part of lung structure
Passive diameter dependent on transpulmonary pressure	Passive diameter dependent on lung volume
Pseudostratified columnar epithelium	Cuboidal epithelium
Submucosal glands	No submucosal glands
Nourished by bronchial circulation	Nourished partly by bronchial and partly by pulmonary circulation

4. There are two pathways to be considered. The bronchial circulation does not ordinarily nourish the alveoli, but when the pulmonary circulation is shut off, sufficient bronchial blood reaches the alveoli to keep the tissue alive. Even though the artery is blocked, the pulmonary veins are open. Because of cardiac contractions and breathing motions, venous blood may reflux into the alveolar wall capillaries.

5. Since 15 liters/min = 15,000 ml/min = 250 ml/sec and since capillary volume is 150 ml, the average residence time for red blood cells is 150 ml/(250 ml/sec) = 0.6 second, which is not much less than at rest.

6. Figure 2-1 shows height in centimeters along the left y-axis. The top of the lung is at 29 cm, 14 cm above the left atrium. Going up the lung, one *subtracts* the height in centimeters (because pressure decreases by 1 cmH$_2$O/cm height) from the pressure in centimeters of water. Thus, $20 - 14 = 6$ cmH$_2$O. At the bottom pressure must be increased by 15 cm; thus, $20 + 15$ cmH$_2$O $= 35$ cmH$_2$O. A quick way to check your answer is to subtract the two pressures. Their difference must equal the difference in height. The calculation for pulmonary venous pressure, taking left atrial pressure as 10 cmH$_2$O at the level of the atrium, yields a negative pressure value, -4 cmH$_2$O at the top. At the bottom, venous pressure $= 10 + 15 = 25$ cmH$_2$O.

7. There are 60,000 terminal respiratory units. Thus, at FRC, 2,400 ml/60,000 = 0.04 ml. At TLC the unit must be larger by a factor of 2.5 (6 liters/2.4 liters); 0.04 ml × 2.5 = 0.10 ml.

CHAPTER 3. SOME FUNDAMENTAL CONCEPTS

1. a. V_A b. $\dot{V}_A$ c. $F_{A_{O_2}}$ d. $\bar{P}pa$
   e. P_L f. $P\bar{v}_{O_2}$ g. Ca_{CO_2} h. P_B
   i. Pao − Palv   j. Ppl
2. a. Pressure at the airway opening
   b. Systemic arterial concentration of oxygen
   c. Fraction of carbon dioxide in expired gas
   d. Volume of dead space
   e. Tidal volume (inspired volume of each breath)
   f. Pressure across the respiratory system
   g. Oxyhemoglobin saturation, or oxygen saturation (hemoglobin implied)
   h. Respiratory exchange ratio
   i. Expiratory time
   j. Pressure difference between alveolar gas and ambient air
   k. Compliance of the chest wall
3. a. STPD; 2.42 liters. The water vapor pressure is zero, therefore condition 1 is *dry*. Temperature is 0°C, which is one of the standard conditions, and the pressure is 760 mmHg, which is also standard. Therefore, condition 1 is standard temperature, pressure, dry. Use Eq. 3-2 for the calculation. Since both temperature and P_{H_2O} are increasing, the second volume will be larger.
   b. ATPD; 5.07 liters. The ambient and water vapor pressures are standard, but the temperature must be ambient, since it is not body temperature.
   c. ATPS; 712 ml. Gas is saturated at ambient temperature.
   d. BTPS; 1.92 liters. Gas is at body temperature and saturated. The barometric pressure is ambient, and normally the alveolar (body) pressure is also.
   e. STPD; 1,492 ml. Standard condition 1 again. The second condition is 2 atm pressure, which reduces the volume by nearly one-half, and the air is saturated with water vapor at a raised temperature.
   f. BTPS; 5.14 liters.
   g. STPD; 6.34 liters. Condition 2 is very cold.
4. R = 298/350 = 0.85. There is no need to convert to STPD, since both measurements were made under the same conditions, namely, ATPS. If you did make the conversion, you should have obtained R = 265/311 = 0.85.
5. Use the Fick principle (Eq. 3-5) after converting $\dot{V}_{O_2}$ to standard conditions. $\dot{Q}$ = (1,200 ml O_2/min converted to STPD)/(200 − 125) ml O_2/liter = 1,044/75 = 13.9 liters/min.
6. Use the Fick equation again. Subjects, patients, and data in questions are not always for a 70-kg adult. The answer, 24 ml/min, may seem too small, but it is for a newborn. The average baby weighs about 3.4 kg (7.5 lb) at birth. Thus, $\dot{V}_{O_2}$ is 24/3.4 = 7 ml O_2/(min × kg), which is double the adult metabolic rate on a per kilogram basis.
7. The data required are the driving pressure and the cardiac output, which are mentioned at several places in the text but are most conveniently found in Appendix 2.
   At rest, PVR = (19 − 11) cmH$_2$O/5.0 liters/min = 1.6 resistance units (cmH$_2$O × min/liters). Millimeters of mercury may also be used: PVR = (14 − 80) mmHg/(5.0 liters/min) = 1.2 units (mmHg × min/liters). If you use cgs units (dynes × sec × cm^{-5}), the factor is 980 (dynes × cm^{-2})/cmH$_2$O × 1 liter/1,000 cm^3 × 60 sec/min = 58.8 dynes × sec × cm^{-5} = 1 cmH$_2$O × min/liter. Thus, PVR = 1.6 units × 58.8 = 94 dynes × sec × cm^{-5}.

In exercise, PVR $= (30 - 15)$ cmH$_2$O $\times$ min/15 liters $= 15/15 = 1.0$ resistance unit; 0.74 if you used mmHg for the pressures; and 58.8 dynes $\times$ sec $\times$ cm^{-5} in cgs units.

8. Although a thorough description of compliance will not be given until Chapter 5, it can be calculated now, since it has been defined as the slope or tangent to the P-V curve. Examine Figure 3.4. By laying a straightedge on the inflation curve you will see that the highest compliance (steepest slope) is in the midrange between 25 and 75% of TLC. The lowest compliances occur at very low and very high volumes, as the slopes decrease toward zero. To make a compliance calculation you need the absolute volume change, ΔV, not a percentage. The question gives 100% volume (TLC) as 4.5 liters. On examining the figure, you will see that lung volume is not zero when P$_L$ (transpulmonary pressure) is zero. The lowest volume is between 10 and 15% of TLC, that is, 0.45 to 0.68 liters. Thus, $\Delta V = 4.5 - 0.45$ (or 0.68) $= 4.05$ (or 3.8) liters. Divide that value by the *change* in P$_L$ over that volume range $\Delta P_L = (30 - 0)$ cmH$_2$O $= 30$ cmH$_2$O. We thus obtain C$_L = 4.05/30 = 0.135$ liters/cmH$_2$O or 3.8/30 $= 0.127$ liter/cmH$_2$O.

CHAPTER 4. LUNG VOLUMES AND VENTILATION

1. Use the alveolar ventilation equation (Eq. 4-4). Check the format of each piece of data before doing the calculation, although in this question the data are in the proper form to use directly.

   a. P$_{ACO_2}$ = 104 mmHg   Hypoventilation
   b. $\dot{V}_A$ = 20 liters/min   P$_{ACO_2}$ low; hyperventilation
   c. $\dot{V}_{CO_2}$ = 370 ml/min   P$_{ACO_2}$ normal; normal ventilation for metabolic state
   d. $\dot{V}_A$ = 1.8 liters/min   P$_{ACO_2}$ high; hypoventilation

2. Use the alveolar gas equation (Eq. 4-5).

   a. P$_{AO_2}$ = 235 mmHg   The correction factor in the brackets works out to be 1.17
   b. P$_{AO_2}$ = 116 mmHg   The correction factor in the brackets equals 1.2
   c. P$_{AO_2}$ = 110 mmHg   Since R $= 1$, the correction factor equals 1
   d. P$_{AO_2}$ = 629 mmHg   Since F$_{IO_2}$ $= 1$, the correction factor equals 1

3. According to the alveolar ventilation equation, if $\dot{V}_{CO_2}$ rises, P$_{ACO_2}$ must also rise unless $\dot{V}_A$ increases. Clearly the tendency will be for P$_{ACO_2}$ to increase. Since the text states that Pa$_{CO_2}$ is closely regulated, you should conclude that ventilation will also rise, to keep P$_{ACO_2}$ as near normal as possible.

4. Since P$_{ACO_2}$ and $\dot{V}_{CO_2}$ are normal, alveolar ventilation must be 4.3 liters/min (alveolar ventilation equation). But V$_D$/V$_T$ = 0.6, by Eq. 4-2, so at the normal frequency of 12 (given), $4.3 = 12 \times V_T (1 - 0.6)$. Then V$_T = 4.3/(12 \times 0.4) = 0.9$ liter.

5. The starting volume of the test breath does not matter; it can be whatever is convenient. What is important is to be sure the subject inspires to TLC and to measure the inspired volume accurately.

6. If some of the dead space gas is included in the expired sample, the *apparent* tracer dilution will be less, so the FRC will appear to be less. Use Eq. 4-1B to see this more formally. Note that V$_I$ is multiplied by the fractional tracer ratio (F$_I$ − F$_A$)/F$_A$. Dead space contamination of the sample will raise F$_A$, decreasing the numerator and increasing the denominator; both effects decrease the ratio and consequently the dilution volume.

7. The calculation is straightforward if you realize that the $F_{A_{O_2}}$ of FRC gas is not zero but 0.143 [see Ch. 3 or calculate it as $102/(760 - 47)$]. Use Eq. 4-1, not the simplified Eq. 4-1A. FRC = 2.6 liters, ATPS, and 2.9 liters, BTPS. The correction to body conditions is to provide some review of Chapter 3.

8. The normal $F_{A_{O_2}}$ is 0.143 at an FRC of 2.4 liters; this amounts to 343 ml O_2. When $P_{A_{O_2}}$ = 30 mmHg, F_A = 30/713) = 0.042, which amounts to 100 ml. The difference $343 - 100 = 242$ ml O_2 removed, BTPS. Since $\dot{V}_{O_2}$ = 250 ml/min and is always given at STPD, convert 242 ml to standard conditions; it equals 200 ml. The time will be $200/250 \times 60$ sec = 48 sec. Of course, as P_{O_2} declines, $P_{A_{CO_2}}$ and Pa_{CO_2} rise. Because R < 1, there is a slow decrease in alveolar volume. The larger tidal volume reaching TLC increases $P_{A_{O_2}}$ slightly, but mainly it increases the O_2 stores in the lung. It also dilutes $P_{A_{CO_2}}$ and delays the rise in Pa_{CO_2}.

9. This is fairly complex. The easiest way to begin is to consider that the alveolar gas is diluted at each breath by a constant fraction $[V_I/(V_I + FRC)]$ of the difference between $F_{I_{O_2}}$ and $F_{A_{O_2}}$ at the beginning of the breath, which corresponds to an exponential step function rise of $F_{A_{O_2}}$. Use the mixing Eq. 4-1 to calculate the $F_{A_{O_2}}$ at the end of each breath. Thus, $(V_I \times F_{I_{O_2}}) + (FRC \times F_{A_{O_2}}, i) = V_{tot} \times F_{A_{O_2}}, f$, where the i and f distinguish between the initial and final alveolar O_2 fractions of each breath, and $F_{A_{O_2}}, f = (V_I \times F_{I_{O_2}} + FRC \times F_{A_{O_2}}, i)/V_{tot}$.

Breath	$F_{A_{O_2}},f$	$P_{A_{O_2}}$, mmHg
0	0.143	102
1	0.395	282
2	0.573	408
3	0.698	498
4	0.787	561
5	0.850	606

Thus, five breaths are needed to reach 600 mmHg. The trick is that V_T is twice normal. Since V_T = 1 liter at normal frequency (12 breaths per minute), $\dot{V}_A$ is increased. $\dot{V}_A = f \times (V_T - V_D) = 12 (1,000 - 150)$ ml = 10.2 liters. Now use the alveolar ventilation equation to compute $P_{A_{CO_2}}$ = 21 mmHg. Then use the alveolar gas equation, which for $F_{I_{O_2}}$ = 1 has a simple form, to obtain $P_{A_{O_2}}$ = 692 mmHg.

CHAPTER 5. MECHANICAL PROPERTIES IN BREATHING: STATICS

1. a. Crs = 0.075 liter/cmH$_2$O, which is slightly less than normal. The C_L is greater than normal but Cw is less.
   b. C_L = 0.2 liter/cmH$_2$O, which is the normal resting value (see Appendix 2). Cw is markedly reduced. Crs is always less than either C_L or Cw even though it is weighted toward the less compliant component.
   c. Ew = 5 cmH$_2$O/liter. These are normal values, although a little lower than in the section on calculating compliance and elastance. Notice how easy it is to work with elastances.

d. Ers = 30 cmH$_2$O/liter, which is much greater than normal. Both the E$_L$ and Ew are increased.

e. C$_L$ = 0.5 liter/cmH$_2$O, which is much greater than normal. These lungs are recoiling from a chest wall with normal elastance (Ew = 5 cmH$_2$O/liter). Thus, the subject's FRC will increase until the lung elastic recoil (P$_L$) exactly equals the chest wall elastic recoil (Pw).

2. This question is about relative pressures. a. The body surface pressure at 100 m = 10,000 cmH$_2$O, which is almost 10 atm of pressure (1 atm = 760 mmHg = 1,033 cmH$_2$O). To have a normal FRC the diver must breathe from a tank that delivers a relative pressure of 10,000 cmH$_2$O at the mouth (Pao). b. Since FRC is normal the pleural pressure will be normal (relatively zero). Then at 100 m depth, the diver's Ppl must be 3.5 cmH$_2$O less than the Pbs. Thus Ppl = 10,000 − 3.5 = 9,996.5 cmH$_2$O. c. The loss of Pao leaves nothing to balance the high Pbs. Instantly, the external pressure will squeeze the abdomen, forcing the diaphragm upward into the chest cavity and compressing the rib cage. FRC will decrease suddenly. All gas-filled cavities in the body will be subjected to the same pressure, but the effect on the nasal sinuses and middle ear will be maximal, and the eardrums will undoubtedly rupture. In addition, much of the blood in peripheral veins will be forced into the thorax, grossly distending the heart and congesting the lungs. Cardiac output will, however, markedly decrease as the high compressive pressures would prevent any flow out of the thorax.

3. Clearly, 0.15 liter/cmH$_2$O is less than the average normal value. But one should resist interpreting data in isolation. At the very least, you should determine the average lung volume over the test range. If the specific compliance is normal, the person is probably small. Another possibility is a loss of lung mass, as when part or all of one lung has been surgically removed for cancer. To make a correct interpretation, more information about the subject is needed, including age, sex, race, body type, and previous pulmonary history.

4. Since the surface tension is high and constant, there will not be much hysteresis. The deflation curve will come very close to the inflation curve, which may be nearly normal. There is no reason for the liquid P-V curve to be altered.

5. a. Since you are given Cw and C$_L$, Crs = 0.1 liter/cmH$_2$O.

b. Use C$_L$ and calculate ΔP from the fact that ΔV = 1 liter between MV and FRC and P$_L$ = 0 at MV; then 0.2 = 1/(P$_L$, FRC − 0). P$_L$ at FRC is 5 cmH$_2$O, which means Ppl is −5 cmH$_2$O because, by definition, P$_A$ = 0 at FRC.

c. and d. Enter the values at FRC in the diagram and then add the information that you have for this part. At the new condition Prs = P$_A$ − Pbs = 0 − (−10) = 10 cmH$_2$O. Since Crs = 0.1 liter/cmH$_2$O, use the compliance formula to calculate ΔV = 1 liter. Use Cw, Pw at FRC, and ΔV to calculate the new Pw = 0 cmH$_2$O. The transdiaphragm-abdominal wall pressure is, by definition, Pw. Fill in the rest of the diagram and make sure all the pressures are reasonable. Note that Ppl = −10 cmH$_2$O at FRC + 1 liter.

e. Since lung volume does not change, none of the relative pressures change, but now P$_A$ = 10 and Pbs = 0.

f. Ppl goes from −10 to 0. Check it out on your model.

6. Use the LaPlace formula (Eq. 5-3), P = 2 × T/r and convert cmH$_2$O to dynes/cm^2; (1 cmH$_2$O = 980 dynes/cm^2). Then 4 × 980 = 2 × T/15 cm, and T = 29,400 dynes/cm.

7. a. A degenerative loss of lung tissue elastic recoil is the most likely cause of the aging effect, either by direct loss of elastic fibers or, more commonly, by a general enlargement of the alveoli due to loss of alveolar wall tissue. Surface tension cannot get lower than it does normally, so it does not have any effect here. b. Whatever happens to chest wall

elastance will not affect your interpretation of lung elastance, since both are independent variables.
8. Point 1 is the only point to the left of the P-V curve, which is the region representing increased compliance (distensibility).
9. Since there is severe expiratory airway obstruction but no lung tissue destruction, the lung static mechanics are probably normal. Therefore, either point 3 or point 5 could be correct, but point 5 is at TLC, making it impossible for the patient to breathe at all. Point 3 correctly shows hyperinflation on a normal P-V curve.
10. As stated in the text, at constant small tidal volumes for a long time, alveolar surface tension approaches its equilibrium value of 28 dynes/cm, which is about midway between the inflation and deflation lines of the P-V curve at FRC. Thus, in normal breathing, the dynamic P-V curve makes a small loop inside the static P-V loop (see Ch. 6).

CHAPTER 6. MECHANICAL PROPERTIES IN BREATHING: DYNAMICS

1. Use the resistance formula, Raw $= (\text{Pao} - \text{P}_A)/\dot{V}$.
   a. $(20 - 5)/4 = 3.8$ cmH$_2$O $\times$ sec/liter. Inspiration, since Pao $>$ P$_A$.
   b. $6 = (0 - 20)/\dot{V}$; $\dot{V} = -20/6 = -3.3$ liters/sec. Expiration because P$_A$ $>$ Pao. Also, flow is negative.
   c. $R = [0 - (-20)]/8 = 2.5$ cmH$_2$O $\times$ sec/liter. Inspiration.
   d. $1.8 = (0 - \text{P}_A)/7$; P$_A = -12.6$ cmH$_2$O. Inspiration.
   e. $5 = (\text{Pao} - 10)/4$; Pao $= 30$ cmH$_2$O. Inspiration.
2. a. Use the equation for resistances in series. R$_T = 1.5 + 0.7 = 2.2$ cmH$_2$O. In series R$_T$ is greater than any individual resistance.
   b. Use equation for resistances in parallel. $1/\text{R}_T = 1/1.8 + 1/1.0 + 1/0.6 + 1/3.5 = 0.56 + 1.0 + 1.67 + 0.28 = 3.51$; R$_T = 1/3.5 = 0.28$ cmH$_2$O $\times$ sec/liter. In parallel R$_T$ is less than any individual resistance.
   c. First calculate the total lung resistance, using the parallel equation, then add airway and lung resistances in series. $1/\text{R}_L = 1/3.5 + 1/1.5 = 0.286 + 0.667 = 0.95$; R$_L = 1/0.95 = 1.05$; R$_T = 1.5 + 1.05 = 2.55$ cmH$_2$O $\times$ sec/liter.
3. The best approach is to use Figure 5-4 starting at TLC and going to RV (not MV) along the deflation P-V curve. You can also use Figure 5-3. The only problem with using Figure 6-1 is that you have to estimate RV. After finding that P$_L = 1$ cmH$_2$O at RV and P$_L = 30$ cmH$_2$O at TLC, VC is found to be 4.8 liters from Table 2-2 or from Figure 5-4. dynC$_L$ $= \Delta V/\Delta P = 4.8/(30 - 1) = 0.16$ liter/cmH$_2$O. Did you mistakenly use the *inflation* P-V curve in Figure 5-4? This is incorrect because to reach RV the lungs must be deflated by forcibly exhaling or by doing the VC maneuver from TLC. Either way requires use of the deflation limb.
4. a. The important point here is that the large breath expanded the alveolar surface area and refreshed the surfactant layer. Thus, FRC is moved back onto the deflation P-V curve or very near it. The dynamic compliance of the next breath will be increased to approximately that of the standard deflation P-V curve in the V$_T$ range, as shown in the figure below.

Answers **219**

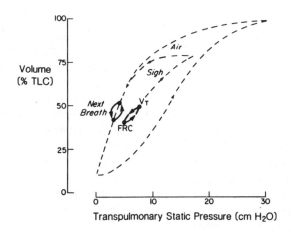

Transpulmonary Static Pressure (cm H_2O)

b. Over the next several minutes at constant V_T, the loop will move to the right and become less steep, until it coincides with the near-equilibrium loop shown in Figure 6-1.

5. a. Dynamic $C_L = \Delta V/\Delta P_L$. At 1 second inspiration, $\Delta V = 0.25$ liter (top graph of V_T in Fig. 6-3). The $\Delta P_L = [-5 - (-6.3)]$, which can be read directly from the bottom graph of Ppl in Figure 6-3. The trick here is to read the correct line. The dashed line gives the correct elastic recoil pressure. The solid line may also be used as long as you realize it is total Ppl from which you must subtract P_A (second graph from bottom) to get P_L equal to the elastic recoil pressure. Either way you should obtain $dynC_L = 0.25/(1.3) = 0.19$ liter/cmH_2O.

b. Dynamic $E_L = 1/dynC_L$. At 1 second deflation, $\Delta V = 0.25$ liter, since the V_T graph is symmetrical. Thus, $dynE_L = 1/0.19 = 5.26$ cmH_2O/liter.

6. There are two main points to consider: end-inspiratory P_L is 10 cmH_2O and the inspiration is rapid. The inspiratory point will be at 3.4 liters and 10 cmH_2O. The inspiratory line will be displaced to the right compared with a normal slow breath. The shaded area is the lost work used to overcome airway resistance. The expiration is passive along a normal trajectory, as shown in the figure below.

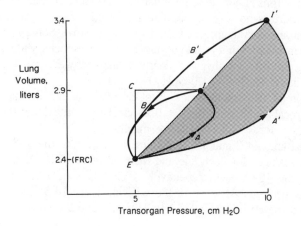

Transorgan Pressure, cm H_2O

7. In this problem, (W) is being done on the lungs *and the chest wall*. If Crs = 0.1 liter/cmH$_2$O and 50% VC = 2.4 liters (Appendix 2 normal values), then P$_L$ = ΔV/Crs = 2.4/0.1 = 24 cmH$_2$O. Since W = P × ΔV, W = 24 cmH$_2$O × 2.4 liters = 60 cmH$_2$O × liters. Since 1 joule = 10 cmH$_2$O × liter, the W = 6 joules and the required power (rate of doing work) equals 6 joules/breath × 1 breath/3 sec = 2 watts.

8. I discussed this important problem in connection with the P-V curve of the chest wall but it needs reinforcement. The lung deflation P-V curve in Figure 5-7 cannot be used because we are dealing with dynamic events. Figure 6-1 could be used if the x-axis were in absolute units. The simplest approach is to recognize that the chest wall P-V curve is the same whether static or dynamic. From Figure 5-7 read FRC = 2.1 liters and Pw = −5 cmH$_2$O.

9. The key point here is that if Ppl is positive at normal FRC, then P$_A$ = 10, since P$_L$ = P$_A$ − Ppl = 5 cmH$_2$O. The subject either is breathing against 5 cmH$_2$O of positive end-expiratory pressure (static) or has a serious expiratory flow limitation such that the airways close while P$_A$ is positive (dynamic).

10. a. Use Eq. 6-4 to compute the total airway resistive pressure. P = 2.4 × $\dot{V}$ + 0.03 × $\dot{V}^2$ = 2.4 × 5 + 0.03 × 5^2 = 12 + 0.75 = 12.75 cmH$_2$O.
    b. Turbulence accounts for 6% of the resistive pressure drop.

CHAPTER 7. PULMONARY AND BRONCHIAL CIRCULATIONS

1. PVR = (Ppa − Pla)/$\dot{Q}$ regardless of zone conditions (relation of P$_A$ to vascular pressures). P$_A$ may affect the flow distribution or Ppa but it is not used in the resistance calculation.
   a. PVR = 2 cmH$_2$O × min/liter. Ppa > Pla > P$_A$: zone 3
   b. PVR = 4 cmH$_2$O × min/liter. Ppa > P$_A$ > Pla: zone 2
   c. $\dot{Q}$ = 2.5 liters/min: zone 3
   d. Ppa = 25 cmH$_2$O. P$_A$ = Pla, which occurs only at the zone 2-zone 3 boundary; in other words, either the bottom of zone 2 or the top of zone 3 (see Fig. 7-9)
   e. PVR = ∞. There is no flow even though there is a positive driving pressure. Zone 1, where P$_A$ > Ppa (that is, >12 cmH$_2$O) (see line 3 in Fig. 7-3). The condition could also be intense pulmonary arterial vasoconstriction, which is equivalent to raising P$_A$ (see line 2 in Fig. 7-3).
   f. Since cardiac output is not zero, P$_A$ must be <70 cmH$_2$O; thus zone 2 or 3 conditions prevail, but there is no way to calculate P$_A$ exactly, as it is an independent variable. PVR and Ppa are very high, but $\dot{Q}$ and Pla are normal. Some type of pulmonary hypertension is involved, but it is not possible to be more specific without more information. In physiology there is not always a clearly defined answer.

2. a. Resistances in series. R$_T$ = 1.0 cmH$_2$O × min/liter.
   b. Resistances in parallel and in series. First calculate the parallel capillary resistances by adding reciprocals, obtaining Rc$_T$ = 0.23 cmH$_2$O × min/liter; then add the three R values in series. R$_T$ = 1.43 cmH$_2$O × min/liter.

3. Note the vertical lines at 3 and 10 liters/min. Read over to the y-axis to find the Ppa − Pla pressure differences for each line and then calculate PVR. At $\dot{Q}$ = 3 the ΔP values are 5.5, 6.5, 11, and 16 cmH$_2$O, respectively. PVR values are 1.8, 2.2, 3.7, and 5.3 cmH$_2$O × min/liter, respectively. At $\dot{Q}$ = 10 the ΔP values are 10.5, 12, 17, and 22.5 cmH$_2$O, respectively, and the PVR values are 1.0, 1.2, 1.7, and 2.2 cmH$_2$O × min/liter, respec-

tively. Note that all the resistances are decreased at the higher flow rate, especially for those curves farthest from the flow axis (abscissa).

4. a. The driving pressure for bronchial blood flow at rest is mean systemic arterial pressure, which equals 90 mmHg minus left atrial or right atrial pressure or their average, since about one-half of bronchial venous flow goes to the left heart and one-half goes to the right heart. Since normal resting cardiac output is 5 liters/min, bronchial flow is 50 ml/min (1% of cardiac output). Thus, bronchial vascular resistance is 1,600 to 1,800 (1,700 mean) mmHg × min/liter.

   b. Bronchial vascular resistance is high because there are many parallel systemic circuits. Since only 1% of cardiac output goes through the bronchial arteries, the bronchial vascular resistance must be 100 times greater than the resistance of the whole systemic circulation (SVR), which it is, since SVR = 17.6 mmHg × min/liter, using right atrial pressure as the downstream pressure.

5. The key to understanding this question is that the coldness of the injectate must be determined relative to normal body temperature, since the injectate is cold blood functioning as a tracer. Thus $(37.5 - 0)°C × 10$ ml = $375°C × $ml is the quantity of cold tracer injected. The cold tracer must all pass the detector during the recording of the temperature change. Thus, flow ($\dot{Q}$, ml/s) times the time (15 sec) for the tracer to pass by the detector times the mean temperature change must equal the amount of cold tracer injected: $\dot{Q} ×$ 15 sec × 0.25°C = 375°C × ml, from which $\dot{Q}$ = 100 ml/sec or 6.0 liters/min.

6. Since all three zones are specified, we need three parallel resistances. The PVR values (in $cmH_2O × $min/liter) are: zone 1, ∞; zone 2, $(24 - 7)/2.2 = 7.7$; zone 3, $(24 - 7)/4.4 = 3.9$. Adding resistances in parallel (reciprocals), $R_T = 2.6$ $cmH_2O × $min/liter.

7. a. We need $C\bar{v}_{O_2}$ to calculate the shunt flow. We begin with systemic arterial blood. Use the HbO_2 curve in Figure 1-2 or Figure 9-1; the latter is easier because all the O_2 data are listed below the graph. At $Pa_{O_2} = 65$ mmHg, $Sa_{O_2} = 85\%$. Thus $O_{2,capacity} = 201 × 0.85 + 65 × 0.03 = 171 + 2 = 173$ ml O_2/liter. Next, use the Fick equation (Eq. 3-5); 7 liters/min = $[380$ ml O_2/min]/$[(173 - C\bar{v})$ ml O_2/min]. $C\bar{v}_{O_2} = 119$ ml/liter. Using the mixing equation (Eq. 7-1) and remembering that flow through the ventilating lung is total flow ($\dot{Q}_T$) minus shunt flow ($\dot{Q}_S$) and that the patient is breathing 100% O_2, we obtain $173 × \dot{Q}_T = (201 + 18) × (\dot{Q}_T - \dot{Q}_S) + (119) × \dot{Q}_S$. Then $\dot{Q}_S = 3.2$ liters/min, or 46% of total cardiac output.

   b. The shunt flow is approximately equal to the mass of consolidated lung, which suggests that in the diseased lung the ability to express hypoxic vasoconstriction has been lost, since there was no flow shift (no reduction of shunt flow).

8. The answer is (b), since a line from the origin to point 2 is closest to the flow axis (x-axis).

9. If you pivot a straightedge around the origin, you will find that points 4 and 7 are the only two lying on the same resistance line. Thus (d) is correct.

10. The question, although vague, is adequate for the purpose, which is to reason about intrathoracic pressure relationships and pulmonary hemodynamics under conditions that differ somewhat from those discussed in the chapter. The increased PA in the left lung would tend to put more of that lung into zone 2 or even into zone 1 if Ppa were low. Either condition will cause Ppa to rise. Thus, (a) is likely to be correct, whereas (b) requires the opposite reasoning and so is highly unlikely, and (c) is not reasonable because the increased PA to the left lung would tend to decrease flow for the same reasons that Ppa would rise. If either (d) or (e) were correct, then Pla or Ppa would have to be <0 or <10 cmH_2O, respectively, at the bottom of the lung; both conditions are extremely unlikely.

CHAPTER 8. MATCHING VENTILATION TO PERFUSION

Of all the problems in respiratory physiology, I believe ventilation/perfusion questions are among the most difficult. Why? Because there is a tendency to overlook the basic requirements of consistency. Consider the $\dot{V}_A/\dot{Q}$ equation (Eq. 8-1). If that is satisfied, then the alveolar ventilation equation (Eq. 4-4) and the Fick equation (Eq. 3-5) are also correct, since these are the sources of the $\dot{V}_A/\dot{Q}$ equation. And if the alveolar ventilation equation is satisfied, then the alveolar gas equation (Eq. 4-5) is correct, as are all other relations concerning breathing and metabolism.

1. a. $\dot{V}_A/\dot{Q} = 0.863 \times 0.8 \times 50)/80 = 0.43$. The low $\dot{V}_A/\dot{Q}$ is due to alveolar hypoventilation because $P_{A_{CO_2}}$ is twice normal. By Eq. 4-4 $\dot{V}_A = 2.1$ liters/min because $\dot{V}_{CO_2}$ should be assumed normal at 200 ml/min. $\dot{Q} = 5$ liters/min.
   b. $\dot{V}_A/\dot{Q} = 0.80$; a normal value. The $P_{a_{CO_2}}$ is 10% below normal, so $\dot{V}_A$ is probably slightly high, but the $(\bar{v} - a) \Delta C_{O_2}$ is 20% below normal, which suggests that $\dot{Q}$ is slightly high. All these numbers, however, are within the normal biologic range among individuals.
   c. $\dot{V}_A/\dot{Q} = 1.6$; that is high. Note that $P_{a_{CO_2}}$ is normal, so $\dot{Q}$ must be low; this is confirmed by the large $(\bar{v} - a)\Delta C_{O_2}$.
   d. $\dot{V}_A/\dot{Q} = 0.79$; normal. Assuming $\dot{V}_{CO_2}$ and $\dot{V}_{O_2}$ are normal ($R = 0.80$), $\dot{V}_A = 4.3$ liters/min and $\dot{Q} = 5.4$ liters/min.
   e. We can use the $\dot{V}_A/\dot{Q}$ equation to calculate either component, given the other. $\dot{V}_A = 14.5$ liters/min and $\dot{V}_A/\dot{Q} = 1.2$, which is high. Since $P_{a_{CO_2}}$ is elevated, there must be hypoventilation relative to the metabolic condition. But $\dot{Q}$ is relatively low, even though it is high in absolute terms. Notice the wide $(\bar{v} - a)\Delta O_2$ difference. These conditions might be found in a person with both ventilatory and cardiac limitations trying to exercise beyond steady-state capabilities.
   f. $\dot{Q} = 5.8$ liters/min. $\dot{V}_A/\dot{Q} = 1.7$, which is high. Persons with these data would be obviously overventilating for their metabolic state, as the low $P_{a_{CO_2}}$ shows.
2. On the surface this problem appears to require a straightforward application of the conservation of mass law. Since all the metabolic and breathing parameters are normal, that approach yields the following result:

$$2.1 \times 0 \quad + \quad 2.1 \times 40 \quad = 4.2 \times P_{A_{CO_2}}$$
(alveolar dead space, lung A)   (normal lung B)
$P_{A_{CO_2}} = 84/4.2 = 20$ mmHg

Since the answer comes out even, you might assume that it is right. However, the answer is wrong. If $P_{A_{CO_2}} = 20$ and $\dot{V}_A$ is normal, then by the alveolar ventilation equation, $\dot{V}_{CO_2}$ must be only one-half of normal. That contradicts the statement that the metabolic state was normal.

Let us rethink the situation. Since all the blood flow is stated to go to lung B (see also the section on other ventilation/perfusion distributions), then all the CO_2 is also delivered there. For that to occur, either $\dot{V}_A$ or $P_{A_{CO_2}}$, for lung B must double. Since the former is fixed by the problem statement, $P_{A_{CO_2}}$ must be 80 mmHg. Thus, recalculation of the expired alveolar gas gives:

$$2.1 \times 0 \quad + \quad 2.1 \times 80 \quad = 4.2 \times P_{A_{CO_2}}$$
(alveolar dead space, lung A)   (normal lung B)

$P_{A_{CO_2}} = 40$ mmHg, which is the correct and only consistent answer.

3. This question is easier than it appears because you are only asked for the P_{O_2} in alveolar gas and pulmonary venous blood of the ventilated unit. It is not necessary to calculate $P\bar{v}_{O_2}$ or Pa_{O_2}, although it would not be wrong to do so.

   This is a straightforward $\dot{V}A/\dot{Q}$ problem, in which all the $\dot{V}A$ goes to lung B but only one-half the $\dot{Q}$ goes there. Thus, $\dot{V}A/\dot{Q}$ is twice normal. Since R, $\dot{V}_{O_2}$, and $\dot{Q}T$ are normal, either Pa_{CO_2} is reduced or $(C\bar{v}_{O_2} - Ca_{O_2})$ is increased. Pa_{CO_2} cannot be reduced, or else $\dot{V}_{CO_2}$ would be reduced (by the alveolar ventilation equation). Thus, $(\bar{v} - a)\Delta C_{O_2}$ is doubled. That information is not needed unless you want to know what $C\bar{v}_{O_2}$ is for calculating Pa_{O_2}. What you do need to know is that Pa_{CO_2} is normal (40 mmHg) and therefore, by the alveolar gas equation, Pa_{O_2} is normal (100 mmHg). This answers the first half of the question. Since there is nothing wrong with lung B except that blood flow is twice normal, there is no reason to think Ppv_{O_2} will be different from normal, that is, equal to Pa_{O_2} (100 mmHg).

4. a. No, static compliance is by definition independent of time and hence of breathing rate. See the definition of statics and the description of the deflation pressure-volume curve in Chapter 5, in which the expiration is to be made "very slowly," which is as close to zero breathing rate as humans can accomplish.

    b. As the breathing frequency increases, dynamic compliance will decrease, because the more slowly filling terminal respiratory units receive less and less of their predicted tidal volume.

5. The resting blood flow varies by a factor of 4 (20/5) between the lower and upper lung. During exercise the flow varies by 30/18, a factor of 1.7. Thus, by increasing flow over the height of the lung, the distribution of flow is more uniform, even though the difference between the top and bottom is nearly the same in absolute flow terms. Obviously, it is the ratio, not the absolute values, that determines the relative uniformity of flow.

6. There are two factors to consider; one is the time constant $(R \times C = \tau)$ and the other is the final equilibrium volume, which is determined by the *static* compliance (C). The former determines the **rate** of filling, the latter the **volume**. The time constants of the two units are equal, so they will fill at the same rate, but the stiff unit will only fill half as much. How is this different from the situation shown in Figure 8-6C? The final unit volume is the same, but in Figure 8-6C the time constant was smaller, so the unit filled faster.

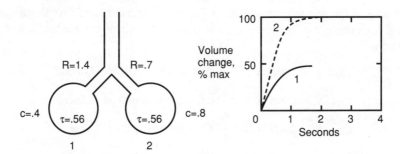

7. Here the curve looks peculiar since ultimately the abnormal lung will fill to 200% of normal volume because its compliance is doubled. The large time constant, however, causes the unit to fill at only one-fourth the rate of the normal unit.

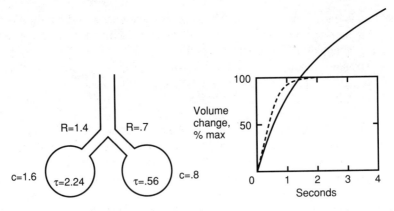

8. The answer is (a). Only hyperventilation (i.e., increased ventilation relative to the metabolic condition) can increase $P_{A_{O_2}}$ and thereby Pa_{O_2}. Decreased ventilation will increase $P_{A_{CO_2}}$ and thus decrease $P_{A_{O_2}}$ by the alveolar gas equation. Changing cardiac output cannot affect $P_{A_{O_2}}$ or Pa_{O_2} as long as $\dot{V}_{O_2}$ is unchanged.

9. a. Use the mixing equation to obtain the mean alveolar gas tensions.

$$P_{A_{O_2}} = \frac{0.2 \times 120 + 0.35 \times 102 + 0.45 \times 93}{1.0}$$

$$P_{A_{O_2}} = 24 + 36 + 42 = 102 \text{ mmHg}$$

$$P_{A_{CO_2}} = \frac{0.2 \times 35 + 0.35 \times 40 + 0.45 \times 41}{1.0} = 7 + 14 + 18 = 39 \text{ mmHg}$$

b. Since the CO_2 equilibrium curve is a straight line and $Pa_{CO_2} = P_{A_{CO_2}}$ for each compartment, the mixing equation applied to arterial blood gives

$$Pa_{CO_2} = \frac{0.10 \times 35 + 0.33 \times 40 + 0.57 \times 41}{1.0}$$

$$Pa_{CO_2} = 3.5 + 13.2 + 23.4 = 40 \text{ mmHg}$$

For arterial oxygen tension one has to use concentration, not partial pressure, as was used in example 2 of the discussion of right-to-left shunt in Chapter 7. For each compartment:

$$Ca_{O_2}, 1 = 0.982 \times 201 + 0.03 \times 120 = 201 \text{ ml } O_2/\text{liter}$$

$$Ca_{O_2}, 2 = 0.975 \times 201 + 0.03 \times 102 = 199 \text{ ml } O_2/\text{liter}$$

$$Ca_{O_2}, 3 = 0.971 \times 201 + 0.03 \times 93 = 198 \text{ ml } O_2/\text{liter}$$

$$\text{Mean } Ca_{O_2} = \frac{0.1 \times 201 + 0.33 \times 199 + 0.57 \times 198}{1.0} = 198.6 \text{ ml } O_2/\text{liter}$$

$$Sa_{O_2} = \frac{198.6 - 3.0}{201} = 97.3\%$$

$$Pa_{O_2} = 98 \text{ mmHg}$$

c. $(A - a)\Delta P_{CO_2} = 39 - 40 = -1$ mmHg, where the minus sign means $Pa > P_A$.

$$(A - a)\Delta P_{O_2} = 102 - 98 = 4 \text{ mmHg}$$

10. a. First, fill in the alveolar CO_2 tensions for each compartment. Compartment 1 has no flow, so $P_{ACO_2} = 0$. For compartment 2, the alveolar ventilation equation gives

$$P_{ACO_2} = \frac{0.863 \times 200}{4.2} = 41 \text{ mmHg}$$

Compartment 3 does not contribute to ventilation. Applying the mixing equation

$$P_{ACO_2} = \frac{1.0 \times 0 + 4.2 \times 41}{1.0 + 4.2} = 33 \text{ mmHg}$$

As for Pa_{CO_2}, it is equal to P_{ACO_2} for each compartment. Compartment 3 drops out because it has no flow. Thus, by the mixing equation

$$P_{ACO_2} = \frac{5.0 \times 41 + 1.0 \times 36}{6.0} = 40 \text{ mmHg}$$

$(A - a)\Delta P_{CO_2} = 33 - 40 = -7$ mmHg. This is a fairly large gradient, even though Pa_{CO_2} is normal. Anytime there is an increased CO_2 difference, there is wasted ventilation.

b. For O_2 start by filling in the alveolar tensions. Compartment 1 is wasted ventilation, so $P_{AO_2} = 0.21 \times (760 - 47) = 150$ mmHg by the alveolar gas equation. In compartment 2

$$P_{AO_2} = 150 - 41 \times \left[0.21 + \frac{(1 - 0.21)}{0.8} \right] = 101 \text{ mmHg}$$

In compartment 3, there is no ventilation, so it contributes nothing. Use the mixing equation

$$P_{AO_2} = \frac{1 \times 150 + 4.2 \times 101}{1.0 + 4.2} = 110 \text{ mmHg}$$

To obtain the arterial P_{O_2} it is necessary to calculate O_2 concentration in the pulmonary venous outflow from each compartment. Since compartment 1 has no flow, it may be ignored. For compartment 2: $Ca_{O_2} = 0.974 \times 201 + 0.03 \times 101 = 199$ ml O_2/liter. In compartment 3, $P_{AO_2} = P\bar{v}_{O_2}$ (shunt); and $Ca_{O_2} = 0.71 \times 201 + 0.03 \times 38 = 143.8$ ml O_2/liter. Applying the mixing equation

$$Ca_{O_2} = \frac{1 \times 143.8 \times 5 \times 199}{1 + 5} = 189.8 \text{ ml } O_2\text{/liter}$$

Then $Sa_{O_2} = 92.8\%$ and the $Pa_{O_2} = 66$ mmHg. $(A - a)\Delta P_{O_2} = 110 - 66 = 44$ mmHg. This is much larger than the P_{CO_2} difference. Although there is a contribution due to the wasted ventilation, the far greater part is due to the venous admixture.

CHAPTER 9. TRANSPORT OF OXYGEN AND CARBON DIOXIDE

1. a. The shift to the left decreases P_{50} from 26 mmHg (normal) to 16 mmHg. Thus, all points on the normal HbO_2 curve must be multiplied by $16/26 = 0.62$. The old P_{O_2} is obtained by dividing the new P_{O_2} by 0.62; old $P_{O_2} = 18.6/0.62 = 30$ mmHg. $S_{O_2} = 57.5\%$ (Fig. 9-1) for the new P_{O_2} is the same as the old P_{O_2}.
    b. This is sneaky. Regardless of the position of the HbO_2 curve the Pa_{O_2} remains the same because PA_{O_2} does not depend on the position of the curve. The changes in Ca_{O_2} and Sa_{O_2} do not affect the answer. Thus, if normal $Pa_{O_2} = 100$ mmHg or any other value, it stays at that value.
    c. The P_{50} increased from 26 to 36 mmHg, a factor of 1.38, so the new P_{O_2}, which equals 55, must be 1.38 times the old P_{O_2}. Thus, the old $P_{O_2} = 55/1.38 = 40$ mmHg. S_{O_2}, as in previous applications, is 75% (Fig. 9-1), and $C_{O_2} = O_2$, capacity $\times 0.75 = 201 \times 0.75 = 151$ ml O_2/liter.
    d. The position of the curve is shifted by $31/26 = 1.19$. Thus, the P_{O_2} goes from 40 mmHg to $40 \times 1.19 = 47.6$ mmHg, which still corresponds to 75% S_{O_2}. However, we must consider what happened to Sa_{O_2} because the question asks about $P\bar{v}_{O_2}$. The PA_{O_2} remains at 100 mmHg—remember, it is not affected. To obtain the new Sa_{O_2} the original P_{O_2} is needed; it is $100/1.19 = 84$ mmHg. The 16-mmHg difference represents a large shift. However, we are using the flat part of the HbO_2 curve; the S_{O_2} associated with 84 mmHg is 96.2%, which is only 1.2% less than normal. This means that mixed venous saturation is reduced to 73.8% for which $P_{O_2} = 39.5$ mmHg on the old curve. The new $P\bar{v}_{O_2}$ is $1.19 \times$ old $P_{O_2} = 39.5 \times 1.19 = 47$ mmHg.
    e. You are asked to determine the new S_{O_2} at a constant $P_{O_2} = 63.5$ mmHg after the position of the HbO_2 curve shifts. Since a *decreased* affinity means a shift to the right, P_{50} increases from 26 to 33 mmHg, a factor of 1.27. The answer requires that you read down along the 63.5 line to obtain the new S_{O_2}. The normal P_{O_2} that when multiplied by 1.27 equals 63.5 mmHg is calculated as $P_{O_2} = 63.5/1.27 = 50$ mmHg. From Figure 9-1, $S_{O_2} = 85.1\%$ (it was 92% originally).
    f. Since the affinity of CO for Hb is 250 times that of O_2, a P_{CO} of 0.4 mmHg is equivalent to a P_{O_2} of $0.4 \times 250 = 100$ mmHg. Since $PA_{O_2} = 100$, the blood leaving the lung will be 50% HbO_2 and 50% HbCO. Thus, $S_{CO} = 50\%$.
2. Since 1 μl $= 10^{-6}$ liters, [Hb] $= 150$ g/liter $= 150 \times 10^{-6}$ g/μl. [Hb]/RBC $= (150 \times 10^{-6}$ g/μl$)/(5 \times 10^6$ RBC/μl$) = 30 \times 10^{-12}$ g/RBC $= 30$ pg/RBC. To convert to moles, divide by 66,500 g Hb/mol. [Hb]/RBC $= 0.45 \times 10^{-15}$ mol/RBC $= 0.45$ fmol/RBC. The molar ratio of O_2 to Hb is 4. Therefore, $4 \times 0.45 = 1.8$ nmol O_2/RBC. If you started with the O_2 capacity of blood equal to 201 ml O_2/liter, then 1 μl contains 201×10^{-6} ml O_2/μl, which when divided by 5 million erythrocytes per microliter gives 40.2×10^{-12} ml/RBC. To show that the two answers are equivalent, divide by 22,400 mlO_2/mol. Thus, $(40 \times 10^{-12}$ mlO_2/RBC$)/(22,000$ mlO_2/ml$) = 0.0018 \times 10^{-12}$ mol/RBC $= 1.8$ mol/RBC $= 1.8$ fmol/RBC.
3. We first calculate that 70 kg $\times 0.07 = 4.9$ kg (4.9 liters). Since 70% of circulating blood volume is in the venous system, the best estimate of emergency O_2 supply is: $S\bar{v}_{O_2} \times$ blood volume $\times O_2$ capacity $= 0.75 \times 4.9$ liters $\times 201$ ml O_2/liter $= 739$ ml O_2. This is about a 3-minute supply at normal resting $\dot{V}_{O_2}$. The correct answer is (b).
4. a. The normal arterial P_{50} is 26 mmHg. After the 3-mmHg right shift, the new P_{50} is 29 mmHg.

b. The simplest approach is to use S_{O_2} because O_2 capacity does not change between arterial and coronary sinus (venous) blood: $Sa_{O_2} = 97.4\%$; $Sv_{O_2} = 47.4\%$. Thus, the mean capillary $S_{O_2} = 72.4\%$. In Figure 9-1, P_{O_2} at the saturation is approximately 38 mmHg (by linear interpolation). The coronary sinus P_{50} is right-shifted by $29/26 = 1.115$. The new mean capillary $P_{O_2} - 38 \times 1.115 = 42$ mmHg. The Bohr shift has increased the P_{O_2} gradient between capillary blood and myocardial mitochondria from $38 - 5 = 33$ mmHg to $42 - 5 = 37$ mmHg, which is an increase of 4 mmHg.

5. Use Figure 9-7 but with the CO_2 arrows reversed. If the conversion of H_2CO_3 to $H_2O + CO_2$ is slow, then the P_{CO_2} of capillary plasma and, consequently, PA_{CO_2} will be lower than in the erythrocytes as the blood leaves the capillaries. The reaction will continue in the pulmonary veins or left heart until an equilibrium is reached. Thus, Pa_{CO_2} must be increased, which will tend to stimulate ventilation. Answer (b) is correct.

6. Anemia means decreased O_2 capacity. If $\dot{V}_{O_2}$ is constant and there is no reason to believe otherwise, either $(a - \bar{v})\Delta C_{O_2}$ or $\dot{Q}$ must rise (Fick equation). The only allowable answer is (b).

7. Since HbCO poisoning is due to the high affinity of CO for Hb compared with O_2, the physiologic treatment of choice is to raise PI_{O_2} by having the patient breathe 100% O_2 (a). By raising PA_{O_2} sixfold, the PA_{CO} necessary to retain 25% S_{CO} is also increased sixfold. That requires more HbCO to dissociate in the lung's capillaries, and the PA_{CO} is washed out by ventilation six times as fast as when the patient is breathing room air. The other answers are probably good advice (b and d) or will slightly increase the rate of CO washout (c and e), but none will decrease the patient's S_{CO} as efficiently as will the increased inspired O_2.

8. In moderate steady-state exercise, Pa_{O_2} and Pa_{CO_2} are normal. Part of the increased transport of O_2 and CO_2 is achieved by increasing the $(a - \bar{v})\Delta C_{CO_2}$ of each. No doubt you know that $C\bar{v}_{O_2}$ is decreased, but by the same reasoning $C\bar{v}_{CO_2}$ is increased. Thus, the HbO_2 curve is shifted to the right and the $S\bar{v}_{O_2}$ is decreased. The only point that fits that description is 7.

9. As stated before, if $\dot{V}_{O_2}$ is normal, neither PA_{O_2} nor Pa_{O_2} is affected by the composition of the blood. Thus, point 1 is correct.

10. Here the curve is shifted to the left but flow, $\dot{V}_{O_2}$, and $C\bar{v}_{O_2}$ are normal. Point 2 is correct.

CHAPTER 10. ACID-BASE BALANCE

1. a. $[H^+] = \dfrac{794 \times 0.03 \times 40}{24} = 40$ nEq/liter; normal

b. $[H^+] = \dfrac{794 \times 0.03 \times 60}{27.2} = 52.5$ nEq/liter; respiratory acidosis. Note that the $[H^+]$

units are *nano*equivalents per liter. The product of the constants is $794 \times 0.03 = 23.8$.

c. $[HCO_3^-] = \dfrac{23.8 \times 15}{25} = 14.3$ mEq/liter

Marked respiratory alkalosis with partial metabolic compensation

d. $[HCO_3^-] = \dfrac{23.8 \times 35}{45} = 18.5$ mEq/liter

Lower left edge of normal range. Slight metabolic acidosis with partial respiratory alkalosis compensation.

e. $P_{CO_2} = \dfrac{30 \times 35.9}{794 \times 0.03} = 45$ mmHg

Metabolic alkalosis with partial respiratory acidosis compensation

2. a. $[H^+]$ = antilog $(-pH)$ = 35 nEq/liter

$$7.45 = 6.10 + \log \dfrac{[HCO_3^-]}{[0.03 \times 35]} = 6.10 + \log [HCO_3^-] - \log 1.05 \log [HCO_3^-]$$

$$= 1.37; [HCO_3^-] = 23.5 \text{ mEq/liter}$$

b. Lower right edge of normal range. Modest respiratory alkalosis; 14% (40/35) hyper-ventilation (Eq. 4-3)

$[H^+]$ = 45 nEq/liter

$$7.35 = 6.10 + \log \dfrac{23.5}{0.03 \times P_{CO_2}}; \log (0.03 \times P_{CO_2}) = 0.121$$

P_{CO_2} = 44 mmHg. Upper left edge of normal range; modest respiratory acidosis and slight metabolic acidosis, since point is to left of the blood buffer line.

c. pH = $-\log [H^+]$ = $-\log 72$ = 7.14.

$$7.14 = 6.10 + \log \dfrac{33}{0.03 \times P_{CO_2}}; \log (0.03 \times P_{CO_2}) = 0.4785$$

P_{CO_2} = 100 mmHg. Severe primary respiratory acidosis.

d. pH = 7.60. $[HCO_3^-]$ = 37.9 mEq/liter. Marked primary metabolic alkalosis.

e. $[H^+]$ = 49 nEq/liter. $[HCO_3^-]$ = 19.5 mEq/liter. Primary metabolic acidosis.

3. a. $[H^+]$ = antilog (-7.40) = 40 nEq/liter. $[H^+]$ = antilog (-6.95) = 112 nEq/liter. $[H^+]$ increased by 72 nEq/liter.

b. pH = $-\log 55$ = 7.26. pH = $-\log 30$ = 7.52. pH changed by 0.26 unit.

4. a. Since $[H^+]$ = 100 mEq/liter = 10^{-1} Eq/liter, pH = $-\log (-1)$ = 1.0.

b. Stomach tissue P_{CO_2} is probably about 50 mmHg. (Remember that P_{CO_2} is one of the three independent variables that determine $[H^+]$.)

c. [SID] is *negative* ([strong anions] > [strong cations]). That's the trick! $[Cl^-]$ is 100 mEq/liter. Thus, [SID] = -100 mEq/liter.

d. $[HCO_3^-]$ must be nearly zero at any P_{CO_2}. Use the Henderson-Hasselbalch equation to calculate $[HCO_3^-]$ = 0.00001 mEq/liter.

5. Answer is (a). [SID] decreases only in metabolic acidosis (Table 10-1).

6. Answer is (b). Adding $NaHCO_3$ increases [SID], which by definition is metabolic alkalosis (Table 10-1). As $[H^+]$ decreases, $\dot{V}_A$ will tend to decrease. Thus, P_{ACO_2} will tend to rise, not fall.

7. The figure below shows the answers.

a. The hyperventilation will decrease P_{CO_2} and $[H^+]$ along the normal blood buffer line, as shown by the arrow A. Since the exact amount of hyperventilation was not given, the final point could be anywhere along the line. To reach P_{CO_2} = 20 mmHg requires that $\dot{V}_A$ be doubled; to reach P_{CO_2} = 10 mmHg means that $\dot{V}_A$ is four times normal.

b. Chronic hyperventilation due to reduced inspired P_{O_2} (hypoxemia). It is partially com-pensated by metabolic acidosis. Thus, the blood will lie within the shaded area B, de-pending on how complete the compensation is. This is the answer required, but just for fun, I have added the complete story (shown by the thin arrow), which will be discussed in Chapter 11. Note that, as the metabolic acidosis develops, ventilation may increase and drive P_{CO_2} even lower.

c. Metabolic alkalosis (to the right along the P_{CO_2} = 40 mmHg line) with some respiratory acidosis compensation (rising as P_{CO_2} rises) by the third day; somewhere in area C.

d. Chronic partially compensated respiratory acidosis at P_{CO_2} = 50 mmHg (25% decreased $\dot{V}_A$). See arrows marked D. Initially, the patient's blood values will lie to the right of the blood buffer line (short arrow parallel to the P_{CO_2} = 50 mmHg line) to show partial compensation for the respiratory acidosis. To this is added an acute metabolic acidosis, as shown by the longer arrow parallel to the P_{CO_2} = 50 mmHg line but pointing to the left. $[H^+]$ is increased. The result implies that the patient's $\dot{V}_A$ cannot be increased, so P_{CO_2} remains constant.

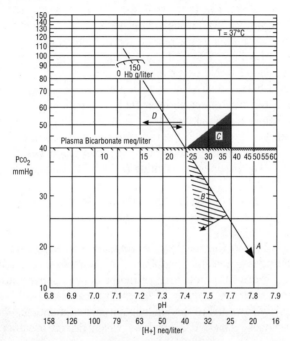

8. As discussed in Chapter 9, increased $[H^+]$ shifts the HbO_2 curve to the right (decreased affinity). This does not affect arterial C_{O_2} significantly, but it raises the P_{O_2} at which O_2 is unloaded. Thus, $P\bar{v}_{O_2}$ will tend to rise (answer d). There is no reason for cardiac output or $\dot{V}_{O_2}$ to change.

9. $[SID]_{CSF}$ is slightly less than in arterial blood because $[H^+]_{CSF}$ is increased ($pH_{CSF} < pH_a$). Since CSF has no protein, thus no $[A_{tot}]$, it is not as good a buffer as is blood (see Fig. 10-3B). Thus, for equal acute changes in P_{CO_2}, $[H^+]$ of CSF changes more than that of blood. But the $[HCO_3^-]$ does not change at all, since the CSF titration (buffer) line is isobicarbonate. The best answer is e.

10. Raising P_{CO_2} by a factor of 3/2 does not increase $[H^+]$ as much because blood has proteins as weak acid buffers. Thus, in Figure 10-3A at P_{CO_2} = 60 mmHg, $[H^+]$ is increased to about 51 nEq/liter and $[HCO_3^-]$ is increased to 28 mEq/liter owing to decreased $[A^-]$. Without any A_{tot}, $[H^+]$ would have increased to 60 nEq/liter (by a factor of 3/2). Thus, the blood acutely buffered nearly one-half the $[H^+]$ increase. The correct answer is b.

CHAPTER 11. CONTROL OF BREATHING

1. d. Since CO_2 is the prime stimulus, with $[H^+]$ a delayed second, the highest Pa_{CO_2} value should be chosen; thus, the answer is (d) instead of (e), which is slightly more acid but has normal Pa_{CO_2}.

2. c. The carotid body chemoreceptors are primarily stimulated by decreased Pa_{O_2}, but Pa_{CO_2} and $[H^+]$ have some effects. The choice is between (b) and (c). Choose (c) because Pa_{CO_2} and $[H^+]$ are higher.

3. b. The alveolar ventilation equation should be used. Since the patient is at rest, it is proper to assume the normal mean resting value of $\dot{V}_{CO_2}$. $\dot{V}_A$ = (0.863 × 200 ml/min)/55 = 3.1 liters/min. The wasted ventilation must be 6.3 − 3.1 = 3.2 liters/min, one-half of the minute ventilation.

4. a. Use the alveolar gas equation (normal R = 0.8) to calculate that the subject has a $P_{A_{O_2}}$ of 58 mmHg if ventilation is not stimulated. According to Figure 11-7, ventilation may be slightly increased, which would lower $P_{A_{CO_2}}$ a little. Changing the inspired P_{CO_2} to 21 mmHg ($F_{I_{CO_2}}$ = 0.03) would stimulate ventilation markedly, not only because of the enhancement of the hypoxic effect on the peripheral chemoreceptors (Fig. 11-7) but also because of the direct effect of CO_2 on the central chemoreceptors (Fig. 11-6). The increased ventilation would occur quickly.

5. b. Without the carotid bodies nearly all hypoxic ventilatory response is lost. The aortic bodies in humans have little effect on breathing. The patient would experience greater than normal hypoxemia at high altitude.

6. a. The arterial blood, CSF, and brain interstitial liquid have reduced P_{CO_2}, owing to the hyperventilation. The fall in P_{CO_2} constricts the brain blood vessels, which decreases cerebral blood flow. The dizziness or fainting is due to inadequate oxygen supply to the brain.

   b. During an episode of acute hysteria breathing is under behavioral control, which overrides the metabolic controller. Thus, minute ventilation is increased in spite of decreased Pa_{CO_2} and increased Pa_{O_2}.

7. Suffocation (asphyxia) means the inability to ventilate the lungs. Thus, $P_{A_{O_2}}$ falls and $P_{A_{CO_2}}$ rises. Both changes stimulate breathing. That is impossible, by definition, but the central controller keeps driving phrenic nerve motor neuron activity in a vain attempt to obtain some alveolar ventilation. In dying of severe hypoxemia due to low inspired oxygen concentration, the ability to ventilate the lungs is not inhibited until just before death when the central controller fails. Thus, $P_{A_{O_2}}$ is low, which drives breathing (Fig. 11-7), so $P_{A_{CO_2}}$ is very low.

8. If T_{tot} is normal, then the frequency of breathing is normal. If T_I is normal, the more vigorously contracting diaphragm will increase tidal volume. $\dot{V}_A$ will rise, $P_{A_{CO_2}}$ will fall, and the larger inspired volume will stimulate the stretch receptors more.

9. In sleep the CO_2 response is depressed. Point 3 is reasonable (see Fig. 11-6).

10. This is somewhat involved. If $P_{I_{O_2}}$ = 71 mmHg, then $P_{A_{O_2}}$ = 22 mmHg if there is no stimulation of breathing (alveolar gas equation). There is no point in the question figure that shows no stimulation, and moreover, such a low P_{O_2} would probably be fatal with Sa_{O_2} < 40% (by Fig. 9-1).

    Figure 11-7 shows that ventilation rises as $P_{A_{O_2}}$ decreases below 60 mmHg. The two points in the question figure showing increased ventilation and decreased $P_{A_{CO_2}}$ are 4 and 5. Point 5 shows a sixfold rise in $\dot{V}_E$, which is too great an effect for 10% inspired oxygen because it would lower $P_{A_{CO_2}}$ to about 5 mmHg. That would make $P_{A_{O_2}}$ = 65 mmHg, so there would be no hypoxic stimulation. Point 4 is the only one that is reasonable. It shows doubled ventilation and $P_{A_{CO_2}}$ decreased by one-half. If you calculate $P_{A_{O_2}}$ for that $P_{A_{CO_2}}$, you get 46 mmHg, which corresponds closely to the O_2 ventilation curve in Figure 11-7.

Appendix 1

Some Standard Symbols and Abbreviations Used in Respiratory Physiology*

MAIN SYMBOLS

Main symbols indicate the nature of the variable and are usually large capital letters. A symbol may be modified by a character over it, such as a bar (−) for a mean value or a single dot (·) for a first derivative (usually a quantity per minute).

MODIFIERS

Main symbols are clarified by the addition of one or more modifiers, usually small capitals for gas phase, standard symbols for chemical species, or lowercase letters for liquids.

GROUP

The respiratory symbols are divided into three groups: alveolar gas exchange and pulmonary circulation, respiratory mechanics, and control of breathing. A few symbols have more than one meaning and must be interpreted in context (usage).

PART I. ALVEOLAR GAS EXCHANGE AND PULMONARY CIRCULATION

Main Symbols

C	Concentration in a liquid
f	Breathing frequency
F	Fraction
P	Pressure, total or partial
Q	Volume of liquid
$\dot{Q}$	Flow of blood, perfusion
R	Gas-exchange ratio
S	Saturation
V	Gas volume
$\dot{V}$	Ventilation

Special Symbols

ATPS, ATPD	ambient temperature, pressure, saturated (S) or dry (D)
BTPS	body temperature, ambient pressure saturated
STPD	standard temperature, pressure dry [760 mmHg, 0°C]

Modifiers

a	Arterial
A	Alveolar
B	Barometric (ambient)
c	Capillary
DS	Dead space
E	Expired
I	Inspired
la	Left atrial
pa	Pulmonary arterial
pv	Pulmonary venous
s	Shunt
t	Time
τ	Total or tidal
ti	Tissue
tot	Total
v	Venous
$\bar{v}$	Mixed venous

---

* All the abbreviations used in this book are from the symbols and abbreviations approved by the International Union of Physiological Sciences (IUPS) Commission of Respiratory Physiology (1980) and used in the American Physiological Society's *Handbook of Physiology: Respiration* (1985–1986).

EXAMPLES

$C\bar{v}_{O_2}$ Concentration of O_2 in mixed venous blood
Pa_{O_2} Partial pressure of O_2 in arterial blood
$\dot{Q}_T$ Cardiac output (generally the T is omitted)
Sa_{O_2} Saturation of hemoglobin with O_2 in arterial blood
$\dot{V}_A/\dot{Q}$ Ventilation/perfusion ratio
$\dot{V}_E$ Expired minute ventilation

PART II. RESPIRATORY MECHANICS

Main Symbols
C   Compliance
E   Elastance
f   Frequency
P   Pressure
R   Resistance
V   Volume
$\bar{w}$ Work

Modifiers
A   Alveolar
ab   Abdomen
ao   Airway opening
aw   Airway
B   Barometric (ambient)
bs   Body surface
di   Diaphragm
dyn   Dynamic
E   Expiratory
el   Elastic
I   Inspiratory
L   Translung or transpulmonary
pl   Pleural
rc   Rib cage
rel   Relaxed or relaxation
rs   Respiratory system
st   Static
ti   Tissue
tm   Transmural
w   Chest wall

EXAMPLES

C_L Lung compliance
E_L Lung elastance, reciprocal of lung compliance; $E = 1/C_L$
P_A Alveolar pressure
Pao   Pressure at the airway opening
$W_{I,L}$ Work done on lung during inspiration ($P \times \Delta V$)

PART III. CONTROL OF BREATHING

T   Time in respiratory cycle

E   Expiratory
I   Inspiratory
T   Total

EXAMPLE

$T_T = T_I + T_E$

Appendix 2

Some Values of Cardiopulmonary Physiologic Variables for a Normal Adult (70 kg body weight) at Rest and During Steady State Exercise

	Units	Rest	Exercise
Constants			
Hemoglobin concentration	g/liter	150	
O_2 capacity of hemoglobin	ml O_2/g Hb	1.34	
Atmospheric pressure (sea level)	mmHg	760	
Water vapor pressure (37°C)	mmHg	47	
Standard conditions (STPD)	K, mmHg, mmHg	273, 760, 0	
Body conditions (BTPS)	K, mmHg, mmHg	310, 760, 47	
Cardiovascular			
Cardiac output	liter/min	5.0	15.0
Heart rate	per minute	60	140
Systemic arterial pressure, mean	mmHg	90	100
Right atrial pressure, mean	cmH$_2$O	2	4
Pulmonary Vascular Pressures (left atrial level)			
Pulmonary arterial, mean	cmH$_2$O	19	30
Left atrial, mean	cmH$_2$O	11	15
Lung Variables, BTPS			
Functional residual capacity	liters	2.4	2.2
Total lung capacity	liters	6	6
Tidal volume	liters	0.5	2.0
Frequency	per minute	12	15
Metabolism, STPD			
Carbon dioxide production	ml/min	200	1,200
Oxygen consumption	ml/min	250	1,500
Respiratory exchange ratio		0.80	0.80
Mechanics			
Pleural pressure, mean	cmH$_2$O	-5	-3.5
Chest wall compliance at FRC	liter/cmH$_2$O	0.2	0.2
Lung compliance at FRC	liter/cmH$_2$O	0.2	0.3
Airway resistance	cmH$_2$O × liters/sec	2.0	1.5

Index

Numbers followed by f indicate figures; those followed by t indicate tables.